This trend-setting book combines information on emerging concepts like free radicals, antioxidants, chronic inflammation, and nitric oxide (NO) with the cutting edge science of telomere length and longevity. Each concept is earmarked with quotable, peer-reviewed scientific evidence. The goal presented in this book is to age-proof the cardiovascular system and keep the vascular network clean and elastic through enhanced NO productivity.

The book includes dozens of easy-to-follow steps and tips to equip the reader with the knowledge to understand the above concepts, to identify the diseases related to those concepts, and to carry out easy-to-perform self-tests to determine one's status regarding the miracle molecule—NO, and to finally steer the reader toward functional foods and supplements to replenish the often depleted NO precursor nitrates.

I shared the key principles of the book with other doctors in our Obesity and Preventive Cardiology clinic. We started using the NO self-test and prescribing proactive functional foods, 'sirtfoods,' a Mediterranean diet, and supplements to our patients as outlined in this book.

If you are either a clinician or an end-user in the domain of cardiovascular disease, inflammatory disorders, immune disorders, and ill health, or simply interested in enhancing your longevity, this book is a game changer.

Naras Bhat, MD, FACP
Concord, CA

This very informative and detailed book on the science of cellular aging and scientifically proven concepts to slow aging is both timely and an essential read for healthcare practitioners and consumers.

This book starts with an easy-to-understand explanation of why we age and explains the mechanisms of aging as well as its clinical consequences. It then describes how to combat and neutralize the causes of aging at the cellular level. The last half of this book focuses on nitric oxide and how the proper diet and select functional foods can provide cellular defense against aging.

With nitric oxide being recognized as one of the most important molecules our body produces to protect our cells and organs, understanding nutritional strategies to enhance nitric oxide is an essential first step for slowing the aging process. Drs. Fried and Nezin present a very complicated science in easy-to-understand language so that every person who reads it can begin tomorrow taking steps to slow their own cellular aging.

At a time when medicine has failed many people with chronic disease, it is time to take control of our own healthcare. After all, it was the 'father of medicine,' Hippocrates, who said "Let food be thy medicine and let medicine be thy food." Drs. Fried and Nezin now provide a scientific mechanism for such and easy-to-follow instructions on how to do-it-yourself.

Nathan S. Bryan, PhD
Baylor College of Medicine
Houston, TX

The authors have done an astoundingly good job in 'translational medicine': They start with crystal clear explanations of the Nobel prize-winning discovery that preserving telomere length significantly extends lifespan and improves quality of life. Then, they 'translate' that ground-breaking research with detailed guidance on the dietary and lifestyle patterns that preserve telomere length and endothelial integrity.

Going far beyond a mere listing of the specific foods that help, the authors give recipes and meal plans. They take the reader from the 'bench' discoveries in laboratories, right into 'clinical practice' on the kitchen table.

This book is a *must* read for people seeking the tools needed to live a long and healthy life, and for the healthcare professionals trying to guide them.

Richard M. Carlton, MD
Psychiatrist and Clinical Nutritionist
New York

Evidence-Based Proactive Nutrition to Slow Cellular Aging is an excellent and timely work on normal aging changes, which should not, however, be viewed as a disease. This is a new concept. This book explains how aging is influenced by the food we consume as we destroy our cells by adverse lifestyle choices, which then results in premature aging.

As a believer in evidence-based medicine, this book, especially the chapter on functional foods, convinced me of the importance of functional foods in our diet as claims are supported by up-to-date scientific references. The mixture of information on the role of functional foods in our aging process and references to evidence-based medicine supporting this role in one book is fantastic and convincing.

Osama Tayeh, M.D., Ph.D., FESC
Professor, Critical Care Medicine
Faculty of Medicine
Cairo University Hospitals
Consultant of Cardiology and Critical Care Medicine
Cairo, Egypt

EVIDENCE-BASED PROACTIVE NUTRITION TO SLOW CELLULAR AGING

Robert Fried

and

Lynn Nezin

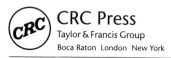

CRC Press

Taylor & Francis Group

Boca Raton London New York

CRC Press is an imprint of the
Taylor & Francis Group, an **informa** business

CRC Press
Taylor & Francis Group
6000 Broken Sound Parkway NW, Suite 300
Boca Raton, FL 33487-2742

Printed on acid-free paper

International Standard Book Number-13: 978-1-138-04332-9 (Paperback)
978-1-138-09227-3 (Hardback)

Library of Congress Cataloging-in-Publication Data

Names: Fried, Robert, 1935- author. | Edlen-Nezin, Lynn, author.
Title: Evidence-based proactive nutrition to slow cellular aging / authors, Robert Fried, Lynn Nezin.
Description: Boca Raton, Florida : CRC Press, 2017. | Includes bibliographical references and index.
Identifiers: LCCN 2017012394| ISBN 9781138043329 (pbk.) 978-1-138-09227-3 (hbk.) | ISBN 9781315173221 (e-book) | ISBN 9781351700221 (adobe reader) | ISBN 9781351700214 (epub) | ISBN 9781351700207 (mobi/kindle)
Subjects: | MESH: Nutrition Therapy--methods | Aging | Nutritional Physiological Phenomena
Classification: LCC QP141 | NLM WB 400 | DDC 613.2--dc23
LC record available at https://lccn.loc.gov/2017012394

Dedication

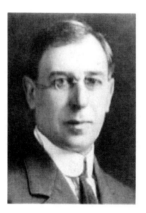

We dedicate this book to Mozes Gomberg (1886–1947), late Professor of Chemistry, University of Michigan.

Dr. Gomberg discovered the existence of organic free radicals and thus became the founder of radical chemistry, a branch of which is helping us to understand how to be healthier and live longer.

The cause of nutrition and growth resides not in the organism as a whole but in the separate elementary parts—the cells.

Theodor Schwann (1810 – 1882)

Contents

Preface

Why do we believe this book is an important addition to the dietary guidance literature? "Evidence-based," the first term in the title of this book, is what distinguishes it from the explosion of dietary programs both on the shelf and online. "Evidence-based" means that (1) every assertion about a relationship between any aspect of the diet that we describe and its health and longevity benefits has been tested and proven and (2) proof was published in a prestigious, conventional basic life-science or medical journal.

Furthermore, the scientific basis of the relationship between diet and health benefits is cited in each instance.

The assertions we make in this book about what supports or endangers longevity are not our own but derived from the research of countless scientists who reported their findings in prestigious medical publications. Our job was to meticulously document all of these theories and conclusions.

This book makes the evidence-based case that a sensible and easy-to-implement nutritional plan can help to prolong cellular life. This is not a claim to prolong lifespan. Lifespan is the number of years available to each individual. It is foremost dependent on hereditary factors over which we have no control, and second, it also depends on environmental and biological factors over which we may or may not have some degree of control. One or more of the environmental and/or biological factors may cause accelerated aging that can compromise our full potential lifespan.

Principal among these factors, and the focus of this book, is the rate at which the cells in our body cycle in reproduction as we constantly "renew." Cycling has consequences: the telomeres, the "caps" at the end of chromosomes in the nucleus of our cells, shorten with each cycle. After about 90 cycles, the typical cell runs out of telomeres and dies. The more quickly our cells cycle, the more quickly we compromise the length of our lifespan.

If our cells reproduce according to the rate we inherited, we have the possibility of achieving our maximum lifespan. If something causes our cells to undergo accelerated cycling, we are at risk of aging prematurely.

This book explains the factors that have been shown to cause accelerated cell reproduction and thus premature aging. Our nutritional plan provides guidance to helps prevent this acceleration, and consequently, helps cells to achieve their hereditary potential.

The strategy that we offer to help prevent premature aging is based on the documented, beneficial effects of the Mediterranean-style diet well-publicized in both the popular and scientific nutrition press. We combine this with so-called sirtfoods and select functional foods as the Proactive Nutrition Program.

We offer the reader the rationale behind these nutritional guidelines based on the scientific findings of thousands of medical researchers worldwide. In many instances, to illustrate the scientific basis of a given demonstrated relationship between diet, and health and longevity outcome, we describe the research that led to a given conclusion. This is our approach to editing down the details and minutia of the scientific research plan and highlighting the results as information that is most pertinent to our readers. In each case, the specific references are also given so that anyone who wishes to do so can readily access the original reports in conventional databases.

We believe this book offers important information that distinguishes it from other books on diet and nutrition. First, it provides a detailed and authenticated scientific explanation for why the Mediterranean diet is so effective in promoting health and longevity. The foods that comprise the Mediterranean diet amply supply the body with nitric oxide (NO) shown to protect the cardiovascular system and the heart, support insulin function, and enhance immune response. We describe a recently developed self-test for NO availability in the body to help the reader track the impact of dietary intake.

Second, low thyroid function is recognized as a major health hazard worldwide. Thyroid deficiency promotes atherosclerosis and jeopardizes insulin function, leading to premature aging. We provide instructions for a simple self-test for basal metabolism, which reflects low thyroid function, and discuss how this can be improved with dietary therapy.

The Proactive Nutrition Plan is substantially supported by the emerging and exciting science that is unraveling the complex process of premature cellular aging. We urge the adoption of our straightforward, evidence-based, and easy-to-implement nutritional guidelines for an enhanced lifetime of enjoyable meals designed to protect health at the cellular level.

Robert Fried
Lynn Nezin

Acknowledgments

We wish to express our profound appreciation first to Ms. Randy Brehm, Senior Editor, Agriculture and Nutrition, Taylor & Francis Group LLC/CRC Press, for her enthusiastic support of the production and publication of this book.

Our sincere appreciation goes to Dr. Naras Bhat, Concord, CA, for his review of the manuscript and his wholehearted endorsement of its scientific basis and proposed applications in the clinical practice of preventive cardiology.

Next, we thank Dr. Nathan S. Bryan, Baylor School of Medicine, for the numerous insights into the metabolic role of nitric oxide and nitrates applicable to proactive nutrition that his many years of research and publications have brought to light. Dr. Bryan was very helpful in shaping our presentation of the use of NO test strips to estimate the functional value of dietary nitrates.

Richard M. Carlton, MD, New York, who is both a psychiatrist and a nutritionist, wrote a very helpful review of the manuscript as it was evolving. Dr. Carlton, as always, made useful suggestions that have made this a better book.

We thank Stuart Nezin, New York, for Figure 4.1. And we wish to express our appreciation to Dr. Jacqueline Perle, Tel Aviv, Israel, for managing the complex task of acquiring permissions for figures and quotes.

We thank our respective families for their patience and support throughout this project.

Authors

Dr. Robert Fried was born in Linz, Austria, immigrated to the United States, and served in the Signal Corps, US Army, supporting radio communications for the Korean Military Advisory Group (KMAG), Seoul, Korea. Following honorable discharge, he entered The City College of New York (CCNY) and then the graduate program at Rutgers University, New Brunswick, New Jersey, earning his PhD in physiological psychology.

Dr. Fried was appointed to the faculty of Hunter College, City University of New York (CUNY), as well as the Doctoral Faculty in Behavioral Neuroscience at the City University of New York (CUNY). He is licensed in clinical psychology in New York State and served for 4 years as Director of the Rehabilitation Research Institute (RRI), International Center for the Disabled (ICD), New York, where he conducted and later published his research on the control of blood gases and blood pH in idiopathic seizure disorders. He was research scientist, Aviation Medical Acceleration Laboratory (Project Mercury); research associate, Eastern Pennsylvania Psychiatric Institute (EPPI), Temple University Medical School, and adjunct assistant professor, The University of Pennsylvania, both in Philadelphia; research psychologist, Atascadero State Hospital for the Criminally Insane Sex Offender, Pasa Robles, California, and visiting professor, California Polytechnic State University, San Luis Obispo; research associate, Department of Community Health, Albert Einstein College of Medicine; and research associate, Payne Whitney Clinic, Cornell University Medical School. He retired from CUNY in 2010 as Professor Emeritus.

Dr. Fried has lectured extensively in the United States and abroad and has conducted numerous workshops on respiratory and cardiovascular psychophysiology and blood gas self-regulation in neurological disorders, cardiovascular function, and stress syndrome. He holds a number of US patents in biomedical instrumentation including one of the earliest ECG-heart rhythm analyzer/computers.

Dr. Fried has authored more than 45 scientific publications in peer-reviewed journals as well as scientific textbooks, including *Erectile Dysfunction As a Cardiovascular Impairment* (Elsevier/Academic Press, 2014) and *The Psychology and Physiology of Breathing in Behavioral Medicine, Clinical Psychology & Psychiatry* (Springer, 1993).

Dr. Fried has also authored several consumer health self-help books including *The Arginine Solution* (Fried and Merrell, Time/Warner Books, 1999) and *Great Food/Great Sex: The Three Food Factors for Sexual Fitness* (Fried and Edlen-Nezin, Balantine Books, 2006). He has been featured in popular health magazines such as *Men's Health* and *Prevention* and interviewed on national and international TV including *Fox News* and *CNN*.

Dr. Fried is Emeritus Member of the American Physiological Society (APS) (Cardiovascular and Respiration division); Fellow, NY Academy of Sciences (NAS); and Diplomate in Behavioral Medicine, International Academy of Behavioral

Medicine, Counseling and Psychotherapy (IABMCP); and he is listed in the "Centennial Edition" of *Marquis Who's Who*. He lives in New York City with his wife Robin, a violinist with the Orchestra of St. Luke's, the Westchester Symphony Orchestra, and the American Ballet Theater (ABT) Orchestra.

Dr. Lynn Nezin is a senior strategic planner for FCB Health in New York City. She completed her doctorate in clinical health psychology in a joint program with the Ferkauf School of Psychology and Albert Einstein College of Medicine, Yeshiva University, and did her predoctoral internship at the St. Luke's Roosevelt Obesity Research Center in New York City.

At the age of 12, Dr. Nezin's family moved to the US Virgin Islands, where she learned to ride horses, sing with a Spanish Christmas carol chorus, and play the flute in the high school marching band. The band went on to perform at the World's Fair and also marched in the Veteran's Day parade in Washington, DC.

Dr. Nezin was among the first personal trainers to be certified by the American College of Sports Medicine. She initiated the employee fitness program at Rockefeller University and was head trainer at the Sports Training Institute, the first one-on-one fitness gym in New York City. A former competitive racewalker, Lynn completed four New York City Marathons.

Dr. Nezin has collaborated on a number of health and nutrition-related federally-funded research programs with the division of epidemiology and social medicine at Albert Einstein and also at the American Health Foundation, under the direction of the late Dr. Ernst Wynder. She has coauthored a number of peer-reviewed journal articles and textbook chapters on behavioral health and nutrition and coauthored *Great Food, Great Sex: The Three Food Factors for Sexual Fitness* (Ballantine Books, 2006) with Dr. Robert Fried.

Dr. Nezin was one of the founding organizers of the Health 2.0 NYC Technology Meetup group, which now numbers more than 1000 members devoted to innovation in public and personal health. She is a member of the American Diabetes Association and has been featured in Cambridge Who's Who.

1 The Science of Longevity

1.1 INTRODUCTION

Our youth-obsessed culture is terrified of aging. This fear has spawned a growing literature claiming that the proper choice of foods, supplements, and caloric restriction can actually stop aging. As seductive as these claims may be, they lack the support of real scientific proof.

In contrast, this book, *Evidence-Based Proactive Nutrition*, describes a new science-based diet program designed to help avert premature body cell aging. This program is not an overpromise but a sensible approach to nutrition that is not only easy to implement but is also backed by reputable, scientific peer-reviewed research.

Aging is a natural cellular process, but premature aging is not a natural process. To understand how nutrition might avert premature aging, here is a brief preview of the process of normal aging. Virtually all cells in the human body will eventually cycle and be replaced by *daughter* cells by a process of cell division called *mitosis*. When the cells divide, the nucleus they contain divides as well and each daughter cell gets its share of the nucleus. There is actually a limit to the number of such cycles for any given cell before it cannot cycle anymore and then it dies. This limit, the "Hayflick limit," (Hayflick 1965) is detailed later in this book. It is estimated that each cell may divide between 50 and 70 times over its lifespan and that were one to add up all such new generations, in ideal circumstances, that would come to about 120 years.

1.2 THE LENGTH OF TELOMERES DETERMINES THE LENGTH OF THE CELL LIFESPAN

The cell nucleus that a daughter cell "inherits" holds the chromosomes, thread-like strands of nucleic acids and protein carrying complex genetic information in the form of genes. Genes determine much about body shape, appearance, skills and talents, how we function, and even what disease we may suffer from or avoid.

The chromosomes are capped at each end with small structures, called telomeres, said to resemble the caps at the ends of shoelaces. It is thought that these prevent the chromosomes from spilling DNA each time a cell cycles. But, each time a cell cycles, the telomeres shorten perceptibly, and when they reach a given length, they are no longer viable and the cell dies.

1.3 FREE RADICALS ACCELERATE AGING

It is current dogma that aging is the aggregate of free-radical damage to body cells and to DNA. This explanation was proposed by Dr. Denham Harman, Emeritus Professor, University of Nebraska, Omaha (Harman 1992). Free radicals are toxic, ubiquitous chemically unstable forms of oxygen that can seriously damage and even destroy cells.

1.4   FREE RADICALS RESULT IN SHORTER TELOMERES

Free radicals typically combine in the body with hydrogen, lipids, or proteins, forming different reactive oxygen species (ROS) that attack cells and damage them, especially the cell membrane that encloses and protects each cell. Under ROS assault, cells cycle more rapidly, thus shortening the telomeres more rapidly with each cycle. The net effect is premature aging. Chapter 2 describes oxygen free radicals in detail, their major sources inside cells and outside, and their impact on telomeres.

1.5   A PROACTIVE NUTRITION PROGRAM CAN PREVENT FREE RADICAL CELL DAMAGE AND PROTECT TELOMERES

The damage to cells caused by free radicals and ROS can be considerably reduced by a diet program that supplies adequate antioxidants. In brief, antioxidants "neutralize" free radicals and reduce the formation of ROS. As will be shown in Chapter 3 on antioxidants, cells make all the antioxidants they need for protecting from the free radicals and ROS that they generate. But first, they need adequate nutrition support in the form of vitamins, minerals, enzymes, and other substances needed to make those antioxidants.

The protection afforded by antioxidants against toxic assaults on cells prevents premature cycling and so preserves telomere length for as long as possible, thereby averting premature aging.

This book will briefly describe elements of the biology of cell aging; detail the nature of free radicals, ROS, and antioxidant functions and interactions; detail the science that supports a nutrition approach to averting premature aging; and provide a list of simple high antioxidant foods, "functional foods," and recipes as means to implement the diet program.

1.6   LIFESPAN CANNOT BE LENGTHENED BUT IT CAN BE SHORTENED

After a number of divisions, and before the chromosomes in a given cell run out of telomeres, the cell can opt to self-repair any damage or even to self-destruct. Otherwise, it will die when it runs out of telomeres. Whichever course it *chooses* when damaged, but while it still has telomeres, may depend to a large degree on nutrition. Curiously, the scientific evidence points to an unexplained "choice" and nutrition can influence that choice.

It is now known that maximum lifespan cannot be lengthened, nor can aging be stopped. However, the lifespan of cells can be significantly shortened by setting the stage for them to make that choice. Lifespan shortens when damage to cells— damage that could have been be avoided—causes them to divide more rapidly, thus abbreviating the telomeres more rapidly, and forcing them to choose division or self-destruction. The more rapidly cells divide, the more rapidly they will run out of telomeres and die, or else they may be so damaged that they will choose to die. This self-destruction is called *apoptosis*.

1.7 SOURCES OF FREE RADICALS

There are two main types of free radicals: exogenous and endogenous. Exogenous free radicals are those that come from the environment. They play an important role but can actually be avoided much of the time. However, the most common free radicals are endogenous, that is, they come from within the cells, and they result, as Dr. Harman pointed out, from *oxidative metabolism* in the *mitochondria* (Harman 1972).

Mitochondria are small structures in the cell that make it possible for it to use oxygen to fuel metabolism. The way that cells use oxygen to create and use energy, however, causes free radicals to form. This source of free radicals and the resulting ROS cannot be avoided, but their impact can be lessened to slow down cell cycling.

1.8 PROACTIVE NUTRITION

The basic purpose and aim of the Proactive Nutrition Program is to slow telomere shortening:

- We can slow telomere abbreviation by slowing the rate of cell division.
- We can slow the rate of cell division by protecting them from free radical and ROS damage.
- We can protect cells from free radical and ROS damage by supporting their antioxidant defense.

There are three components to the Proactive Nutrition Program:

- It is basically a Mediterranean type-food plan that is rich in plant-based sources of antioxidants, vitamins, amino acids, etc.
- It is inherently a modestly restricted calories diet. Restricted calories activate longevity-promoting genes in the sirtuin family involved in energy management and storage (as fat) in the body.
- It is supplemented with so-called "sirtfoods" that activate the SIRT1-related longevity-promoting gene.

1.9 DOCUMENTATION

In most cases, popular diets aim at weight loss. This diet is aimed at longevity regardless of one's weight: a later section of this chapter will report that a study recently published in the *Journal of the American Medical Association* (*JAMA*) shows that baring extremes, overweight is not an obstacle to long life.

Much of what is in this book is quite new science. For that reason, the scientific sources supporting assertions or findings about the information presented here are thoroughly documented by citations of highly regarded conventional clinical/medical and other biological science sources. The information presented is based on conventional medical laboratory research methods, with the results published in prestigious, conventional medical journals, and accepted by the scientific community. Those rare cases where there is controversy will be indicated.

1.10   THE PLAN OF THE BOOK

Chapter 1 explains that one cannot prolong life but that it can be shortened. It describes how metabolism is the prime source of the oxygen free radicals that can cause accelerated cell division, telomere abbreviation, and therefore, premature aging. It also explains that normal, ordinary aging is not a disease, but that one can expect a natural age-related decline in function that is unavoidable. However, it is also pointed out that one can accelerate that decline by adverse lifestyle and diet choices causing premature aging.

Chapter 2 explains how metabolism results in the formation of toxic radical oxygen molecules, especially in *mitochondria*, and how these affect cell function and telomere length. The chapter also details how faced with oxygen radical attacks and the ensuing damage, cells may opt out by self-destruction.

Chapter 3 explains the nature of antioxidants and their action in combating toxic radicals that lead to telomere abbreviation. The chapter differentiates the antioxidants made by the body (endogenous) from those obtained through nutrition and the environment (exogenous), and it also provides information on United States Department of Agriculture (USDA) sources that list the antioxidant capacity of common foods.

Chapter 4 focuses on organelles in the cell in addition to mitochondria and shows how these are subject to radical attack that leads to cell damage and telomere abbreviation.

Chapter 5 discusses the gas nitric oxide (NO). The winners of the 1998 Nobel Prize in Medicine identified NO as a powerful antioxidant and as the "miracle molecule" that keeps the heart and blood vessels free of atherosclerotic sludge and keeps them "humming." While the primary aim of this book is to describe how telomeres can be protected, it also focuses on nutritional factors known to help avert aging of the cardiovascular system and the heart by drawing on the experience of the authors with nutrition that is rich in common NO-donor foods (Fried and Nezin 2006).

This chapter also introduces the reader to the use of the HumanN™ (formerly) Neogenis® N-O Test Strips. These are easy to use little saliva test strips that indirectly assess NO availability from the concentration of nitrites in saliva.

Chapter 6 traces the evolution of US government policy concerning consumer nutrition, which ultimately led to failure to guide Americans away from an unhealthy Western pattern diet due to the intrusion of corporate agriculture interests. It also describes attempts to improve diet via the heart-healthy diet of the American Heart Association (AHA) and ends by endorsing an enhanced Mediterranean diet pattern as being the best nutrition plan to preserve telomeres.

Chapter 7 details high-antioxidant diet plans and supplies sample recipes for both the Mediterranean diet component of the Proactive Nutrition Program and the supplementation of that food plan with so-called sirtfoods.

Chapter 8 presents selected relevant "functional foods" and supplements and documents their contribution to preserving telomere length. For instance, ginger is a powerful antioxidant and anti-inflammatory agent, which is superior to aspirin and much safer to consume. Likewise, sea vegetables (seaweed) are a handy source of iodine to add to the conventional diet to avert low thyroid function, which is now reaching epidemic proportions in the American population.

The nature, action, and source of free radicals are detailed in Chapter 2, but here is a brief introduction to the very important cell organelles, the *mitochondria*, that play such an important role in determining lifespan.

1.11   IN THE BEGINNING

Millions of years ago, science now reveals, a single cell swimming in the ocean gobbled up a bacterium that happened to pass by. This certainly would not have been a solitary occurrence as bacteria were apparently the common stuff these cells consumed. However, what made this fateful event different and propitious is that instead of being digested by the cell, the bacterium managed to set up residence in the cell where it replicated by division and populated it. And then it divided again when the cell divided so that the daughter cells of the bacterium migrated inside the daughter cells of the original cell.

This prototypical cell colonized then differentiated, and the bacterium inside the cell—now called a *mitochondrion*—accompanied the evolution of more and more complex cellular life so that its descendants now inhabit all biological forms that depend on oxygen for their metabolism. In fact, were it not for that initial event, there would be today no life as we know it because that first mitochondrion brought the cell new technology, a new way to form and manage energy based on oxygen.

1.11.1   MITOCHONDRIA

The mitochondrion had a life-enhancing advantage over the cell. It had developed the use of the increasing concentration of oxygen in the atmosphere to create energy. The host cell had never acquired this technology—its energy formation was relatively crude by comparison—and so the association between the mitochondrion and the cell benefited both: the mitochondrion got a host, and the host cell got the benefit of the newly acquired efficient "oxidative metabolism."

Mitochondria are small structures (organelles) found in large numbers in most cells (Figure 1.1). They are commonly called the cell "powerhouse" because they are involved in cell respiration and energy production in the form of adenosine triphosphate (ATP). (Mitochondria are illustrated in the context of a cell in Figure 4.1, in Chapter 4.)

ATP transports chemical energy within cells to power metabolism. ATP captures chemical energy obtained from the breakdown of food molecules and releases it to fuel other cellular processes. Some cells which use a lot of energy (muscles, for instance) have thousands of mitochondria, whereas other cells may have only a few hundred.

Mitochondria even have their own DNA and protective "cell" membrane. They are essentially "cells within cells" that help meet all of the body's basic energy needs. However, free-radical attacks on mitochondrial DNA damage them, causing the host cells to divide more quickly, thus shortening telomeres. Alternately, free radicals may damage them beyond repair, signaling them to self-destruct.

Protecting the cell cycle and, thus, the telomeres can be accomplished by (a) supporting the formation of antioxidants by the mitochondria to counter the free

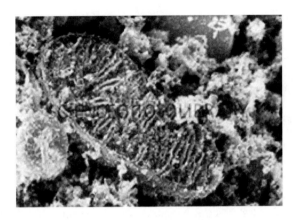

FIGURE 1.1   (See color insert.) Mitochondrion. Colored scanning electron micrograph (SEM) of a mitochondrion in a nerve cell. (Courtesy of Furness, D., Keele University/Science Photo Library, http://www.sciencephoto.com/media/77027/view.)

radicals that their metabolism generates, and (b) supplying an additional antioxidant-rich nutrition program such as the Proactive Nutrition Program.

1.12   AGING IS NOT A DISEASE

Science really does not know what actually *causes* aging. But, it knows the *biology of aging*: the biology of aging details what takes place as we age, that is, changes in body structure/shape and in physiological body functions.

It is clear that barring some rare exceptions, it is not possible to reliably estimate how long one would live based solely on observation of structure and function. "Longevity" and "life expectancy" are statistical concepts that rely on observing and calculating averages. However, science now finally has a window into individual longevity. Amazing as that may seem, this knowledge allows assessment of the length of telomeres at the ends of chromosomes to reveal how much time may be left on one's biological clock.

1.13   BIO 101

The chromosomes in the nucleus of each cell are little X- or Y-shaped structures that contain the hereditary information that controls cell growth, function, and reproduction. They contain the DNA conformed in genes that holds all the information required for creating, sustaining, and replicating the life of the cells. DNA is a sort of encrypted blueprint for every aspect of individual life. Until fairly recently, only cells could read this blueprint.

The mitochondria, as noted above, are organelles located inside the cell, in the gelatinous cytoplasm but outside the nucleus. They are responsible for energy production. They provide the power needed for metabolism, and they ventilate the cell. They are also responsible for cell growth and the cell life cycle including, in some cases, its self-destruction—a sort of cell suicide that scientists call *apoptosis*.

Both of these structures inside the cell respond to the factors that can cause premature aging. Telomeres can be thought of as the "face" of the clock that actually reveals the rate at which one is aging. Knowledge of telomere function can lead to simple nutritional strategies to avert premature aging. Chapter 7 will detail these science-based strategies, and how to effectively and efficiently incorporate them into daily life to help avoid premature aging.

It is important to understand that there is nothing in science that actually reveals how to *stop* or *reverse* aging. However, there is valid scientific evidence that one can prematurely *accelerate* aging with faulty lifestyle choices.

Here follow examples of natural changes in body function and shape that coincide with aging. These natural, expected, progressive changes do not, in and of themselves, constitute diseases. But, they can become diseases if they occur sooner than they would normally occur, or if they occur to a significantly greater degree than expected as a result of simple age progression.

1.14   CAN AGING BE TREATED BY MEDICINE?

For the most part, "anti-aging" books propose that aging is in some way abnormal—some sort of "deficiency disease." For example, *scurvy* plagued the world until the diet of British sailors was supplemented with citrus fruits by the Royal Navy physician, James Lind, in the mid-1700s. Subsequently, Albert Szent-Gyorgyi showed that scurvy, once a worldwide and often fatal epidemic disease, was due to a deficiency of vitamin C, and could be cured by supplementing with citrus fruits that are high in this vitamin. This discovery earned Szent-Gyorgyi the Nobel Prize in Medicine in 1937. Some years earlier, in 1923, Dr. Frederick G. Banting was awarded the Nobel Prize in Medicine for successfully treating type 1 diabetes with injections of insulin, after discovering that patients with this disease were deficient in this hormone produced by the pancreas.

There are many other examples of deficiency diseases and early medical findings set the stage for the growing belief that the concept of *deficiency diseases* also explains aging. This created an industry, claiming to be based on science, that various medicine and nutritional supplements could "turn back the clock" in the *disease* of aging.

"Aging-as-disease" is an accepted concept even today in conventional medical science circles. Many medical authorities maintain that aging is essentially the aggregate of diseases and medical conditions acquired during one's lifetime. In other words, aging is about being diseased. But the question then must be, does disease *cause* aging, or does aging *cause* disease?

Researchers from the prestigious Buck Institute, Novato, CA, the nation's first independent research facility focused solely on understanding the connection between aging and chronic disease, underscored the aging–causes–disease theme:

> Aging is the single most important risk factor in human disease.... Moreover, if aging causes multiple diseases then it is reasonable to think that pharmacological agents that slow aging could be also effective in preventing or slowing a wide spectrum of diseases. (Alavez and Lithgow 2011)

Their argument is that if aging can be cured, then diseases can be prevented.

On the other hand, a study recently appearing in the journal *Medical Reports*, titled "Age-related changes in clinical parameters and their associations with common complex diseases" (Murakata et al. 2015), approached the question from the opposite direction: What goes wrong as we age?

The investigators aimed to observe what they thought to be age-related changes in 13 clinical conditions, and how these conditions contributed to common diseases in their population sample. In other words, they began the study by assuming that to age is to become diseased, and here are the major diseases that one will get, and one will see them worsen with age: in brief, in men and women (with some minor differences), body mass index (BMI) and waist circumference rise with age and many become obese; blood pressure rises with age and many develop hypertension; type 2 diabetes mellitus increases gradually with age; dyslipidemia develops as all forms of bad serum cholesterols rise, while the good ones decline; and the kidneys gradually malfunction and the risk of chronic kidney diseases rises. This is just a small sample of their depressing observations. It is not surprising that they confirmed their belief that aging is the product of the accumulation of diseases and they concluded that if aging is about being diseased, then it should be medically treatable.

Of course, the conditions described in the study mentioned above do actually occur in almost all of us. But they are quite natural lifetime events, albeit the label "disease" is often applied even when these conditions are relatively trivial and do not really indicate a health hazard.

This book challenges the premise that aging is about being diseased. In fact, although it is obvious that life functions change with age, that does not have to lead to the conclusion that, in all cases, the changes spell "disease."

If it is held that aging is tantamount to disease, then it is reasonable to ask medicine to treat it. But, there was a time when medicine said that aging is not a disease but a natural event in human life. As medical science progressed to modern times, even relatively minor discomforts have come to be considered disease. The public demanded cures and medicine gave it to them: natural changes such as weight gain, the metabolic shift from fat to sugar, the increase in blood pressure, the loss of bone and muscle mass with hormone cycles, and many more became "diseases" at epidemic levels, and these diseases are now often treated with prescription medicines.

1.15   HOW DOES THE BODY CHANGE NATURALLY WITH AGE?

Body shape and functions change progressively with age. The changes that take place are natural, well known, and predictable, and they occur in all organs, even in individual cells (Masoro 2012; Baynes 2014).

1.15.1 Blood Pressure

On average, both systolic and diastolic blood pressure rise progressively in maturing men and women. Beginning in middle age, systolic blood pressure continues to rise, but diastolic blood pressure declines in both men and women. This is considered a function of normal aging. Diastolic blood pressure in people in their early 50s declines somewhat more steeply in men than in women at about the time when sex hormones decline (testosterone in men and estrogen in women) (Burt et al. 1995; Franklin et al. 1997; McEniery et al. 2005).

It is likely that the continuous rise in systolic blood pressure with age is related to a progressive increase in arterial stiffness (Mackenzie et al. 2002). Arterial stiffness is a measure of what medicine calls "compliance," or the elasticity of blood vessels. That arterial stiffness may, or may not, reflect the extent of atherosclerosis which progresses with age. Alternatively, it may reflect compensation for the lower volume of blood in the aging body (Minaker 2011).

There are two principal measures of blood vessel "elasticity": the *augmentation index* and arterial *pulse wave velocity*. Both of these measures indicate that as we age, our blood vessels become progressively more rigid (Mackenzie et al. 2002; McEniery et al. 2005; Djelić et al. 2013).

1.15.2 HEART FUNCTION AND BLOOD VESSELS

As we age, the heart tends to enlarge slightly, developing thicker walls and slightly larger chambers. The increase in size is mainly due to an increase in the size of individual heart muscle cells. The walls of the arteries and arterioles become thicker, and the space within the arteries, the *lumen*, widens slightly. Also, the amount of elastic tissue within the walls of the arteries and arterioles starts to shrink. Together, these changes make the vessels somewhat stiffer and less resilient as noted also in the elasticity/compliance measures cited above.

During rest, the older heart functions in almost the same way as a younger heart except that the heart rate is slightly lower. However, during exercise, the older heart cannot increase the volume of blood pumped out quite as much as a younger heart can, and this can limit performance.

As the arteries and arterioles become less elastic with age, they cannot relax as quickly during the rhythmic pumping of the heart. As a result, with aging, blood pressure increases more when the heart contracts during systole than it does in younger people (Shea 2016).

A team of researchers at Johns Hopkins University School of Medicine found that each year, as people age, the time it takes for their heart muscles to squeeze and relax increases by 2–5% (Lima 2007). Progressive detrimental age-related changes in heart function have been attributed in part to an insulin-like growth factor, peptide IGF-1 (Shioi and Inuzuka 2012), which is also associated with diseases that develop with age such as atherosclerosis (Higashi et al. 2012).

All in all, resting healthy young and old hearts are not all that different. The volume of blood pumped through the heart each minute (cardiac output) does not change much with age. However, there is at least one important difference between a healthy resting young heart and an older one: when a person is lying down, the pulse rates of a young and old heart remain about the same, but when sitting, heart rate is slower in older people compared with that in younger men and women. This difference is not known to have any clinical significance.

Medical research studies of structures of the heart have failed to find any evidence of microscopic changes that can be ascribed to aging alone. However, there appear to be age-related changes in both the anatomy and physiology of major arteries (Klausner and Schwartz 1985).

Atherosclerosis, commonly known as hardening of the arteries, increases with age as seen by the increase in plaque formation in blood vessels. Plaque formation begins when free radical–oxidized cholesterol is taken up by immune system cells—macrophages usually—and deposited in the wall of a blood vessel. Thereafter, the macrophages disintegrate leaving debris that injures the site where they are deposited. The injury is recognized by blood platelets that rush to repair it. In the process, they release *serotonin* that promotes the formation of a fiber structure that envelops the debris and ultimately accumulates calcium to form rigid plaque.

Writing in the journal *Circulation Research*, the journal of the AHA, in 2012, Wang and Bennett paint a pretty dismal picture:

> Atherosclerosis is classed as a disease of aging... and telomere shortening and dysfunction. Not only is cellular senescence (aging) associated with atherosclerosis, there is growing evidence that cellular senescence promotes atherosclerosis. (Wang and Bennett 2012)

What they are saying is that as we age we accumulate plaque and accumulating plaque ages us. Note especially that the process shortens *telomeres*. The purpose of the Proactive Nutrition Program is to help prevent this premature shortening that will help slow down the aging process.

1.15.3 Blood Sugar and Insulin Function

Serum blood sugar (glucose) levels vary with metabolism and level of activity and, in turn, also vary with sleep/wake cycles. It is commonly measured after overnight fasting. But, in order to get a clearer picture of blood sugar level and insulin function, there are measures that estimate average blood sugar level over a greater time span.

One such measure is the A1C test, and the other is the similar estimated average glucose (eAG) test that will soon replace A1C in conventional routine medical test procedures. The A1C test estimates the average level of glucose bound in hemoglobin in blood cells over a 3-month period. The eAG test changes the A1C percentage to conventional mg/dl units. A1C levels rise progressively with age even in non-diabetic populations (Pani et al. 2008).

The Framingham Heart Study conducted by the National Heart, Lung, and Blood Institute (NHLBI) of the National Institutes of Health (NIH), and Boston University, beginning in 1948, first showed progressive age-related rising trends in blood sugar levels in men and women. But it actually revealed more: it was found that participants with the lowest blood glucose levels lived longer than those with higher blood glucose levels (Yashin et al. 2009).

The reason for this difference in survival rate may be related to the age-related shift from fat as the primary fuel of metabolism to sugar as the primary fuel. Burning (oxidizing) these different fuels causes the formation of different quantities of free radicals. Sugar produces the most free radicals which results in *oxidative stress*, the damage caused by "free radical oxidation."

Oxidative stress is the principal culprit in premature aging.

1.15.4 DECREASED INSULIN VERSUS RESISTANCE TO INSULIN

The metabolism of carbohydrates depends on the secretion of insulin by cells in the pancreas. Secretion of insulin helps keeps the blood sugar level from getting too high (hyperglycemia) or too low (hypoglycemia). No one questions that blood sugar in excess of metabolic needs is harmful. Elevated blood sugar is *diabetes*. Type 1 diabetes, which most commonly affects children and young adults, occurs when insulin secretion is insufficient due to dysfunction of cells in the pancreas. Type 2 diabetes, thought to be due either to insulin insufficiency or to "resistance" to insulin, more commonly develops in adults. But, it is now increasingly seen in children, and it is associated with the growing rate of obesity.

According to investigators reporting in the journal *Diabetes*, impaired tissue sensitivity to insulin is the primary factor responsible for the decrease in glucose tolerance observed with advancing age. Since liver glucose production is normally suppressed by insulin in older individuals, the site of insulin resistance must be in other organs such as muscles. The response of pancreatic beta cells to glucose cannot account for the age-related decline in glucose metabolism (DeFronzo 1979).

1.15.5 BLOOD LIPIDS

Cholesterol is one of the lipids found throughout the body in all tissues including blood. It is an important component of living cells. Together with carbohydrates and proteins, lipids are the main constituents of plant and animal cells. Cholesterol plays a central role in the formation of cell membranes, and is required for the formation of bile acid in the liver and the production of hormones, such as steroid hormones in the adrenal glands. The blood and liver make all the cholesterol needed and circulate it through the blood.

Serum LDL cholesterol and HDL cholesterol first rise progressively with age in men and women. Then they both decline with age (Ferrara et al. 1997). The rate of decline is affected by cardiorespiratory fitness (Park et al. 2015). Furthermore, while serum cholesterol progressively rises with age, the rise is steepest in those men and women with cardiovascular heart disease (Gertler et al. 1950).

In the early 1980s, the Lipid Research Clinics Program Prevalence Study sponsored by the NHLBI also reported that plasma lipid and lipoprotein concentrations in men and women rise with age. Higher total cholesterol values in men, compared with those in women, appear between the ages of 20 and 50 years, and higher LDL cholesterol levels were observed in the same age span. HDL cholesterol, thought to protect the heart, was higher in women than in men throughout the age range considered (Heiss et al. 1980).

This progressive age-related rise in serum cholesterol is so well defined and constant that it is even maintained when total population serum cholesterol values decline. This was illustrated in a report published in the *Annals of Internal Medicine* in 1996. This report compared data trends in serum cholesterol levels for different 5-year age ranges beginning at 25 years old to 64 years old.

The trends were virtually parallel from the first year observed, 1972, to the last year observed, 1992, even though the serum cholesterol levels declined with each sampled year. This seems to reflect an inherent age-related progressive increase in serum cholesterol level regardless of the overall level (Jousilahti et al. 1996). The study, conducted in Finland, reported data indistinguishable from those reported in American men in the study by Heiss et al. (1980), cited above.

1.15.6   Body Fat Percentage and Body Mass Index

Most people will gain weight with age, and the body fat percentage (BFP) increases with age both in men and in women (Mills 2005; St-Onge and Gallagher 2010). BFP correlates reasonably well with BMI, a weight to height ratio. The major reason for the increase in body fat in older persons appears to be weight gain rather than a true age-related increase in percentage of body fat (Silver, et al. 1993). BFP rises with age in both men and women, from 15% to 45% in women and from 8% to 35% in men.

Figure 1.2 comes from a study that evaluated the effect of smoking *and* obesity on mortality (Berrington de Gonzalez et al. 2010). Looking only at risk of death from obesity, it seems that in white adults, overweight and obesity (and possibly underweight) are associated with increased all-cause mortality. All-cause mortality is generally lowest with a BMI of 20.0–24.9. But, being in the underweight category (<18.5) is actually more hazardous than being in the overweight category (25–29.9). A significant increase in the risk of death only begins with moderately obese people.

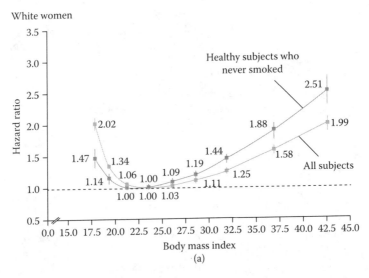

FIGURE 1.2   **(See color insert.)** Estimated hazard ratios for death from any cause according to body mass index (BMI) for all study participants and for healthy subjects who never smoked. Hazard ratios and 95% confidence intervals are shown for white women (a). The hazard ratios were adjusted for alcohol intake (grams per day), educational level, marital status, and overall physical activity. (From Berrington de Gonzalez, A., et al., *N. Engl. J. Med.*, 363, 2211–2219, 2010. With permission.)   *(Continued)*

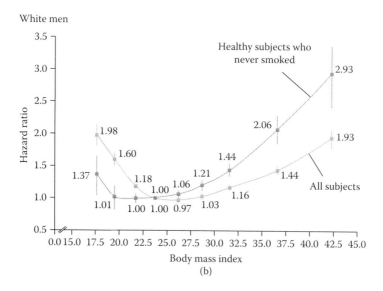

FIGURE 1.2 (Continued) (See color insert.) Estimated hazard ratios for death from any cause according to body mass index (BMI) for all study participants and for healthy subjects who never smoked. Hazard ratios and 95% confidence intervals are shown for white men (b). The hazard ratios were adjusted for alcohol intake (grams per day), educational level, marital status, and overall physical activity. (From Berrington de Gonzalez, A., et al., *N. Engl. J. Med.*, 363, 2211–2219, 2010. With permission.)

1.15.7 THYROID FUNCTION

There is progressive age-related decline in thyroid function. Parenthetically, thyroid dysfunction due to dietary iodine deficiency is considered to be the second most prevalent deficiency disease in the United States (see Chapter 8). Subclinical thyroid dysfunction, as measured by clinical test, is found in up to 10% of women over the age of 50 (Stockigt 2011).

The thyroid gland produces two principal hormones, thyroxine (T4) and the more active triiodothyronine (T3). T3 and T4 are synthesized from iodine and tyrosine. The thyroid also produces calcitonin, which plays a role in calcium homeostasis. Hormonal production by the thyroid is regulated by thyroid-stimulating hormone (TSH), produced by the pituitary gland.

A 2011 report in *The Journal of Clinical Endocrinology & Metabolism* tells us that aging is associated with increased serum TSH concentrations with no change in free T4 concentrations. The largest TSH increase is in people with the lowest TSH at baseline. This suggests that the TSH increase arises from age-related alteration in the TSH set point or reduced TSH bioactivity rather than thyroid disease per se (Bremner et al. 2012).

Insufficient iodine is one of the reasons for thyroid deficiency. But, another reason is that dopamine availability progressively declines with age by about 46% over the age range of 18 to 88 years, or 6.6% per decade. This decline is largely due to the gradual failure of the process by which dopamine is transported in the brain, that is, by the striatal dopamine transporter (DAT), for example (van Dyck et al. 2002). Decreased dopamine availability has implications for many "reward"-sustained functions including how we eat.

Note: Earlier, it was pointed out that atherosclerosis is a progressive age-related medical condition. Hypothyroidism is likewise a progressive age-related medical condition. There is reason to believe that the parallel progress of these conditions is not coincidental. In fact, a report in *The Journal of Clinical Endocrinology & Metabolism* informs us that it has been known for some time that a relationship exists between hypothyroidism and atherosclerosis. Apparently, thyroid hormone regulation of lipids and homocysteine metabolism contribute an explanation for how hypothyroidism raises the risk of cardiovascular disease (Cappola and Ladenson 2003). Perhaps, at least in some cases, conditions that are "known" to be age-related may be ameliorated, where possible, by the management of the one or the other.

1.15.8   KIDNEY FUNCTION

When kidneys are working well, they filter out wastes and excess fluid that become part of the urine the body makes each day. When kidneys are not working well, they do not remove enough wastes and fluids to maintain health and to make important hormones needed for blood and bones. The age-related loss of kidney function resulting in progressive decline in filtration rate and blood flow to the kidneys varies widely in the population (Weinstein and Anderson 2010).

There are three routine blood test estimates of how well kidneys work. *Creatinine* is a waste byproduct of muscle metabolism. It rises steadily with age (Tiao et al. 2002). Blood urea nitrogen (BUN) that forms when protein breaks down also rises progressively with age. The glomerular filtration rate (GFR) estimates how much blood passes through the tiny structures in the kidneys that filter waste from the blood. GFR declines progressively with age (Glassock 2009; Glassock and Winearls 2009).

Now, the good news. According to Dr. R.J. Glassock writing in the *Nephrology Times* about the decline in GFR observed to occur as we age,

> [It] is a normal and expected phenomenon that does not in and of itself confer any selective disadvantage upon the individual unless other diseases are superimposed.... GFR decline is independent of hypertension or cardiovascular impairment, occurring even in indigenous native societies where hypertension is completely absent. (Glassock and Winearls 2009)

1.15.9   STEROID HORMONES

There are two classes of steroid hormones: corticosteroids formed in the adrenal glands and sex steroids formed in the gonads or the placenta. Steroid formation progressively declines with age and the lower levels tend to potentiate other functions that decline with age in parallel.

1.15.9.1   The Immune System

Dehydroepiandrosterone (DHEA), the most abundant steroid in the bloodstream, is formed in the adrenal glands early in the day. It is converted to androgens, estrogens, and other hormones that regulate fat, metabolism, sexual and reproductive function, and energy levels. Levels gradually decline with age, falling as much as 90% by age 60 (Danenberg et al. 1995).

DHEA has consistently been shown to boost beneficial interleukin-2 and suppress damaging interkeukin-6 levels. Interleukins are proteins that regulate the activities of white blood cells in our immune system. Interleukin-6 tends to be overproduced in the aging, which may contribute to autoimmune disease, immune dysfunction, osteoporosis, slower healing, breast cancer, B-cell lymphoma, and anemia (van Vollenhoven et al. 1998).

1.15.9.2   Blood Sugar Metabolism/Weight Management

DHEA helps to maintain insulin growth factor (IGF). However, aging causes a decline in IGF level that contributes to the loss of lean body mass, as well as excess fat accumulations, neurological impairment, and age-associated immune dysfunction (Morales et al. 1998; Ribeiro and Garcia-Segura 2002).

1.15.9.3   Heart Disease

DHEA inhibits abnormal blood platelet aggregation, a major factor in the development of sudden heart attack and stroke (Jesse et al. 1995).

1.15.9.4   Estrogen/Testosterone Levels

On average, men and women produce predictable levels of both male (testosterone) and female (estrogen) sex hormones. These levels fluctuate regularly with changing age-related body conditions over the lifespan. All sex hormones progressively decline with age.

Testosterone in men rises sharply at puberty and then progressively declines over the lifespan. Estrogen in men rises gradually at puberty and remains more or less constant at much lower levels over the lifespan. Estradiol (an estrogen made by women) rises sharply at puberty and then declines in the late 40s as women approach menopause. Testosterone rises somewhat in the mid-20s in women and then gradually declines over the lifespan. Sexual desire (libido) is driven primarily by testosterone in men and in women, and it declines as testosterone levels decline (van Anders 2012).

1.15.10   BONES, MUSCLES, AND JOINTS

Bone mass (density) is lost as we age. In particular, women lose bone mass with loss of estradiol at menopause due to loss of calcium and other minerals. In both men and women, bone mass begins to decline at about age 30. Women lose more bone mass, and do so more quickly than do men, starting at about 50 years of age, the approximate age at which women go through the menopause. Not only do their menstrual periods lessen and eventually cease, but their ovaries also reduce in size and then cease producing estrogen.

The spinal vertebrae are separated by a gel-like cushion (disk). With age, the trunk becomes shorter as the disks gradually lose fluid and become thinner. Likewise, vertebrae lose mineral content making each bone thinner. The spinal column curves somewhat and it compresses. The foot arches become less pronounced, contributing to a slight loss of height. The arm and leg bones do not change length and this makes them appear longer when compared with the shortened trunk. The joints become stiffer and less flexible.

Hip and knee joints may show degenerative cartilage changes. The finger joints lose cartilage and the bones thicken slightly. Finger joint changes are more common in women. Some joints, such as the ankle, typically change very little with aging.

Lean body mass decreases in part due to muscle tissue atrophy. Muscle changes often begin in the 20s in men and in the 40s in women.

Lipofuscin, an age-related pigment, and fat are deposited in muscle tissue as muscle fibers shrink. Muscle tissue may be replaced by a tough fibrous tissue that is most noticeable in the hands, making them look thin and bony. Muscles may become rigid with age and may lose tone, even with regular exercise.

Bones become more brittle and may break more easily. Overall height decreases, mainly because the trunk and spine shorten. Breakdown of the joints may lead to inflammation, pain, stiffness, and deformity. Joint changes affect almost all elderly people with conditions ranging from minor stiffness to severe arthritis.

Stooping may occur and knees and hips may become more flexed. The neck may tilt and shoulders may narrow while the pelvis becomes wider. Movement slows and may become limited. Gait may become slower and shorter, and the individual gets tired more easily (Anonymous, No date; MedlinePlus 2016).

1.15.11 ANTIOXIDANT DEFENSES

It was previously noted that there is considerable scientific support for a free radical theory of aging that proposes that we age prematurely because our body cells fail to prevent *oxidative stress*, the accumulation of damage caused by free radicals over time. The good news is that scientific evidence leads to the conclusion that the body can combat free radicals with antioxidants that it naturally makes to *passivate* (make passive or inactivate) free radicals.

However, over time, the body progressively loses the ability to form these antioxidants. The age-related loss of antioxidant formation is detailed in Chapter 3.

Investigators writing in the journal *Experimental Biology and Medicine* in 2002 report that as we age, respiratory function declines, and that tends to cause enhanced production of free radicals in mitochondria. In addition, with age, there occur changes in the ability of antioxidants to neutralize free radicals in the mitochondria. The net result is that oxidative stress rises in the mitochondria and their ability to produce the energy for metabolism is jeopardized.

Given sufficient oxidative damage, mitochondria can self-destruct (apoptosis), impairing the life function of the cell that they inhabit. Oxidative damage leading to destructive changes in mitochondria was found to increase with age in various human tissues (Wei and Lee 2002). Some investigators proposed that endogenous (body-formed) antioxidants such as lipoic acid and L-carnitine are specifically intended to target free radicals formed by, and found in, mitochondria (Savitha et al. 2005).

It is clear that all endogenous antioxidant formation declines with aging, and the evidence for this decline will be detailed in Chapter 3. But, it should be noted that glutathione peroxidase (GPx), one of our most important sources of protection from free radicals and ROS, shows the most prominent age-related decline (Kasapoglu and Ozben 2001).

As noted earlier, Dr. D. Harman was the first scientist to propose in 2007 that we age prematurely because of oxidative stress. He wrote:

> In order to achieve healthy aging the older people should be encouraged to acquire healthy life styles which should include diets rich in antioxidants. (Rahman 2007)

The proposed Proactive Nutrition Program is intended to follow that advice.

REFERENCES

Alavez, S., and G. G. Lithgow. 2011. A new look at old compounds. *Aging*, 3(4): 338–339.

Anonymous. *Exercise, Nutrition, Hormones, and Bone Tissue*. http://oerpub.github.io/epubjs-demo-book/content/m46305.xhtml

Baynes, J. W. 2014. Aging. In: Baynes, J. W., and M. H. Dominiczak, eds. *Medical Biochemistry*. 4th ed. Philadelphia, PA: Elsevier Saunders, pp. 592–601.

Berrington de Gonzalez, A., P. Hartge, J. R. Cerhan, et al. 2010. Body-mass index and mortality among 1.46 million white adults. *New England Journal of Medicine*, 363: 2211–2219.

Bremner, A. P., P. Feddema, P. J. Leedman, et al. 2012. Age-related changes in thyroid function: A longitudinal study of a community-based cohort. *The Journal of Clinical Endocrinology & Metabolism*, 97(5): 1554–1562.

Burt, V. L., P. Whelton, E. J. Roccella, et al. 1995. Prevalence of hypertension in the US adult population. Results from the Third National Health and Nutrition Examination Survey, 1988–1991. *Hypertension*, 25(3): 305–313.

Cappola, A. R., and P. W. Ladenson. 2003. Hypothyroidism and atherosclerosis. *The Journal of Clinical Endocrinology & Metabolism*, 88(6): 2438–2344.

Danenberg, H. D., A. Ben-Yehuda, Z. Zakay-Rones, et al. 1995. Dehydroepiandrosterone (DHEA) treatment reverses the impaired immune response of old mice to influenza vaccination and protects from influenza infection. *Vaccine*, 13(15): 1445–1458.

DeFronzo, R. A. 1979. Glucose intolerance and aging: Evidence for tissue insensitivity to insulin. *Diabetes*, 28(12): 1095–1101.

Djelić, M., S. Mazić, and D. Žikić. 2013. A novel laboratory approach for the demonstration of hemodynamic principles: The arterial blood flow reflection. *Advances in Physiology Education*, 37(4): 321–326.

Ferrara, A., E. Barrett-Connor, and J. Shan. 1997. Total, LDL, and HDL cholesterol decrease with age in older men and women. The Rancho Bernardo Study 1984–1994. *Circulation*, 96: 37–43.

Franklin, S. S., W. Gustin, 4th, N. D. Wong, et al. 1997. Hemodynamic patterns of age-related changes in blood pressure. The Framingham Heart Study. *Circulation*, 96(1): 308–315.

Fried, R., and L. Nezin. 2006. *Great Food—Great Sex*. New York: Ballentine Books.

Gertler, M. M., S. M. Garn, and E. F. Bland. 1950. Age, serum cholesterol and coronary artery disease. *Circulation*, 2: 517–522.

Glassock, R. J. 2009. Viewpoint. The GFR decline with aging: A sign of normal senescence, not disease. *Nephrology Times*, 2(9): 6–8.

Glassock, R. J., and C. Winearls. 2009. Ageing and the glomerular filtration rate: Truths and consequences. *Transactions of the American Clinical and Climatological Association*, 120: 419–428.

Harman, D. 1972. A biologic clock: The mitochondria? *Journal of the American Geriatrics Society*, 20(4): 145–147.

Harman, D. 1992. Free radical theory of aging. *Mutation Research/DNAging*, 275(3–6): 257–266.

Hayflick, L. 1965. The limited in vitro lifetime of human diploid cell strains. *Experimental Cell Research*, 37(3): 614–636.

Heiss, G., I. Tamir, C. E. Davis, et al. 1980. Lipoprotein-cholesterol distributions in selected North American populations: The lipid research clinics program prevalence study. *Circulation*, 61(2): 302–315.

Higashi, Y., S. Sukhanov, A. Anwar, et al. 2012. Aging, atherosclerosis, and IGF-1. *Journal of Gerontology Series A Biological Science & Medical Science*, 67(6): 626–639.

Jesse, R. L., K. Loesser, D. M. Eich, et al. 1995. Dehydroepiandrosterone inhibits human platelet aggregation in vitro and in vivo. *Annals of the New York Academy of Sciences*, 774: 281–290.

Jousilahti, P., E. Vartiainen, J. Tuomilehto, et al. 1996. Twenty-year dynamics of serum cholesterol levels in the middle-aged population of eastern Finland. *Annals of Internal Medicine*, 125(9): 713–722.

Kasapoglu, M., and T. Ozben. 2001. Alterations of antioxidant enzymes and oxidative stress markers in aging. *Experimental Gerontology*, 36(2): 209–220.

Klausner, S. C., and A. B. Schwartz. 1985. The aging heart. *Clinics in Geriatric Medicine*, 1(1): 119–141.

Lima, J. A. C. 2007. *Aging Heart Changes Shape, Shrinks And Loses Pumping Function Too.* http://www.hopkinsmedicine.org/news/media/releases/aging_heart_changes_shape shrinks_and_loses_pumping_function_too.

Mackenzie, I. S., I. B. Wilkinson, and J. R. Cockcroft. 2002. Assessment of arterial stiffness in clinical practice. *Quarterly Journal of Medicine*, 95: 67–74.

Masoro, E. J. 2012. The physiology of aging. In: Boron, W. F., and E. L. Boulpaep, eds. *Medical Physiology*. 2nd ed. Philadelphia, PA: Elsevier Saunders, pp. 1281–1292.

McEniery, C. M., I. R. Yasmin Hall, A. Qasem, et al. 2005. Normal vascular aging: Differential effects on wave reflection and aortic pulse wave velocity: The Anglo-Cardiff Collaborative Trial (ACCT). *Journal of the American College of Cardiology*, 46: 1753–1760.

MedlinePlus. 2016. *Medline.* NIH National Library of Medicine. https://www.nlm.nih. gov/medlineplus/ency/article/004015.htm

Mills, T. C. 2005. Predicting body fat using data on the BMI. *Journal of Statistics Education*, 13(2). www.amstat.org/publications/jse/v13n2/datasets.mills.html

Minaker, K. L. 2011. Common clinical sequelae of aging. In: Goldman, L., and A. I. Schafer, eds. *Goldman's Cecil Medicine*. 24th ed. Philadelphia, PA: Elsevier Saunders, pp.104–109.

Morales, A. J., R. H. Haubrich, J. Y. Hwang, et al. 1998. The effect of six months treatment with a 100 mg daily dose of dehydroepiandrosterone (DHEA) on circulating sex steroids, body composition and muscle strength in age-advanced men and women. *Clinical Endocrinology*, 49(4): 421–432.

Murakata, Y., T. Fujimaki, and Y. Yamada. 2015. Age-related changes in clinical parameters and their associations with common complex diseases. *Biomedical Reports*, 3(6): 767–777.

Pani, L. N., L. Korenda, J. B. Meigs, et al. 2008. Effect of aging on A1C levels in individuals without diabetes: Evidence from the Framingham Offspring Study and the National Health and Nutrition Examination Survey 2001–2004. *Diabetes Care*, 31(10): 1991–1996.

Park, Y.-M. P, X. Sui, J. Liu, et al. 2015. The effect of cardiorespiratory fitness on age-related lipids and lipoproteins. *Journal of the American College of Cardiology*, 65(19): 2091–2100.

Rahman, K. 2007. Studies on free radicals, antioxidants, and co-factors. *Clinical Interventions in Aging*, 2(2): 219–236.

Ribeiro, M. F., and L. M. Garcia-Segura. 2002. Dehydroepiandrosterone regulates insulin-like growth factor-1 system in adult rat hypothalamus. *Endocrine*, 17(2): 129–134.

Savitha, S., J. Tamilselvan, M. Anusuyadevi, et al. 2005. Oxidative stress on mitochondrial antioxidant defense system in the aging process: Role of dl-α-lipoic acid and l-carnitine. *Clinica Chimica Acta*, 355(1–2): 173–180.

Shea, M. J. 2016. *Effects of Aging on the Heart and Blood Vessels, Merck Manual*. Kenilworth, NJ: Merck Sharp & Dohme.

Shioi, T., and Y. Inuzuka. 2012. Aging as a substrate of heart failure. *Journal of Cardiology*, 6(6): 423–428.

Silver, A. J., C. Guillen, M. J. Kahl, et al. 1993. Effect of aging on body fat. *Journal of the American Geriatric Society*, 41(3): 211–213.

St-Onge, M.-P., and D. Gallagher. 2010. Body composition changes with aging: The cause or the result of alterations in metabolic rate and macronutrient oxidation? *Nutrition*, 26(2): 152–155.

Stockigt, J. 2011. Clinical Strategies in the Testing of Thyroid Function. *Thyroid Disease Manager*. South Dartmouth, MA: Endocrine Education.

Tiao, J. Y., J, B. Semmens, J. R. Masarei, et al. 2002. The effect of age on serum creatinine levels in an aging population: Relevance to vascular surgery. *Cardiovascular Surgery*, 10(5): 445–451.

van Anders, S. M. 2012. Testosterone and sexual desire in healthy women and men. *Archives of Sexual Behavior*, 41(6): 1471–1484.

van Dyck, C. H., J. P. Seibyl, R. T. Malison, et al. 2002. Age-related decline in dopamine transporters analysis of striatal subregions, nonlinear effects, and hemispheric symmetries. *American Journal of Geriatric Psychiatry*, 10: 36–43.

van Vollenhoven, R. F., L. M. Morabito, E. G. Engleman, et al. 1998. Treatment of systemic lupus erythematosus with dehydroepiandrosterone: 50 patients treated up to 12 months. *Journal of Rheumatology*, 25(2): 285–289.

Wang, J. C., and M. Bennett. 2012. Aging and atherosclerosis. Mechanisms, functional consequences, and potential therapeutics for cellular senescence. *Circulation Research*, 111: 245–259.

Wei, Y.-H., and H.-C. Lee. 2002. Enzymes in aging oxidative stress, mitochondrial DNA mutation, and impairment of antioxidant. *Experimental Biology and Medicine*, 227: 671–682.

Weinstein, J. R., and S. Anderson. 2010. The aging kidney: Physiological changes. *Advances in Chronic Kidney Diseases*, 17(4): 302–307.

Yashin, A., S. V. Ukraintseva, K. G. Arbeev, et al. 2009. Maintaining physiological state for exceptional survival: What is the normal level of blood glucose and does it change with age? *Mechanisms of Ageing and Development*, 130(9): 611–618.

2 Free Radicals Damage Cells

2.1 INTRODUCTION

The first chapter documented the pattern of age-related decline in function as a normal and, indeed, a natural progressive change. What's more, as much as it may be desirable, there is no scientific proof that one can lengthen lifespan. The changes are perceived as erosion of functions, but in some respects, some can also be viewed as adaptive changes. Yet, there is a long history of evolution on this planet and what was adaptive "then" may not necessarily be adaptive now. Just two examples are given below.

For instance, age-related changes in the preponderance of sugar as a fuel versus fat as a fuel for metabolism, and fat storage in the body for consumption in "leaner" times, as noted in the previous chapter, may have favored the survival of our Paleolithic ancestors, but it does little except lead to obesity and type 2 diabetes now—both health disasters.

Theories of age-related changes and adaptation may explain how lifespan plays out, but it would still be desirable to delay the inevitable end as much as possible. There is a way to do that and the Proactive Nutrition Program is the way to go: this proactive diet singles out and combats the proven main culprit in premature aging: free radicals and ROS. Free radicals are the dark side of oxygen that we cannot avoid but that we can combat.

2.2 WHY DO WE AGE?

Chapter 1 made the case that for the most part, age-related changes over the lifespan are not "disease" per se. In fact, these age-related changes are natural, despite being mostly undesirable. On average, these changes follow a biologically programmed plan that is inscribed in DNA. This programming determines the aging rate of the individual lifespan of the 50–70 billion cells that make up the body.

Right from the start of life, most of these cells divide in repetitive division cycles. At the same time, the body sheds cells to more or less maintain its appropriate shape and function as the body develops. What cells divide and what cells are shed is preprogrammed but is influenced by free radicals.

Gerontologists from a university research institute in Madrid, Spain, estimate that when all the cells in the body have divided to make daughter cells, and some are shed, and those daughter cells divide again, and those are shed, and so on, the maximum lifespan including all those generations is estimated to be 120 years (Ruiz-Torres and Beier 2005). Curiously, this coincides with scripture: "The Lord said, 'My breath shall not abide in man forever, since he too is flesh; let the days allowed him be a hundred and twenty years'" (Genesis 6:3).

This raises two questions: first, why doesn't the population live to 120 years and, second, why only 120 years?

No one seems to know the answer to either of these questions. It is known that the average lifespan of men and women in the United States is now 79.68 years according to the Centers for Disease Control and Prevention (CDC) (Xu et al. 2016), whereas just over 100 years ago, in 1916, it was 54.3 years (Anonymous No date). What accounts for the increase? Changes in nutrition should definitely be considered as one possible factor.

The body, by analogy, is a community with various degrees of organization from single cells, to tissues, to organs, etc. What happens at any level is a consequence of what happens at all lower levels. For this reason, to understand the "biological clock," it is necessary to look at the biological clock of all the cells that make up our body. The sum of those cellular clocks determines our cellular clock. This chapter will examine how this clock might be inadvertently sped up, and alternatively, how that could be prevented.

2.3   WHAT IS THE BIOLOGICAL CLOCK?

Aging is observable and the rate at which it takes places can vary considerably in different people. Clearly, we all have a different clock and genetically, while it may not seem that way, we are all more similar than we are different. For that reason, science can derive some general rules about what factors contribute to aging, but not what causes it. Science has shown that the clock can be sped up, and what remains to be understood is how that can be avoided. Free radicals age us. We can speed up aging by feeding *free radicals* to the clock.

The genetics of aging has made substantial strides, but it has been confined primarily to the study of animals. There really are differences in individual longevity. There are *longevity genes* but, as luck would have it, that knowledge does not help us to predict anything. A researcher from the Department of Biochemistry and Molecular Biology, Louisiana State University Health Sciences Center, New Orleans, reports that these longevity genes (about 35 or so) encode a wide array of cellular functions, leading to the conclusion that there are also multiple mechanisms of aging.

Some generalizations are already emerging as processes in aging: metabolic control, resistance to stress, gene deregulation, and genetic stability. The first two concern caloric restriction, which has been shown to postpone aging and increase lifespan in rodents. Many of the human longevity homolog genes found in different organisms have been identified (a homolog gene is inherited in two different species by a common ancestor) (Jazwinski 2000).

2.4   WHAT JEOPARDIZES LONGEVITY?

Why would people with genes inscribed for a long lifespan fail to reach it, barring an accident, a hostile environment, or fatal disease, for instance? In general, longevity results from the cells dividing into the maximum number of generations, estimated to be between 50 and 70. But, why would cell division accelerate? The short answer is damage caused by free radicals, that is, oxidative stress.

2.4.1 What Are Free Radicals?

When an oxygen atom loses an electron to another atom that has one missing, the first atom will try to attract one from another atom nearby. This results in a cascade of atoms trying to attract electrons from each other as they, in turn, lose one. This destabilizes the whole chemical environment.

Free radicals are atoms, or groups of atoms, most often oxygen, with one unpaired electron—a radical—or something combined with oxygen in that form. Figure 2.1 shows both environmental (exogenous) and intracellular metabolic (endogenous) sources of free radicals including radiation, UV radiation from the sun, smoking, pollution, etc.

The metabolism of cells, in particular the mitochondria, is largely responsible for the endogenous free radicals—those we make within our bodies. There are also many other sources of free radicals in the body. Figure 2.1 shows that a major target of free radicals is usually the DNA in chromosomes in the cells.

2.4.2 Free Radical Sources from Cell Metabolism

There are numerous mitochondria in *eukaryote* cells, which constitute most of our cells and also have a nucleus (see Chapter 4, Figure 4.1). Mitochondria are the power plants of our cells that provide them with the capability of oxidative metabolism, that is, burning

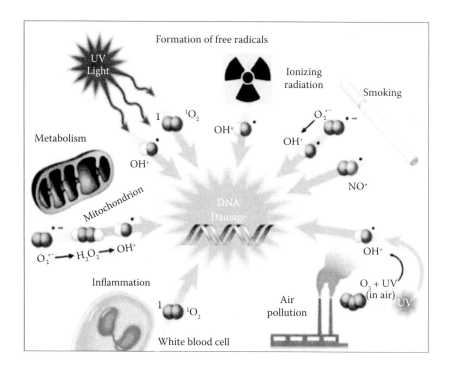

FIGURE 2.1 **(See color insert.)** Environmental and metabolic sources of free radicals. (From Pendyala et al., *J. Indian Soc. Periodontol.*, 12, 3, 79–83, 2008. With permission.)

food/fuel with oxygen that the cells otherwise lack. In the process, they generate free radicals.

This might not matter much except that cells are made up of many different types of component substances including proteins and phospholipids that form the basic flexible structure of the cell bilayer membrane. Scattered in the lipid bilayer are cholesterol molecules that help to keep the membrane fluid consistent.

Free radical oxygen combines with lipids to form *lipid peroxide*. It is not simply a matter of cholesterol combining with oxygen to form oxidized cholesterol, but a radical oxygen forming what eventually turns out, through an intermediate process, to be *hydrogen peroxide*. Hydrogen peroxide is used to bleach hair, and it is a prime component of rocket fuel and, in some cases, explosives. It is not helpful to have it circulating in the blood stream in any quantity.

Lipid peroxidation is a major culprit in many diseases, especially atherosclerosis leading to cardiovascular and heart disease. It is generated naturally in relatively small amounts in the body, mainly by the effect of several reactive oxygen species including hydrogen peroxide.

2.5 WHAT ARE REACTIVE OXYGEN SPECIES?

In scientific journals, scientists usually do not talk much about free radicals as they do about *reactive oxygen species*. What are they? The combination of free radical oxygen with other molecules forms different types (species) of reactive, destructive compounds. These reactive oxygen species (ROS) readily attack the cholesterol in the cell membrane, initiating a self-propagating chain reaction. The adverse alteration of cell membrane lipids and the end-products of such lipid peroxidation reactions can do serious damage to cells, and even to tissues.

For the most part, ROS are formed by the free radicals generated by the oxidative metabolism of the cell power plant, the mitochondria. However, while a cell cannot avoid producing free radicals, it has its own defense system consisting of natural antioxidants (catalases).

2.5.1 ANTIOXIDANTS

An antioxidant is a molecule that prevents the oxidation of other molecules. Oxidation means "combining with oxygen."

Exogenous antioxidants are outside the body, while *endogenous* antioxidants are made in the body. There are enzymatic antioxidants such as catalase and superoxide dismutase (SOD), and nonenzymatic antioxidants such as vitamin A and vitamin E. They make up our antioxidant defense against free radicals and ROS. Lipid peroxidation has been implicated in disease states such as atherosclerosis, asthma, Parkinson's disease, kidney damage, preeclampsia, and many others. (Mylonas and Kouretas 1999).

In order to prevent *premature aging*, it is important to understand that in terms of oxygen, there can be too much of a good thing. On the one hand, life as we know it cannot exist without oxygen; on the other hand, excess oxygen, which can be in the form of free radicals, rapidly damages body cells. In fact, oxygen burns everything.

It is so dangerous that the body has a mechanism in hemoglobin, in red blood cells, that limits how much of it gets into tissues.

The more oxygen in the body, the more free radicals there will be. This fact is well known to medical science: the journal *Experimental Cell Research* reported in 1995 that "Mild hyperoxia shortens telomeres and inhibits proliferation of fibro-blasts: A model for senescence?" (von Zglinicki et al. 1995). A fibroblast is a type of connective tissue cell that forms the structural framework of our tissues.

Oxygen is stressful to the body and the more taken in above what is needed, the more rapid will be the process of aging. Even a mild excess oxygen (hyperoxia) rapidly shortens *telomeres* and, in addition, reduces the body's capacity to repair itself.

2.6 ACCELERATED CELL DIVISION, REPAIR, OR SELF-DESTRUCTION

When free radicals or ROS attack and damage DNA in the chromosomes in the nucleus of the cells, or in the mitochondria that power them, cells may either divide ahead of schedule in order to repair the damage, or they may opt to self-destruct. In the case of accelerated division, telomeres will shorten more rapidly. Short telo-meres is said to be the hallmark of accelerated aging.

2.7 EXOGENOUS FREE RADICALS

2.7.1 EXAMPLE 1: ULTRAVIOLET RADIATION IN SUNLIGHT SHORTENS TELOMERES

Aging of the skin on the face can be accelerated by overexposure to free radicals generated by ultraviolet (UV) radiation in sunlight. When directly exposed to solar radiation, the skin can generate free radicals as well as ROS from targeted cell metabolism. It is estimated that among all environmental factors, UV radiation may contribute up to 80% of free radical damage when their formation exceeds the antioxidant defense capacity of the irradiated cells.

The primary mechanism whereby UV radiation damages human skin is the photochemical generation of ROS (including hydrogen peroxide). The only protec-tion afforded to our skin is by endogenous antioxidants (melanin and enzymatic) and exogenous antioxidants consumed in food (vitamin A, C, E, etc.) (Poljšak and Dahmane 2012).

The wrinkling of the skin is not even the worst outcome of overexposure to UV radiation. In fact, UV radiation shortens lifespan by accelerating cell division and, therefore, telomere abbreviation. Researchers writing in the *Journal of International Medical Research*, in 2012, compared cells irradiated with UV light to comparable non-irradiated cells. In non-irradiated cells, telomeres were longer, consistent with a fewer number of cell division cycles. In cells exposed to UV, telomeres were signifi-cantly shorter than in non-irradiated comparison control individuals (Ma et al. 2012). In other words, radiation sped up cell division and faster cell division means shorter telomeres, and shorter telomeres mean faster aging.

Human chromosomes contain a gene, TP53, that carries instructions for making a tumor protein, p53, bound directly to DNA, that regulates cell division and is therefore tumor suppressing. It does that by keeping cells from growing and dividing too fast or in an uncontrolled way. When the DNA in a cell becomes damaged by UV rays from the sun, for instance, this protein plays a critical role in determining whether the DNA will be repaired or the damaged cell will self-destruct (*apoptosis*).

If the DNA can be repaired, p53 activates other genes to fix the damage and if not, prevents the cell from dividing and signals it to self-destruct. By stopping cells with mutated or damaged DNA from dividing, p53 helps prevent the development of tumors. Because p53 is essential for regulating cell division and preventing tumor formation, it has been nicknamed the "guardian of the genome." Investigators from the Department of Dermatology, Boston University School of Medicine, Boston, MA, reported that in "photo-damage" aging, p53 is involved in telomere protection or abbreviation (Kosmadaki and Gilchrest 2004; Panich et al. 2016).

2.7.2 Sirtuins and Photodamage

Chapter 4 examines the importance and impact of the recently discovered "sirtuins." The term stands for "silent mating-type information regulation." So far seven of them have been found, forming a "family," and they act basically as cell regulation enzymes. They have recently received a considerable amount of attention because it was shown that certain foods activate a gene that forms some of them, SIRT1 in particular, with implications for weight loss. Specifically, SIRT1 is involved in managing metabolism and energy storage as fat in times of food shortage.

It has been shown that the activity of the SIRT1 gene is increased following gene damage in a number of different cell types (Wang et al. 2006). This study, reported by the Molecular Oncology Program, H. Lee Moffitt Cancer Center and Research Institute, Tampa, FL, is the first report of increased SIRT1 gene activation after damage to *keratinocytes*, the predominant cell type in the outermost layer of the skin (epidermis), constituting 90% of the cells found there. Studies in other cell types suggested that SIRT1 functions in DNA repair and maintaining DNA integrity (Wang et al. 2008). New evidence also points to a possible mechanism where SIRT1 facilitates repair (Fan and Luo 2010). The Proactive Nutrition Program also entails promoting sirtuin activation.

Wang et al. 2006 suggested that these data support the hypothesis that SIRTs play an important role in resistance to UV overexposure (photo-damage) and identify specific SIRTs that respond to photo-damage and may possibly be targets for skin cancer prevention (Benavente et al. 2012).

It also follows from this research that niacin, part of the activation process, is a critical factor in resistance to photo-damage. Niacin deficiency has long been known to be associated with skin sensitivity to sunlight. Niacin is also known as vitamin B3 or nicotinic acid. Supplementation has been recommended for protecting the skin from UV light from the sun (Lin et al. 2012).

2.7.3 Example 2: "Smoke! Smoke! Smoke! (That Cigarette)"

The noted bandleader, Phil Harris (1904–1995, who made famous a song called "Smoke! Smoke! Smoke! That Cigarette)," was not a smoker and lived to be

91 years old. Another Phil Harris, captain in *Deadliest Catch*, was a heavy smoker and died of a heart attack at the age of 53. Every puff of a cigarette contains about 100 trillion free radical molecules.

Researchers reported in the journal *Environmental Health Perspectives*, in 1985, that cigarette smoke contains two very different types of free radicals: one type is in the tar and the other one is in the smoke/gas. The tar contains free radicals that react with DNA. The gas phase of cigarette smoke contains small oxygen- and carbon-centered radicals that are much more reactive than the tar radicals.

The gas-phase radicals do not arise in the flame but rather are produced in a steady state by the oxidation of nitric oxide (NO) to nitrogen dioxide (NO_2), a toxic gas that fouls the air when concentrated in air pollution. The investigators suggested that the active oxidants are NO and NO_2. They also report the toxicological implications of the radicals in smoke for a number of radical-mediated disease processes, including emphysema and cancer (Church and Pryor 1985).

According to investigators reporting in the journal *Carcinogenesis*, in 2001, the major cause of lung cancer is cigarette smoking and p53 gene mutations are common in lung cancers from smokers but less common in non-smokers. p53 mutations are frequent in tobacco-related cancers, and the mutational load is often higher in cancers from smokers than from non-smokers. The "mutational load" is the total genetic burden in a population resulting from accumulated harmful mutations. In lung cancers, the p53 mutation patterns are different in smokers and non-smokers, with considerable evidence of DNA damage in smoking-associated cancers. The investigators concluded that p53 gene mutations in lung cancers can be attributed directly to DNA damage from cigarette smoke-formed free radicals (Hainaut and Pfeifer 2001; Pfeifer et al. 2002).

2.7.4 SMOKING CIGARETTES SHORTENS TELOMERES

A study published in the *European Respiratory Journal*, in 2006, reported the effects of tobacco smoking on telomere shortening in circulating lymphocytes. Lymphocytes are a type of white blood cell, part of the immune system protecting us from bacteria, viruses, fungi, and parasites. The aim of the study was to determine whether telomere abbreviation was further amplified in smokers who develop chronic obstructive pulmonary disease (COPD).

Telomere length was determined in circulating lymphocytes from never-smokers, smokers with normal lung function, and smokers with moderate-to-severe airflow obstruction. In contrast to never-smokers, telomere length decreased significantly with age in smokers. There was also a dose–effect relationship between the cumulative long-life exposure to tobacco smoking (pack/years) and telomere length. The presence and/or severity of chronic airflow obstruction did not modify this relationship.

The authors concluded that smoking exposure enhances telomere shortening in circulating lymphocytes with a direct dose–effect relationship between exposure to tobacco smoking and telomere length—the longer the duration of smoking, the shorter the telomeres. This effect was not increased in smokers who develop COPD (Morlá et al. 2006). Other studies also supported the finding of shorter telomeres in different cell types proportional to the duration of smoking (Babizhayev et al. 2011).

2.7.5   EXAMPLE 3: FREE RADICALS FROM SMOG AND AIR POLLUTION

In extreme cases, air pollution typically means smog, produced by the chemical reaction between sunlight, nitrogen oxides, and volatile organic compounds in the atmosphere. This mix produces airborne particles and ground-level ozone. There are two types of smog: photochemical smog due to the interaction of sunlight with air pollution, and industrial smog. The main difference is that it is the photochemical smog that produces ground-level ozone. Ozone is not a free radical but it can produce them. Here is what is mostly in smog according to a report in the *American Journal of Respiratory and Critical Care Medicine* (Volume 153, 1996) on recent research on the effects of ambient outdoor air pollution on health in Canada:

- Volatile organic compounds derived from automobile tailpipe emissions, evaporation of gasoline at service stations, surface coatings such as oil paints, solvents such as barbecue starters, and fuel combustion products
- Nitrogen oxides such as nitric oxide (NO) and nitrogen dioxide (NO_2) derived from automobile tailpipe emissions, industrial manufacturing processes, electric power stations, fossil fuel powered plants, oil refineries, pulp and paper plants, and incinerators
- Sulphur dioxide (SO_2) derived from non-ferrous metal smelting, oil refineries, pulp and paper plants, incinerators
- Particulate matter derived from automobile tailpipe emissions, volcanic eruptions, forest fires, and fossil fuel–powered plants

2.7.6   HEALTH CONSEQUENCES OF SMOG

Ozone (O_3) is formed naturally in the atmosphere and protects us from damaging UV rays from the sun. However, at ground level, ozone is a harmful invisible air pollutant damaging also animals, plants, and man-made materials (rubber, for instance).

Nitrogen oxides are produced by burning fossil fuels such as coal, oil, gas, and diesel in motor vehicles, industrial plants, power plants, and homes. Volatile organic compounds are carbon-based chemicals that evaporate easily at room temperature. They include carbon-containing gases that are created when gasoline and oil-based solvents are burned.

Photochemical smog is caused by a free-radical chain mechanism that converts nitric oxide (NO) to nitrogen dioxide (NO_2). Then, in a further reaction, nitrogen dioxide produces ozone (O_3) and other potentially harmful substances (Uen et al. 1998).

2.7.7   AIR POLLUTION DAMAGES TELOMERES

In a study published in 2009, in the journal *Environmental Health*, researchers aimed to determine whether traffic officers exposed to car fumes commonly containing benzene and toluene suffered from exposure to free radicals. They compared the length of telomeres in the conventional target, white immune system blood cells (leukocytes), in traffic workers and in indoor office workers.

Their results showed that leukocyte telomere length was significantly shorter in traffic officers than in office workers. Telomere length was found to decrease also with the age of the participant, an index of the length of exposure, in both groups but it was shorter still in the traffic workers in all age categories. Telomere length varied also in accordance with whether a traffic officer worked in higher or lower traffic density areas. In short, telomere length decreased with increasing levels of personal exposure to benzene and toluene. The authors concluded that leukocyte telomere length is shortened in subjects exposed to traffic pollution, suggesting early biological aging and increased risk of disease (Hoxha et al. 2009).

In another study, leukocyte telomere length (LTL) was measured repeatedly approximately every 3 years from 1999 through 2006 in never-smoking men, and compared to the black carbon airborne particle concentration at their residence. The authors reported that telomere attrition linked to biological aging may be associated with long-term exposures to airborne particles, particularly those rich in black carbon, that are primarily related to automobile traffic (McCracken et al. 2009)

2.7.8 EXAMPLE 4: INFLAMMATION CAUSES OXIDATIVE STRESS

Systemic inflammatory response syndrome (SIRS) is a state of inflammation affecting the whole body. Oxygen free radicals contribute to the development of this condition. In the early stages of the process, free radicals exert their actions by activating components in the cell nucleus that induce the formation of *cytokines*. These aid cell-to-cell communication in immune responses and stimulate the movement of immune system cells toward sites of inflammation. Free radicals also exert their toxic effects at the site of inflammation by reacting with different cell components, inducing loss of function and cell death.

In contrast to SIRS, localized inflammation is a protective response that is generally tightly controlled by the body at the site of injury. However, loss of this local control or an overly activated immune response results in an exaggerated effect on distant organs which can then become SIRS. The authors propose that antioxidant therapies may be appropriate to prevent cell damage (Closa and Folch-Puy 2004) Investigators writing in the journal *Free Radical Biology & Medicine*, in 2010, went one step further, concluding that oxidative stress, chronic inflammation, and cancer are closely linked (Reuter et al. 2010)

2.7.9 EXAMPLE 5: IMMUNE RESPONSE AND ROS

There is another source of ROS, where inflammation causes their rapid production, leading to oxidative stress. Immune cells actually "use" ROS in order to support their functions and therefore adequate levels of antioxidants are needed in order to avoid the harmful effect of this excessive production of ROS.

Oxidative stress is a major cause of the high mortality rates associated with several diseases such as sepsis and endotoxic shock. This condition can be controlled to a certain degree by antioxidant therapies. Victor et al. 2004 suggest the potential clinical use of antioxidants in the treatment of severe immune reactions such as is the case in septic shock.

2.8   ENDOGENOUS FREE RADICALS

There are many organelles and other structures and processes inside cells that are sources of free radicals. As noted above, prime among these are the mitochondria. Ordinarily, mitochondria generate relatively modest amounts of ROS and the damage they cause is limited by the antioxidant action of SOD. However, there are circumstances when large amounts of ROS can be produced.

In a study published in *Trends in Biochemical Sciences*, in 2000, human skin fibroblasts were exposed to hydrogen peroxide and other damaging substances and were then examined for damage to telomeres. DNA damage was observed in all cases and, except in the case of hydrogen peroxide, the damage was quickly repaired. However, damage induced by exposure to hydrogen peroxide was not repaired: telomere length was reduced significantly by peroxide-induced damage, indicating that ROS directly attack telomere DNA and cause increased attrition. DNA loss from the telomeres was increased significantly with each cell doubling cycle.

That study suggests here also that there is a basic aging mechanism governed by telomere shortening in mitochondria that can appear to be affected by the lifetime production rates of oxygen free radicals.

When ROS are responsible for such damage, the breaks cannot easily be repaired and telomere shortening is accelerated. The authors further contend that dietary restriction lowering basal metabolic rate and thus free radical formation could decelerate telomere shortening and thus extend lifespan (Raha and Robinson 2000).

2.9   THEORY: FREE RADICALS CAUSE AGING

In 2007, Dr. Harman published a very controversial theory that, basically, aging is due to the accumulated damage to mitochondrial DNA caused by oxidative stress. His theory appearing in the journal *Clinical Interventions in Aging* essentially laid out the scenario for the damaging effects of free radicals.

According to Dr. Harman, free radicals, antioxidants, and co-factors interact in important ways in maintaining health, aging, and age-related diseases. Free radicals cause oxidative stress that is counteracted by the body's endogenous antioxidants plus co-factors, and by the addition of exogenous antioxidants.

If the generation of free radicals is greater than the protection antioxidants can provide, the resulting oxidative stress can overwhelm cells. This damaging effect accumulating during the life cycle of the cells is implicated in aging and age-dependent diseases such as cardiovascular disease, cancer, neurodegenerative disorders, and other chronic conditions.

Dr. Harman contended that as the life expectancy of the world population rises, this aging process will lead to an increase in the number of older people acquiring age-related chronic diseases, placing greater financial burdens on health services and high social costs for individuals and society. Thus, in order to achieve healthy aging, older people should be encouraged to acquire a healthy life style that should include nutrition rich in antioxidants (Rahman 2007).

Not everybody is on board. In 2008, the journal *Current Aging Science* published a rebuttal in a "critical review." The authors disagree with the *mitochondrial free radical theory of aging* (MFRTA) that proposes that mitochondria free radicals produced as by-products during normal metabolism cause oxidative stress damage. Furthermore, they disagree that the accumulation of this oxidative damage is the main driving force in the aging process.

They held that although this theory is widely accepted, it remains unproven. For example, while long-lived animals produce fewer free radicals and evidence lower oxidative stress damage in their tissues, this, per se, does not prove that free radical generation determines lifespan. In fact, the longest living rodent, the naked mole-rat (*Heterocephalus glaber*) produces high levels of free radicals and has significant oxidative damage levels in proteins, lipids, and DNA.

According to the authors of this critique, Drs. A. Sanz and R.K. Stefanatos from the Mitochondrial Gene Expression and Disease Group, Institute of Medical Technology, University of Tampere, Finland, at best, the MFRTA proposes that these free radicals damage mitochondrial DNA (mtDNA) and in turn provoke mutations that alter mitochondrial energy production. Therefore, oxidative stress damage to mitochondrial DNA (mtDNA) is inconsistent with maximum lifespan in mammals. However, in contrast to the MFRTA predictions, high levels of oxidative damage in mtDNA do not decrease longevity in mice. Moreover, mice with alterations in a critical mitochondrial DNA enzyme accumulate 500 times more mutations in mtDNA and yet do not seem to age prematurely.

Dietary restriction is the only non-genetic treatment that clearly increases *mean* and *maximum lifespan*. According to the MFRTA, caloric-restricted animals produce fewer mitochondrial reactive oxygen species (mtROS). However, dietary restriction alters more than just free radical production. For one thing, it decreases insulin function and therefore the increase in longevity cannot be exclusively attributed to a decrease in mtROS generation (Sanz and Stefanatos 2008).

2.10 BENEFICIAL EFFECTS OF FREE RADICALS IN IMMUNE DEFENSE

It turns out that there is also another side to free radicals. On the one hand, they can be harmful, and on the other hand, they can be beneficial. In fact, they play an important role in immune defense. The journal *Annals of Clinical & Laboratory Science* in 2000 detailed the role of oxygen free radicals in both "natural" and "acquired" immune responses.

Natural immunity is inborn, whereas acquired immunity results from the development of antibodies in response to exposure to an antigen, as from vaccination or an infectious disease, or from the transmission of antibodies from the mother to the fetus through the placenta. Free radicals are important in both natural and acquired immunity. They are used by immune system cells as a sort of *bullet* that they shoot at bacteria and other invaders (Knight 2000).

At low or moderate levels, ROS are vital to human health. In low concentrations, ROS are necessary for the maturation of cells and can act as weapons for the host defense system. In fact, many of our immune system cells such as phagocytes and macrophages release free radicals to destroy invading harmful microbes as part of the body's defense mechanism against disease (Droge 2002; Young and Woodside 2001).

For example, nitric oxide (NO) also controls blood flow and prevents blood clots (Fried 2014; Pacher et al. 2007; Pham-Huy et al. 2008).

Nitric oxide is derived in the body from two principal sources: (a) the amino acid L-arginine and (b) nitrates, both derived from food sources. It plays a major role in supporting immune function and cardiovascular and heart health. Because it is crucial in maintaining health, and because it is derived from foods that are readily part of our proposed Proactive Nutrition Program, it has earned its own chapter (see Chapter 7).

REFERENCES

Babizhayev, M. A., E. L. Savel'yeva, S. N. Moskvina, et al. 2011. Telomere length is a biomarker of cumulative oxidative stress, biologic age, and an independent predictor of survival and therapeutic treatment requirement associated with smoking behavior. *American Journal of Therapeutics*, 18(6):e209–e226.

Benavente, C. A., S. A. Schnell, and E. L. Jacobson. 2012. Effects of niacin restriction on Sirtuin and PARP responses to photodamage in human skin. *PLoS One*, 7(7):e42276.

Church, D. F., and W. A. Pryor. 1985. Free-radical chemistry of cigarette smoke and its toxicological implications. *Environmental Health Perspectives*, 64:111–126.

Closa, D., and E. Folch-Puy. 2004. Critical review: Oxygen free radicals and the systemic inflammatory response. IUBMB *Life*, 56(4):185–191.

Droge, W. 2002. Free radicals in the physiological control of cell function. *Physiological Review*, 82:47–95.

Fan, W., and J. Luo. 2010. SIRT1 regulates UV-induced DNA repair through deacetylating XPA. *Molecular Cell*, 39:247–258.

Fried R. 2014. *Erectile Dysfunction as a Cardiovascular Impairment.* San Diego, CA: Academic Press.

Hainaut, P., and G. P. Pfeifer. 2001. Patterns of p53 G→T transversions in lung cancers reflect the primary mutagenic signature of DNA-damage by tobacco smoke. *Carcinogenesis*, 22(3):367–374.

Hoxha, M., L. Dioni, M. Bonzini, et al. 2009. Association between leukocyte telomere shortening and exposure to traffic pollution: A cross-sectional study on traffic officers and indoor office workers. *Environmental Health*, 8:41. doi: 10.1186/ 1476-069X-8-41. 9 pages.

Jazwinski, S. M. 2000. Aging and longevity genes. *Biochimica Polonica*, 47(2):269–279.

Knight, J. A. 2000. Review. Free radicals, antioxidants, and the immune system. *Annals of Clinical & Laboratory Science*, 30(2):145–158.

Kosmadaki, M. G., and B. A. Gilchrest. 2004. The role of telomeres in skin aging/photoaging. *Micron*, 35(3):155–159.

Lin, F., W. Xu, C. Guan, et al. 2012. Niacin protects against UVB radiation-induced apoptosis in cultured human skin keratinocytes. *International Journal of Molecular Medicine*, 29(4):593–600.

Ma, H. M., W. Liu, P. Zhang, et al. 2012. Human skin fibroblast telomeres are shortened after ultraviolet irradiation. *Journal of International Medical Research*, 40(5):1871–1877.

McCracken, J., A. Baccarelli, M. Hoxha, et al. 2009. *Annual Ambient Black Carbon Associated with Shorter Telomeres in Elderly Men: Veterans Administration Normative Aging Study.* Bethesda, MD: National Institutes of Health, U.S. Department of Health and Human Services, National Institute of Environmental Health Science (NIEHS).

Morlá, M., X. Busquets, J. Pons, et al. 2006. Telomere shortening in smokers with and without COPD. *European Respiratory Journal*, 27(3):525–528. doi: 10.1183/09031936.06. 00087005.

Mylonas. C., and D. Kouretas. 1999. Lipid peroxidation and tissue damage. *In Vivo*, 13(3):295–309.

Pacher, P., J. S. Beckman, and L. Liaudet. 2007. Nitric oxide and peroxynitrite in health and disease. *Physiological Review*, 87(1):315–424.

Panich, U., G. Sittithumcharee, N. Rathviboon, et al. 2016. Ultraviolet radiation-induced skin aging: The role of DNA damage and oxidative stress in epidermal Stem cell damage mediated skin aging. *Stem Cells International*, 2016:7370642. doi: http://dx.doi.org/10.1155/2016/ 7370642.

Pendyala, G., B. Thomas, and S. Kumari. 2008. The challenge of antioxidants to free radicals in periodontitis. *Journal of Indian Society of Periodontology*, 12(3):79–83.

Pfeifer, G. P., M. F. Denissenko, M. Olivier, et al. 2002. Tobacco smoke carcinogens, DNA damage and p53 mutations in smoking-associated cancers. *Oncogene*, 21(48):7435–7451.

Pham-Huy, L. A., H. He, and C. Pham-Huy. 2008. Free radicals, antioxidants in disease and health. *International Journal of Biomedical Science*, 4(2):89–96.

Poljšak, B., and R. Dahmane R. 2012. Free radicals and extrinsic skin aging. *Dermatology Research and Practice*, 2012:135206. doi: http://dx.doi.org/10. 1155/2012/135206.

Raha, S., and B. H. Robinson. 2000. Mitochondria, oxygen free radicals, disease and ageing. *Trends in Biochemical Sciences*, 25(10):502–508.

Rahman, K. 2007. Studies on free radicals, antioxidants, and co-factors. *Clinical Interventions in Aging*, 2(2):219–236.

Reuter, S., S. C. Gupta, M. M. Chaturvedi, et al. 2010. Oxidative stress, inflammation, and cancer: How are they linked? *Free Radical Biology & Medicine*, 49(11): 1603–1616.

Ruiz-Torres, A., and W. Beier. 2005. On maximum human life span: Interdisciplinary approach about its limits. *Advances in Gerontolology*, 16:14–20.

Sanz, A., and R. K. Stefanatos. 2008. The mitochondrial free radical theory of aging: A critical view. *Current Aging Science*, 1(1):10–21.

Uen, I., M. Hoshino, T. Miura, et al. 1998. Ozone exposure generates free radicals in the blood samples in vitro. Detection by the ESR spin-trapping technique. *Free Radical Research*, 29(2):127–135.

Victor, V. M., M. Rochab, and M. de la Fuente. 2004. Immune cells: Free radicals and antioxidants in sepsis. *International Immunopharmacology*, 4(3):327–347.

von Zglinicki, T., G. Saretzki, W. Döcke, et al. 1995. Mild hyperoxia shortens telomeres and inhibits proliferation of fibroblasts: A model for senescence? *Experimental Cell Research*, 220(1):186–193.

Wang, C., L. Chen, X. Hou, et al. 2006. Interactions between E2F1 and SirT1 regulate apoptotic response to DNA damage. *Nature Cell Biology*, 8:1025–1031.

Wang, R. H., K. Sengupta, C. Li, et al. 2008. Impaired DNA damage response, genome instability, and tumorigenesis in SIRT1 mutant mice. *Cancer Cell* 14:312–323.

Xu, J., S. L. Murphy, K. D. Kochanek, et al. 2016. Deaths: Final data for 2013. *National Vital Statistics Reports*, 64(2):1–119.

Young, I., and J. Woodside. 2001. Antioxidants in health and disease. *Journal of Clinical Pathology*, 54:176–186.

3 Antioxidants Neutralize Free Radicals

3.1 INTRODUCTION

The typical lifespan is dictated by hereditary inscription in genes. Unless it is accelerated by lifestyle factors or disease, aging is a natural, normal, process of "declining" functions. These declining functions do not constitute disease. This functional decline cannot be treated by conventional medicine unless it is actually related to premature aging due to lifestyle choices.

What causes premature aging? The short answer is free radicals, a toxic by-product of cell metabolism. They cause *oxidative stress* of the cell organelles, especially the mitochondria that power cell metabolism. Free radicals damage the cells that form them and make the cells speed up division. The evidence is in the rapid shortening of telomeres.

Excess free radical formation, both from inside cells and from the environment, damages DNA, shortens telomeres, and accelerates aging. But free radical formation is also essential to immune defense. So, there is a thin line between the need to reduce free radical damage and the need to preserve immune defense. Health and longevity depend on this "juggling act."

Here we examine the nature and function of antioxidants (also known as free radical scavengers), their sources, how their concentration is measured, and their function and benefits. With aging, endogenous antioxidants, those that the body makes, rapidly decline. This results in dwindling protection from free radicals and reactive oxygen species (ROS).

3.2 WHAT ARE ANTIOXIDANTS?

An oxidant is a substance that readily combines with oxygen. In other words, an oxidant oxidizes. Examples of this are the rust that forms on iron when exposed to oxygen and butter turning rancid if left uncovered on the table. An antioxidant is a substance that inhibits or prevents oxidation. Many sources define antioxidants as substances that prevent cell damage. This is true, but that is not actually the definition of antioxidants, it only explains their use.

Antioxidants are also sometimes called "free radical scavengers." This definition refers to the disappearance of free radicals by some sort of *mopping up* action. There are endogenous free radicals (made by the body) and exogenous free radicals (that come from the environment). There are also endogenous antioxidants (made by the body) and exogenous antioxidants (those that we usually get from foods or beverages).

The possible mechanisms of action of antioxidants were first explored when it was discovered that any substance with antioxidant activity is likely to be one that is itself readily oxidized.

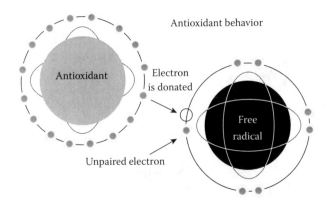

FIGURE 3.1   The antioxidant gives up an electron to a free radical. (From Block, K.I., et al., *Int. J. Cancer*, 123(6), 1227–1239, 2008. With permission.)

Figure 3.1 represents antioxidant action. The antioxidant is a molecule stable enough to give up an electron to a free radical molecule to pair electrons in the formerly free radical molecule. This action stabilizes the formerly free radical molecule. This reduces the free radical chain reaction of attracting electrons from nearby molecules before damage to cell structures and to DNA can take place (Halliwell 1995). Two principal mechanisms of antioxidant action have been proposed (Rice-Evans and Diplock 1993).

3.3   LEVELS OF ANTIOXIDANT ACTION

Antioxidants in the defense systems have *preventive*, *radical scavenging*, and *repair* properties. The first line of defense is preventive antioxidants that suppress free radical formation. The second line of defense is free radical scavenging to suppress the chain initiation and/or break the chain propagation reactions.

The third line of defense is repair and de novo (newly formed) antioxidants. Proteolytic enzymes are present in mitochondria. Proteolytic enzymes break down proteins into smaller units, amino acids. They degrade and remove ROS and prevent the accumulation of oxidized proteins. The DNA repair systems also play an important role in the total body defense system against oxidative damage. There is an additional adaptation function involved in forming the signal for the production and transporting the appropriate antioxidant to the site where it is needed (Niki 1993).

3.4   THE ANTIOXIDANTS THE BODY MAKES

Endogenous antioxidants are made in and by the body in the course of normal metabolism (Shiet al. 1999). They act as free radical scavengers, working to detoxify ROS in both the cell and in its surrounding environment (Frie 1988). The body makes five basic types of endogenous antioxidants: superoxide dismutase (SOD), alpha-lipoic acid (ALA), coenzyme Q10 (CoQ10), catalase (CAT), and glutathione peroxidase (GPx).

3.4.1 SUPEROXIDE DISMUTASE(S) (SODs)

Superoxide (O_2^-) is a by-product of oxygen metabolism and can cause many types of cell damage. Superoxide dismutases (SODs) are a class of closely related enzymes that enhance the breakdown of the superoxide (O_2^-) radical into either ordinary oxygen (O_2) or hydrogen peroxide (H_2O_2). Hydrogen peroxide is also damaging, but less so, and is further degraded by other enzymes such as CAT.

SODs provide important antioxidant defense in nearly all living cells exposed to oxygen. We have three forms of SOD depending on the metal cofactor:

- SOD1 is formed and located in the cell cytoplasm.
- SOD2 is formed and located in the mitochondria.
- SOD3 is extracellular.

SOD1 and SOD3 contain copper and zinc, whereas SOD2, the mitochondrial enzyme, has manganese in its reactive center.

3.4.2 BUYER BEWARE

A number of health supplement–related websites recommend supplementation with formulations that incorporate trace elements. These supplements are intended to enhance antioxidant formation. However, this should be considered with caution because few data on humans are available concerning the effective dosages, safety, and adverse side effect of such supplementation. In some cases, it is a minefield. For instance, the *Journal of Biological Chemistry* reported in 2013 that a manganese-rich environment increases the activity of the Lyme disease bacterium *Borrelia burgdorferi* (Aguirre et al. 2013).

3.4.3 CATALASE (CAT)

Catalase (CAT) is a common enzyme found in nearly all living organisms that are exposed to oxygen. It breaks down hydrogen peroxide into oxygen and water. The term "catalase" is derived from its chemical action, that is, to *catalyze* or to cause an action or a process to begin.

Hydrogen peroxide is a harmful by-product of many normal metabolic processes. To prevent damage, it must be quickly converted into other less dangerous substances. Catalase is used by cells to speed up the breakdown of hydrogen peroxide into less reactive oxygen and water molecules.

It was previously thought that glutathione peroxidase was largely responsible for eliminating hydrogen peroxide. However, a study published in the journal *Blood*, in 1996, showed that glutathione peroxidase removed hydrogen peroxide from red blood cells at a rate of only 17% of the rate that catalase disposed of it (Gaetani et al. 1996).

In addition to its action as a super antioxidant, catalase also can use hydrogen peroxide to oxidize other toxic substances including methanol, ethanol, formaldehyde, and nitrite. For instance, catalase reduces blood alcohol concentration over time.

This is only considered a minor metabolic process of alcohol oxidation, except in the fasting state (Handler and Thurman 1990). It has been shown that chronic alcohol consumption (in an animal model using rats) results in increased hydrogen peroxide and increased catalase activity (Misra et al. 1992).

3.4.4   GLUTATHIONE (GSH) SYSTEM: GLUTATHIONE PEROXIDASE(S) (GPX)

Glutathione (GSH) is often considered the "master antioxidant" of the body. It can be found in virtually every cell of the human body. It is made up of three amino acids: cysteine, glycine, and glutamate. The highest concentration of GSH is in the liver, where it plays a critical role in detoxification processes. The principal function of GSH is to prevent oxidative stress, but it is also an essential part of the natural defense system. Depletion of GSH has been associated with impaired immune function and increased vulnerability to infection due to reduced ability of the liver to detoxify. Free radical damage to healthy cells depletes glutathione. This increases susceptibility to viruses, bacteria, heavy metal toxicity, radiation, certain medications, and even affects the normal process of aging.

Direct attack by free radicals and other oxidative agents can also deplete GSH. However, an internal (homeostatic) balance system works to keep GSH resupplied even as it is being used up. Oxidative depletion can outpace GSH synthesis because amounts available from foods are limited (less than 150 mg/day) (Essential Nutraceuticals™ 2012; Lushchak 2012).

The glutathione system includes glutathione and glutathione peroxidases (GPx). GPx is an enzyme that helps break down hydrogen peroxide to water. Glutathione peroxidase 1 is the most abundant form and is a very efficient scavenger of hydrogen peroxide. Levels of these enzymes are especially high in the liver and also serve in detoxification metabolism (Hayeset et al. 2005) and regulating mitochondrial function (Handy et al. 2009). It has also been shown that low serum levels of glutathione peroxidase may be a contributing factor to type 2 diabetes (Sedighi et al. 2014).

3.4.5   UBIQUINONE, ALSO KNOWN AS COENZYME Q10 (CoQ10)

Ubiquinone, also known as coenzyme Q10 (CoQ10), is similar to a vitamin and is found in every cell of the body, primarily in the mitochondria. It functions as an antioxidant, protecting the body from damage caused by free radicals and ROS. CoQ10 is naturally present in small amounts in a wide variety of foods, but levels are particularly high in organ meats such as heart, liver, and kidney, as well as beef, soybean oil, sardines, mackerel, and peanuts. It participates in mitochondrial oxidative metabolism to generate energy. Ninety-five percent of our energy is generated by this process (Dutton et al. 2000; Ernster and Dallner 1995).

There are three forms of CoQ10. Ubiquinol is the most important for its antioxidant property. When consuming a "reduced" CoQ10 supplement (ubiquinol), the body can convert it to the oxidized form, ubiquinone, and vice versa. This conversion takes place to maintain a state of equilibrium between reduced CoQ10 (ubiquinol) and oxidized CoQ10 (ubiquinone).

Note: The formation of CoQ10 can be impaired by interfering with serum cholesterol levels in the body. The main source of CoQ10 in humans is a complex 17-step process requiring at least seven vitamins (vitamin B2 [riboflavin], vitamin B3 [niacinamide], vitamin B6, folic acid, vitamin B12, vitamin C, and pantothenic acid) and several trace elements, making it highly vulnerable. Many authorities hold that average or "normal" levels of CoQ10 are suboptimal in a large segment of the population and that the low levels observed in advanced disease states represent only the tip of a deficiency "iceberg." Furthermore, these levels normally drop anyway after the age of 40.

Both cholesterol-lowering statins and blood pressure–reducing beta-blockers can further lower CoQ10 formation (Kishi 1977; Mortensen et al. 1997). Statins can reduce serum levels of CoQ10 by up to 40% (Ghirlanda et al. 1993).

In fact, in a report to the Federal Drug Administration (FDA) titled "Cardiovascular diseases research in biomedical aspects of Coenzyme Q10," the cardiologist Dr. P. H. Langsjoen suggested a *black box* warning in the labeling for all statins sold in the United States to read as follows:

> Warning: HMG CoA reductase inhibitors block the endogenous biosynthesis of an essential cofactor, coenzyme Q10, required for energy production. A deficiency of coenzyme Q 10 is associated with impairment of myocardial function, with liver dysfunction and with myopathies (including cardiomyopathy and congestive heart failure). All patients taking HMG CoA reductase inhibitors should therefore be advised to take 100 to 200 mg per day of supplemental coenzyme Q10. (Langsjoen 2002)

Not everyone agrees, but the issue is not about whether statins inhibit formation of CoQ10, but whether supplementation actually works, at least in restoring muscle function attributed to low CoQ10 (Deichmann 2010).

3.4.6 ALPHA-LIPOIC ACID (ALA)

Alpha-lipoic acid is used by the body to break down carbohydrates and to make energy for organs in the body. It is also a vitamin-like, potent, and protective antioxidant that is both fat and water soluble. This means it can penetrate virtually all body tissues, including the brain and nerves. It also acts as a heavy metal chelator that bonds with metal ions, helping the body rid itself of toxic metals such as lead and mercury. ALA helps maintain levels of glutathione.

ALA is used to treat diabetes and the nerve-related symptoms of diabetes, including burning pain and numbness in the legs and arms. High doses of ALA are approved in Germany for the treatment of these symptoms.

3.5 TELOMERES SHORTEN WHEN ENDOGENOUS ANTIOXIDANTS FAIL

According to a report in the *American Journal of Physiology*, appearing in 2006, it is unclear why women live longer than men, and why men are more likely subject to kidney disease. It is known, however, that cell aging (senescence) plays a major role in kidney disease. The authors examined the levels of the major antioxidants, SOD, glutathione peroxidase 1 (GPx1), and glutathione reductase, in an animal model (rats). They found age-related telomere shortening was more pronounced in males than in females.

SOD expression was elevated in the kidneys of females compared with males. GPx1 and glutathione reductase levels were also increased in older females compared with males. These findings indicate that a reduction in oxidative damage protection may be responsible for accelerated telomere shortening over time. This resulted in increased cellular senescence (aging), loss of renal function, and death in male rats (Tarry-Adkins et al. 2006).

Enzymes are proteins that initiate and facilitate chemical reactions. They generally help to break down a substance into its constituents. However, telomerase is a "reverse transcriptase" enzyme that does the opposite: it helps lengthen telomeres.

A report published in 2004 in the *Journal of Biological Chemistry* examined the impact of high intracellular concentrations of glutathione on the regulation of telomerase activity in fibroblast cells in culture. Fibroblasts are the main connective tissue cells in the body. When these cells have decreased glutathione levels, telomerase activity decreases by 60% and cell growth is delayed; glutathione concentration parallels telomerase activity. These results underscore the main role of glutathione in the control of telomerase activity and the cell cycle (Borrá et al. 2004).

In another study on the impact of antioxidants on telomeres in fibroblasts, exogenous SOD significantly reduced both the production of ROS and the rate of subsequent telomere shortening (Serra et al. 2003). There is also a report that cells that are approaching senescence (aging out) can be "cleared" by SOD-initiated conversion on the road to self-destruction (apoptosis) (Deruy et al. 2010).

3.6 AGE-RELATED DECLINE IN ENDOGENOUS ANTIOXIDANTS

Numerous studies report that endogenous antioxidants protect telomere length. The problem, however, is that our ability to form these antioxidants also declines with age. For instance, a study published in the journal *Biomedical Research*, in 2008, compared the antioxidant defense status in elderly individuals (aged 60 ± 10 years) with that in young people (aged 25 ± 7 years) by measuring total antioxidant activity in both groups.

A significant reduction in total antioxidant activity was found in the elderly people compared with young individuals. This reduction was thought to imply a defect in the antioxidant system, perhaps due to a reduction in individual antioxidants (Adiga and Adiga 2008). Another study published in the journal *Clinical Chemistry*, in 1991, examined the biological variability of blood levels of superoxide dismutase (SOD), glutathione peroxidase (GPx), and catalase (CAT) in a large sample of apparently healthy people ranging in age from 4 to 97 years. Antioxidants were assayed in plasma red blood cells (erythrocytes).

Except for GPx levels that were significantly higher in women compared with men, no other significant variations in these antioxidant enzyme levels were found by gender. Antioxidant activity appeared to be stable in adults under 65 years of age, but was decreased in most of the elderly (Guemuri et al. 1991).

Similar data have been reported in the elderly in India. Advanced age is associated with an accumulation of free radical damage that leads to physiological and clinical modifications. Age-related changes caused by free radical reactions include increasing levels of lipid peroxides and alterations in enzyme activities. The study found an increase in lipid peroxidation and a decrease in antioxidants in normal elderly people (Akila et al. 2007).

A study appearing in the *Journal of Gerontology Series A: Biological Sciences and Medical Sciences*, in 2008, was the first to examine the association between age and glutathione peroxidase (GPx) activity in a cohort of older women with disability and chronic disease: after age 65, GPx activity declines with age in women with disability. This decline did not appear to be related to any diseases that have been previously reported to alter GPx activity (Espinoza et al. 2008). The first three graphs in Figure 3.2 are taken from different studies depicting age-related levels of the endogenous antioxidant enzymes, catalase, SOD, and glutathione, and show that the levels have already decreased by about half by age 40. Furthermore, Figure 3.2d shows that CoQ_{10} declines as well.

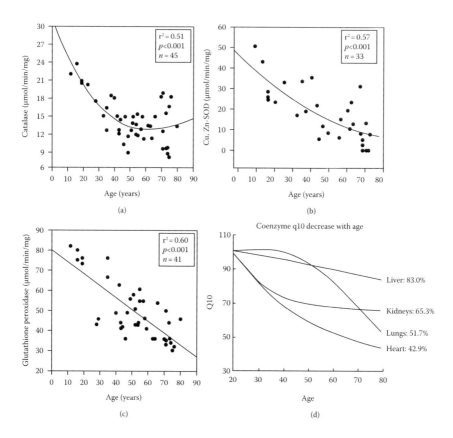

FIGURE 3.2 Age-dependent changes in the activities of free radical scavenging enzymes in fibroblasts from normal human subjects: (a) catalase; (b) Cu, Zn-SOD; (c) glutathione peroxidase. (From Lu, et al., *Mutat. Res.*, 423(1–2), 11–21, 1999. With permission.) (d) Age-related decrease in coenzyme Q10. (Adapted from Kalen., A., et al., *Lipids*, 24, 579–584, 1989, http://www.alsearsmd.com/your-power-to-defend-against-cancer/. With Permission.)

The authors of the report from which these data were taken, writing in the journal *Mutation Research*, in 1999, suggested that the decline in antioxidants and the resulting elevation in oxidative stress may play an important role in damage to mitochondrial DNA (mtDNA) and even mutations affecting the aging process (Lu et al. 1999).

A report in the *Indian Journal of Clinical Biochemistry*, in 2007, tells us to expect free radical damage to accumulate as we age. Age-related changes include increasing levels of lipid peroxides and alterations in enzyme activities. The investigators found an increase in lipid peroxidation and a decrease in antioxidants in normal elderly people. Diabetes and hypertension increased the burden. They proposed supplementation with antioxidants to prevent further oxidative injury in elderly people (Prashan et al. 2007). A Spanish study reported that the SOD activity level was 9% higher in a young urban population than in older adults (De la Torre et al. 1990).

The natural aging process results in sarcopenia, loss of muscle tissue. A report in *BioMed Central (BMC) Geriatrics*, in 2013, strongly suggested that ROS had an adverse effect in sarcopenia. It also suggested that hydrogen peroxide plays a key role in the onset of sarcopenia. The decline in antioxidant protection by catalase and GPx is indicative of antioxidant dysfunction and may therefore be a major contributing factor to the development or onset of sarcopenia (Sullivan-Gunn and Lewandowski 2013).

3.7   EXOGENOUS ANTIOXIDANTS

Exogenous antioxidants are those that cannot be made by the body. These antioxidants must be obtained from antioxidant-rich foods or commercial antioxidant supplements. Science tells us that as terrestrial plants emerged from the ocean, they gradually began to produce substances with antioxidant properties such as ascorbic acid (vitamin C), polyphenols, and tocopherols. The evolution of antioxidants as chemical defenses against ROS, particularly during the Jurassic period, became a steady by-product of photosynthesis (Benzie 2003).

Medicine is interested in the potential of antioxidants to prevent premature telomere shortening. But first, can the capacity of antioxidants to neutralize free radicals and ROS be measured in any given substance?

3.8   QUANTITATIVE MEASURES OF ANTIOXIDANT CAPACITY

It is not enough to assert that something is an antioxidant. The claim that a given substance is an antioxidant requires a measure of that antioxidant activity to make the observation useful. Science is about objective observation. However, free radicals are invisible and have never been observed to disappear in reaction to an antioxidant. An objective, verifiable, reproducible measure of antioxidant activity is needed for useful applications. There are several laboratory methods that can actually measure antioxidant activity and others that can help us assay antioxidant impact on ROS in our body.

3.8.1   THIOBARBITURIC ACID REACTIVE SUBSTANCES (TBARS)

Can laboratory techniques measure the *number* or *concentration* of free radicals? What units apply? How about number of free radicals produced per unit time in a given cell or tissue? That must be in the billions of trillions even in small samples, and in small time lapses. And then, there is the question of how many free radicals per unit time does it take to actually cause any kind of damage, or even how many free radicals per unit time do we need to mop up to avert damage?

One of the most commonly reported clinical signatures of lipid peroxidation is a substance known as malondialdehyde (MDA). It is a secondary by-product of lipid peroxidation and is widely used a measure of damage to cells. When MDA reacts with thiobarbituric acid (TBA), it turns pink, but this is not sufficiently specific to be clinically useful. However, a specific and reliable method for MDA determination in plasma by high-performance liquid chromatography has been validated (Grotto et al. 2007; Moselhy et al. 2013).

It was further shown that TBARS (thiobarbituric acid reactive substances) method as a marker of oxidative stress coincides with other such markers and with clinical disorders as well. A study published in the journal *Atherosclerosis*, in 2007, reported that the presence of impaired glucose tolerance (IGT), diabetes, and increased TBARS levels appear to be significant determinants of telomere shortening (Adaikalakoteswari et al. 2007).

Another study appearing in the journal *Molecular and Cell Biochemistry*, in 2012, reported that oxidative stress as determined by lipid peroxidation (TBARS) was significantly higher in patients with type 2 diabetes compared with a group with normal glucose tolerance. The mean telomere length was shorter in patients with type 2 diabetes compared with those individuals with normal glucose tolerance (Monickaraj et al. 2012).

These studies reveal that we can use a derived measure like TBARS to indicate the concentration of ROS in the body, or at least the adverse effects of ROS concentration. This measure correlates with clinical disorders where ROS are known to play a major role. What is more, level of TBARS supports the theory that ROS play a major role in telomere shortening. TBARS methodology tells us something about oxidative stress levels in the body that helps us understand the impact of ROS.

3.8.2 OXYGEN RADICAL ABSORBANCE CAPACITY (ORAC)

Writing in the journal *Free Radical Biology & Medicine*, in 1993, three researchers from the Agricultural Research Service (ARS) of the US Department of Agriculture (USDA) reported that they had developed a relatively simple, sensitive, and reliable method of measuring the oxygen radical absorbance capacity (ORAC) of antioxidants in serum (Cao et al. 1993). The method of obtaining ORAC units is based on comparison of a test sample to the net antioxidant protection provided by a standard quantity of Trolox, a water-soluble analog of vitamin E.

TBARS assess the damage done by ROS by measuring a by-product of ROS. ORAC assesses the antioxidant capacity of any substance by comparing it with a known antioxidant.

In February 1999, the Human Nutrition Research Center on Aging, a branch of the Agricultural Research Service (ARS) of the US Department of Agriculture (USDA), announced that "High-ORAC Foods May Slow Aging." What does this actually mean? (McBride 1999). It means that measuring the *oxygen radical absorbance capacity* of foods (ORAC) is now feasible, and consuming foods with a high ORAC value may help to avert accelerated aging.

The report went on to state that studies of animal and human blood show that foods that score high in their ORAC antioxidant analysis may protect cells and organelles from oxidative damage. What is more, eating plenty of high ORAC fruits and vegetables, such as spinach and blueberries, may help slow aging. The studies showed that eating "plenty" of high ORAC value foods raised the antioxidant power of the human blood by 10–25%. According to administrator Floyd P. Horn:

> If these findings are borne out in further research, young and middle-aged people may be able to reduce risk of diseases of aging—including senility—simply by adding high-ORAC foods to their diets.

And according to Guohua (Howard) Cao, a physician and chemist who developed the ORAC assay:

> It may be that combinations of nutrients found in foods have greater protective effects than each nutrient taken alone.

In November 2007, Rosaline M. Bliss, also from the ARS, released a report titled "Data on food antioxidants aid research" (Bliss 2007). This report included the ORAC values of 277 selected foods, some of which are shown in Table 3.1,

---

TABLE 3.1

Estimates of Antioxidant Capacity in Selected Foods (Micromole TE per household measure and grams)

Household measure	Food	ORAC value
1 am, 149 g	Apple, red delicious, w/skin	6370
1 oz, 28 g	Chocolate, dark	5903
1/2 c, 87 g	Plums, dried	5700
5 fl oz, 147 g	Wine, red	5693
1/2 med, 60 g	Artichokes, ocean mist, boiled	5650
1 oz, 28 g	Pecans	5023
1/2 c, 74g	Blueberries, fresh	4848
1 oz, 28 g	Walnuts, English	3791
1/2 c, 83 g	Strawberries, sliced	2969
1 med, 114 g	Sweet potato, baked	2411

Source: US Department of Agriculture Research Service, USDA National Nutrient Database for Standard Reference, Release, 2007, Nutrient Data Laboratory home page, https://www.ars.usda.gov/nutrientdata.

and stated that the database can be used to help guide ongoing research into how antioxidants may contribute to health benefits.

For example, many fruits and vegetables are known to be good sources of antioxidant vitamins, such as C and E, and beta-carotene, a form of vitamin A. But these natural foods also contain other compounds, collectively known as phytonutrients, that may contribute to health and so it is not entirely clear how much the antioxidant properties contribute. Nevertheless, there had initially been a recommendation by the USDA of a minimum of 5000 ORAC units/day.

Then, the USDA dramatically reversed its position on recommending ORAC because there seemed to them no way to avoid its abuse in marketing health foods and related products. In 2010, ARS issued the following repudiation of ORAC, cited in part here,[*] titled "Oxygen radical absorbance capacity (ORAC) of selected foods, Release 2 (2010)":

> In 2012 USDA's Nutrient Data Laboratory (NDL) removed the USDA ORAC Database for Selected Foods from the NDL website due to mounting evidence that the values indicating antioxidant capacity have no relevance to the effects of specific bioactive compounds, including polyphenols on human health.
>
> There are a number of bioactive compounds which are theorized to have a role in preventing or ameliorating various chronic diseases such as cancer, coronary vascular disease, Alzheimer's, and diabetes. However, the associated metabolic pathways are not completely understood and non-antioxidant mechanisms, still undefined, may be responsible. ORAC values are routinely misused by food and dietary supplement manufacturing companies to promote their products and by consumers to guide their food and dietary supplement choices....
>
> There is no evidence that the beneficial effects of polyphenol-rich foods can be attributed to the antioxidant properties of these foods. The data for antioxidant capacity of foods generated by in vitro (test-tube) methods cannot be extrapolated to in vivo (human) effects and the clinical trials to test benefits of dietary antioxidants have produced mixed results. We know now that antioxidant molecules in food have a wide range of functions, many of which are unrelated to the ability to absorb free radicals.
>
> For these reasons the ORAC table, previously available on this web site has been withdrawn. (http://www.ars.usda.gov/nutrientdata/ORAC)

The stated basis for this reversal was that no systematic peer-reviewed clinical studies had shown that a given ORAC unit value, or range of values, provides any health benefit or reverses illness. In all fairness, it may be said that the statements in the last paragraph do not exactly fit the facts: the benefits of antioxidants have been repeatedly reported in human participants. What makes it even more difficult to make recommendations is that clinical trials to test any treatment can result in conflicting published reports.

The position reversal and conclusion of the 2010 USDA document appears to rely heavily on a publication in the journal *Free Radical Biology & Medicine* that questions the validity of ORAC on the grounds that it seems that consuming foods rich in flavonoids results in only low concentrations in human plasma. Furthermore, fruits and vegetables contain many macro- and micronutrients, in addition to flavonoids,

---

[*] We have omitted here only the technical description of the ORAC procedure chemistry.

that may directly or through their metabolism affect the total antioxidant capacity of plasma. The authors conclude their critique by pointing out that:

> the large increase in plasma total antioxidant capacity observed after the consumption of flavonoid-rich foods is not caused by the flavonoids themselves, but is likely the consequence of increased uric acid levels. (Lotito and Frei 2006)

3.8.3 TROLOX EQUIVALENT ANTIOXIDANT CAPACITY (TEAC)

In support of ORAC, the journal *Food Chemistry* reported a study comparing ORAC and another measure of antioxidant activity related to Trolox, termed TEAC (Trolox equivalent antioxidant capacity), to measure the antioxidant capacity of milk, orange juice, and a milk/orange juice combination. It was found that ORAC is an accurate way to measure food antioxidant capacity and is actually better than TEAC (Zuluet ael. 2009).

The choice of a valid and reliable measure of antioxidant capacity is not settled, for a number of reasons. Despite modification of the TEAC assay to improve agreement with the ORAC method, correlation of the two assays was not found to be high, as reported in the journal *Clinical Chemistry* in 2004. The coincidence was greater at higher TEAC and ORAC values. However, it was thought also that poor correlation may have resulted from the use of different free radical sources in the two methods: the TEAC assay used exogenous ABTS radicals (decolorization assay; Pellegrini, Proteggente et al. 1999), whereas the ORAC assay used peroxyl radicals. But, since peroxyl radicals are the most common radicals found in the human body, ORAC measurements should be more appropriate. There were also other differences including variations between TEAC and ORAC in "inhibition time" (Wang et al. 2004).

That said, out of context, it must be admitted that there is no indication that a better assessment of the antioxidant capacity of foods says anything about their contribution to better health or to combating illness. However, a recent clinical study published in the *Nutrition Journal* reported that dietary total antioxidant capacity is inversely related to C-reactive protein (CRP) concentration (a marker of inflammation) in young Japanese women (Kobayashi et al. 2012) (see Chapter 8 on functional foods for more information).

In yet another recent study, the total antioxidant capacity of two coffees of different strengths was compared in human volunteers over a period of 4 weeks. Plasma total antioxidant status (TAS), oxygen radical absorbance capacity (ORAC), oxidized LDL, erythrocyte superoxide dismutase (SOD), glutathione peroxidase (GPx), and CAT activity were measured at baseline and after the interventions.

The authors reported that ORAC increased after consumption of MLR (mild light roast) coffee. No significant alteration in lipid peroxidation biomarkers was observed. Both coffees had antioxidant effects. Although MLR contained more chlorogenic acids, similar antioxidant effects were seen with both treatments. The authors concluded that effects may be important in the risk of diseases caused by oxidative stress (Corrêa et al. 2012).

There seems to be little disagreement about the beneficial effects of certain antioxidants. It remains to be seen whether a unit value such as ORAC can be a helpful benchmark for measuring the health benefits of certain foods. ORAC at present tells us little more than that a given ORAC unit value represents a greater or smaller antioxidant free-radical-absorbing capacity than another ORAC unit value. For example, 1800 ORAC units are twice 900. But can we say that 1800 units are twice as beneficial to health as 900 units? We also do not know what is the lowest ORAC unit value that has any health benefits or what is the highest unit value that has adverse—even toxic—effects.

That said, the USDA Database for the Oxygen Radical Absorbance Capacity (ORAC) of Selected Foods, Release 2 is nevertheless accessible online now at

http://www.orac-info-portal.de/download/ORAC_R2.pdf.

A small sample of ORAC unit values for common foods is given in Table 3.2.

Keep in mind that a high ORAC value food is more "antioxidant" than a low ORAC value food, but that there is no way for the typical lay consumer to interpret ORAC value in any more meaningful terms. Furthermore, there is no way to determine what one's antioxidants needs are at any given moment and what ORAC value food(s) would satisfy that need.

3.9 MAINTAINING A HEALTHY BALANCE

Nature is not known for overlooking details vital to survival. For the most part, humanity survived many years without glaring evidence of widespread corrosion by free radicals. Furthermore, as noted above, there are protective processes inside most cells that adjust cell antioxidants capacity to meet free radical density: It is an endogenous antioxidant defense involving an *antioxidant response element* (ARE). Research informs us that excess antioxidant intake can lead to reducing that ARE. By consuming more antioxidants than needed, a dependence on them develops and the ability to detoxify reduces.

TABLE 3.2
ORAC Unit Values for Selected Fruits

Rank	Food Item	Serving Size	Total Antioxidant Capacity per Serving Size
1	Wild blueberry	1 cup	13,427
2	Blueberry (cultivated)	1 cup	9019
3	Cranberry	1 cup (whole)	8983
4	Blackberry	1 cup	7701
5	Prune	Half cup	7291
6	Raspberry	1 cup	6058
7	Strawberry	1 cup	5938
8	Red delicious apple	1 whole	5900
9	Granny Smith apple	1 whole	5381
10	Sweet cherry	1 cup	4873

Source: USDA, https://www.ars.usda.gov/nutrientdata/ORAC.

Cells exposed to oxidative stress, or drugs and toxins, respond by triggering up-regulation of genes that contain a DNA-regulating element that promotes the ARE (for more detail, see Nguyen et al. 2003).

3.10　PLANT AND OTHER FOOD-BASED ANTIOXIDANTS

3.10.1　POLYPHENOLS

Polyphenols are substances in plants believed to have evolved to protect them from attack by insects and pathogens, and even to protect them from solar UV radiation. They are part of the plant defense system. However, polyphenols also have antioxidant activity. Furthermore, it is clear that long-term consumption of a diet rich in plant polyphenols may offer protection against many common health conditions including cardiovascular and heart disease, diabetes, and even cancer.

Polyphenols occur naturally in fruits, vegetables, cereals, and certain beverages. Fruits such as grapes, apples, pears, cherries, and berries contain up to 200–300 mg of polyphenols per 100 g fresh weight. Typically, a glass of red wine or a cup of tea or coffee contains about 100 mg of polyphenols. Cereals, dry legumes, and dark chocolate also contribute to the polyphenolic intake.

However, the exact outcome of antioxidant intake and biomarkers of their benefit are still basically unknown; we need accurate measures of their dietary intake to verify their health benefits. Current methods that rely mainly on food records and on food composition tables, are not particularly useful in measuring total and effective antioxidant intake (Spence et al. 2008). There are many thousands of polyphenolic compounds in various plant species. They all arise from a common intermediate, phenylalanine, or a close precursor. They can be classified into different groups, including:

- Phenolic acids, found abundantly in foods, are divided into two classes: derivatives of benzoic acid and derivatives of cinnamic acid.
- Flavonoids come in more than 4000 varieties, many of which are responsible for the attractive colors of flowers, fruits, and leaves. Flavonoids may be divided into six subclasses:
  - Flavonols.
  - Flavones.
  - Flavanones.
  - Flavanols.
  - Anthocyanins, particularly abundant in brightly colored fruits such as berry fruits and concord grapes and grape seeds, are responsible for the colors in fruits. They have been shown to have potent antioxidant and anti-inflammatory activity, as well as the capacity to inhibit lipid peroxidation and other inflammatory mediators.
  - Isoflavones.
- Quercetin and catechins, examples of common flavonoids, are found in all plant products including fruits, vegetables, cereals, fruit juices, tea, wine, etc.
- Stilbenes in plants are mostly antifungal compounds that are synthesized only in response to infection or injury. Resveratrol is one of the best-studied naturally occurring polyphenol stilbenes. It is found largely in grapes and

in Japanese knotweed. The active form is trans-resveratrol. It is fragile and there is virtually none of it in red wine.

*   Lignans are considered to be phytoestrogens. Their richest dietary source is linseed.

Many factors influence the antioxidant activity of these substances. It is reported that phenolics are more concentrated in the outer layer of plants, and therefore, ripeness at the time of harvest affects the concentrations and proportions of various constituents. It has also been observed that phenolic acid content decreases during ripening, whereas anthocyanin concentrations increase.

Note on anthocyanins: A later chapter (Chapter 5 on nitric oxide) will detail the dual role of nitric oxide (NO) in inflammation, a significant source of ROS as well as an antioxidant. Flavonoids have been reported to lower oxidative stress and to possess beneficial effects on chronic inflammatory diseases associated with the biological activity of the gas, nitric oxide (NO), that they can form. Common phenolic compounds, including anthocyanins, present in fruits, were investigated for their effects on NO formation in macrophages in the inflammatory process in a report in the *Journal of Agricultural and Food Chemistry* in 2002.

NO is essential in macrophage defense function in inflammation: macrophages can release considerable amounts of NO that, being a free radical, can worsen local tissue injury. In some cases, anthocyanins were shown to have strong inhibitory effects on NO production. This was the first study to report the inhibitory effects of anthocyanins and berry phenolic compounds on NO production (Wang and Mazza 2002). This finding may explain why blackberry extract shows strong anti-inflammatory activity. This is thought to be due to the suppression of NO formation by macrophages (Pergola et al. 2006) (see Chapter 8 on functional foods).

Cooking also has a major effect on polyphenol concentration. Onions and tomatoes lose 75–80% of initial quercetin content after boiling for 15 minutes, 65% after cooking in a microwave oven, and 30% after frying (Crozier et al. 1997).

During absorption, polyphenols undergo extensive modification by microflora in the intestines, such as bacteria and microscopic algae and fungi, and later in the liver. Therefore, the forms of the substances reaching the blood and tissues are different from those present in food. It is very difficult to identify and evaluate all the metabolites and their biological activity (Setchell et al. 2003). Most important to remember is that it is the chemical structure of polyphenols and not their concentration that determines the rate and extent of absorption and the nature of the metabolites circulating in the plasma.

The most common polyphenols in our diet are not necessarily those with the highest concentration of active metabolites in target tissues; consequently, the biological properties of polyphenols greatly differ from one polyphenol to another.

3.10.2   ANTI-AGING EFFECT OF POLYPHENOLS

It is now generally recognized that the rate of accumulation of oxidative damage increases with age and, what is worse, the efficiency of antioxidants and repair mechanisms decreases with age (Rizvi and Maurya 2007a, 2007b).

The antioxidant/anti-inflammatory polyphenolic compounds found in fruits and vegetables when consumed may be effective as anti-aging compounds (Cao et al. 1998; Joseph et al. 2005).

Fruit and vegetable extracts that have high levels of flavonoids also display high total antioxidant activity. These include spinach, strawberries, and blueberries. A recent study demonstrated that tea catechins have strong anti-aging activity. Drinking green tea, rich in these catechins, may reduce chronic inflammation and delay the onset of aging (Maurya and Rizvi 2008; Pandey and Rizvi 2009) (see Chapter 8 on functional foods).

3.11 CAROTENOIDS

Carotenoids are a class of naturally occurring pigments that have powerful antioxidant properties. They are the compounds that give foods their vibrant colors. There are over 700 naturally occurring carotenoids. They can be classified into two groups:

- Carotenes include lycopene (found in red tomatoes) and beta-carotene (found in orange carrots) which is converted by the body into vitamin A.
- Xanthophylls lutein, canthaxanthin (the gold in chanterelle mushrooms), zeaxanthin, and astaxanthin. Zeaxanthin is the most common carotenoid that naturally exists in nature and is found in peppers, kiwi fruit, maize, grapes, squash, and oranges.

3.11.1 Examples of Carotenoid Sources

- Carrots: Carotenoids help give orange vegetables their color. Carrots are a good source of beta-carotene. A one-half cup serving of raw carrots provides 184% of the adult recommended daily intake (RDI) of vitamin A. An 8 oz serving of canned carrot juice provide 451%. Cooked carrots, fresh carrot juice, and carrot soup are additional valuable sources.
- Sweet potatoes: One medium-sized baked sweet potato (unpeeled) provides more than 400% of the adult RDI of vitamin A.
- Dark leafy greens: Because carotenoids also promote the vibrant color of green vegetables, dark green leafy vegetables, such as kale, spinach, turnip, and mustard greens, are valuable carotenoid sources. One cup of fresh spinach provides 56% of the adult RDI of vitamin A. Freezing and cooking condense vegetables, thus providing more nutrients per serving. One half cup serving of frozen spinach provides more than 200% of the adult RDI of vitamin A.
- Tomatoes: Carotenoids also contribute color to the redness of plant foods, tomatoes included. Tomato products, including juices and sauces, are a very good source of lycopene. Tomatoes and tomato products also provide beta-carotene. One cup of canned tomato juice provides 22% of the adult RDI of vitamin A.

3.11.2 Additional Vitamin Antioxidants: Vitamins A, C, E

Vitamins serve largely as antioxidants. There is a critical equilibrium between oxidation and antioxidation that we believe is necessary for the maintenance of a healthy biological system. The basic cellular antioxidant defense system including superoxide dismutase (SOD), catalase (CAT), glutathione peroxidase (GPx), glutathione (GSH), and others, as noted above, effects the elimination of excess ROS. However, the endogenous antioxidant defense system is only part of the picture. There is also reliance on exogenous antioxidants such as vitamin C, vitamin E, carotenoids, and polyphenols to prevent oxidative stress (Bouayed and Bohn 2010).

3.11.2.1   Vitamin A

Vitamin A, found in liver, full-fat dairy products, spinach, broccoli, tomato juice, peppers, and watercress, is an antioxidant. It is also known as retinol and is essential to vision and also to healthy skin, healthy bone growth, and immune function. Contrary to the common belief, there is no vitamin A in carrots, but consistent with other yellow and orange vegetables, carrots contain beta-carotene that the body can convert to vitamin A.

In sufficient quantity, vitamin A can be dangerously toxic. For that reason, some sources caution against supplementation with cod liver oil that has high levels of vitamin A. In addition, a report in the *Annals of Otolaryngology, Rhinology, & Laryngology*, in 2008, states that, in one clinical context, large doses of vitamin A may actually counter the beneficial effects of vitamin D (Cannell et al. 2008).

3.11.2.2   Vitamin C

Vitamin C is an antioxidant and essential for normal growth and development. The body can neither make nor store vitamin C so it needs to be routinely replenished by nutrition. All fruits and vegetables contain some amount of vitamin C. Fruits with the highest sources of vitamin C include:

- Cantaloupe
- Citrus fruits and juices, such as orange and grapefruit
- Kiwi fruit
- Mango
- Papaya
- Pineapple
- Strawberries, raspberries, blueberries, and cranberries
- Watermelon

Vegetables with the highest sources of vitamin C include:

- Broccoli, Brussels sprouts, and cauliflower
- Green and red peppers
- Spinach, cabbage, turnip greens, and other leafy greens
- Sweet and white potatoes
- Tomatoes and tomato juice
- Winter squash

3.11.2.3   Vitamin E

There are eight forms of vitamin E with antioxidant activity. However, only alpha-tocopherol is transported in the blood bound to a lipoprotein. Therefore, it is the predominant form of vitamin E found in the blood and tissues.

3.11.2.3.1 Antioxidant Activity of Vitamin E

Alpha-tocopherol functions primarily as a fat-soluble antioxidant. As noted in the previous chapter, fats are integral to all cell membranes and are, therefore, vulnerable to damage by ROS. Alpha-tocopherol can prevent a chain reaction of lipid peroxidation that works to maintain the viability of the cell membrane and protect the fats in the low-density lipoproteins (LDLs) that transport fats through the bloodstream. Oxidized LDLs have been implicated in the development of cardiovascular disease (Trpkovic et al. 2015).

3.11.2.3.2 Food Sources of Vitamin E

Major sources of alpha-tocopherol in the American diet include vegetable oils (olive, sunflower, and safflower oils), nuts, whole grains, and green leafy vegetables and fish. More specific information about food composition and constituents can be found at the website of the USDA Food Composition Databases (https://ndb.nal.usda.gov/).

3.12 WHEN IT COMES TO VITAMINS, MORE IS NOT ALWAYS BETTER

A study in adults with normal coagulation (clotting) status appearing in *The American Journal of Clinical Nutrition*, in 2004, warned that daily supplementation with 1000 IU (670 mg) of RRR-alpha-tocopherol for 12 weeks decreased a vitamin K–dependent factor required for blood coagulation. Individuals taking anticoagulant drugs like aspirin and warfarin, and those who are vitamin K deficient should not take vitamin E supplements without medical supervision because of the increased risk of severe bleeding (Booth et al. 2004; Pastori et al. 2013).

According to the Mayo Clinic Vitamin E Dosing webpage (http://www.mayo-clinic.org/drugs-supplements/vitamin-e/dosing/hrb-20060476), the recommended daily intake for adults over 14 years of age is 15 mg (or 22.5 IU). For adults older than 18 years, pregnant women, and breastfeeding women, the maximum dose is 1000 mg daily (or 1500 IU).

Impaired blood clotting may increase the likelihood of hemorrhage in some individuals. One study concluded that vitamin E raised the risk of hemorrhagic stroke by 22% but reduced the risk of ischemic stroke by 10%. This differential risk pattern is said to be "obscured" when total stroke is examined. Given the relatively small risk reduction of ischemic stroke and the generally more severe outcome of hemorrhagic stroke, "indiscriminate widespread use of vitamin E should be cautioned against" (Schürks et al. 2010).

3.13 RESVERATROL

The grape polyphenol, resveratrol, is a recently discovered antioxidant and anti-aging agent. Resveratrol has been reported to consistently "prolong the life span" by its link to caloric restriction or partial food deprivation (Harikumar and Aggarwal 2008). It has been shown that the target of resveratrol is a sirtuin. Seven sirtuins have been identified in mammals, with SIRT1 believed to mediate the beneficial effects on health and longevity of both caloric restriction and resveratrol (Markus and Morris 2008) (see Chapter 7 on proactive nutrition).

3.14 QUERCETIN

Recently, quercetin has also been reported to exert a preventative effect on aging, but on a yeast and not a human. The *Journal of Agricultural and Food Chemistry* reported, in 2007, that hydrogen peroxide resistance increased in cells pretreated with quercetin. Cellular protection was correlated with a decrease in the oxidative stress markers including increased levels of ROS. Quercetin increased the chronological lifespan of this cell type by 60% (Belinha et al. 2007). It is probable that quercetin may be very beneficial to health, but so far there have been no long-term studies to show that.

3.15 BLACK/GREEN TEA, COFFEE, AND COCOA

Tea is one of the most commonly consumed beverages in the world and is rich in the antioxidant polyphenolic flavonoid compounds. A study appearing in the *International Journal of Food Science & Nutrition*, in 2000, aimed to evaluate the possible effects of different preparation methods on the antioxidant properties of green and black tea.

Green tea, black leaf tea, and black tea in tea bags were infused with water at 90°C for time periods ranging from 0.25 minutes to 15 minutes. Green tea had an approximately 2.5-fold greater antioxidant capacity than both types of black tea. Both green and black teas released quantities of antioxidants into the hot water within 2 minutes of infusion. Preparation of teas in the temperature range of 20–90°C revealed that although antioxidants were liberated from the leaves into the water in cooler infusions, increasing the temperature could increase antioxidant potential by 4- to 9.5-fold.

Black tea prepared using tea bags had significantly lower antioxidant capacity than black leaf tea at temperatures between 20°C and 70°C, suggesting that tea bag materials may prevent some extraction of flavonoids into the tea solution. The addition of milk appeared to diminish the antioxidant potential of black tea preparations. This effect was greatest where whole cow's milk was used and appeared to be primarily related to the fat content of the added milk.

The author concluded that maximum antioxidant capacity may be derived from green tea or from black leaf tea prepared by infusion with water at 90°C for up to 2 minutes and taken with the addition of either fat-free milk, or better yet, without adding milk (Langley-Evans 2000).

3.15.1 BLACK TEA VERSUS GREEN TEA VERSUS RED WINE VERSUS COCOA

These beverages may be high in phenolic phytochemicals, including theaflavin, epigallocatechin gallate, resveratrol, and procyanidin. A study in the *Journal of Agricultural and Food Chemistry* (2003) compared the phenolic and flavonoid contents and total antioxidant capacities of cocoa, black tea, green tea, and red wine.

It was found that cocoa contained much higher levels of total phenolics and flavonoids per serving than black tea, green tea, or red wine. The relative total antioxidant capacities of the samples in both assays were as follows in decreasing order: cocoa > red wine > green tea > black tea. These results suggest that cocoa is more beneficial to health than tea and red wine in terms of its higher antioxidant capacity (Lee et al. 2003).

3.16 ANTIRADICAL VERSUS ANTIOXIDANT

There is a difference between "antiradical" and "antioxidant" activity. Antiradical activity is the ability of components to react with free radicals (in a single free radical reaction), whereas antioxidant activity is the ability to inhibit the process of oxidation (which usually involves a set of different reactions).

A review appearing in the journal *Antioxidants*, in 2013, compared the determination of antioxidant as well as antiradical activity in AA Arabica and Robusta coffee roasted at different temperatures as well as by different methods. The assays were done using the ORAC and TEAC methods (detailed below). The authors found that the most antioxidant-rich beverages are:

- Coffee: 200–550 mg/cup
- Tea: 150–400 mg/cup
- Red wine: 150–400 mg/glass

Coffee and cocoa are comparable to tea in antioxidant capacity. Cocoa has the highest antioxidant activity because it contains both water-soluble and lipid-soluble antioxidants. It has also been shown that solutions of green and roasted coffee have significant antiradical activity against ROS (Daglia et al. 2004).

One source reporting in the journal *Antioxidants*, in 2013, held that drinking two or three cups of coffee made with roasted beans supplies the recommended daily amount of antioxidants. In recent decades, instant coffee grades have been widely applied. True coffee lovers likely prefer natural roasted coffee because it has a unique taste and aroma, but, due to concentration during the extraction procedure, some varieties of instant coffee may actually contain greater amounts of antioxidants than roasted coffee (Yashin et al. 2013).

In yet another report in the *Journal of Agricultural and Food Chemistry*, in 2001, the relative antioxidant activity of tea, coffee, and cocoa on a cup-serving basis was assessed. Under standard cup-serving conditions, milk did not alter the antioxidant activity. The influence of coffee bean source and degree of roasting was further investigated. Robusta coffee made with green coffee beans exhibited 2-fold higher antioxidant activity than Arabica coffee, but, after roasting, this difference was no longer significant. In conclusion, these commonly consumed beverages have significant antioxidant activity, the highest being found in instant coffee on a cup-serving basis (Richelle et al. 2001).

3.17 RED WINE

Many constituents in wine have potentially healthful antioxidant activity. However, it must be borne in mind that the consumption of alcoholic beverages in any quantity, and at any frequency, is a potential health hazard and, therefore, the authors of this book neither endorse nor recommend it.

There are many varieties of grapes and each variety is different from the others in antioxidant constituents. For instance, Malbec has a thick skin and is said to have a high resveratrol content. Grapes grown in cooler climates have higher resveratrol levels than those from warmer regions. It is said that the varieties with the most resveratrol in the wine include Malbec, Petite Sirah, St. Laurent, and Pinot Noir. Tannins in wine are natural antioxidants that protect the wine.

3.17.1 Resveratrol in Red Wines

When plants come under attack by bacteria or fungi, they produce substances, phytoalexins, that have antibacterial activity, in order to defend themselves. Resveratrol is a phytoalexin produced naturally by several plants, including vines.

There are two forms of resveratrol, trans-resveratrol and cis-resveratrol. Wine contains mostly cis-resveratrol, but only the trans-resveratrol offers health benefits. In fact, trans-resveratrol is a fragile substance that is readily damaged by exposure to light. What is more, the cis form can actually nullify the effects of trans-resveratrol.

Wine plants, grape skin, and seeds also contain proanthocyanidins that are essentially flavonoids, such as catechins. These are also known as oligomeric proanthocyanidins, or OPCs.

Anthocyanidins and proanthocyanidins are powerful antioxidants. Some research indicates that the vascular benefits of red wine depend on the presence of OPCs. Studies have shown that OPCs may prevent cardiovascular disease by mitigating the negative effects of high cholesterol on the heart and blood vessels (Feldman et al. 1996).

A note on proanthocyanidins (OPCs): OPCs are said in the study cited above (Feldman et al. 1996) to "prevent cardiovascular disease by mitigating the negative effects of high cholesterol on the heart and blood vessels."

There is evidence that now questions whether high cholesterol, per se, damages blood vessels and the heart. In fact, OPCs promote the formation of nitric oxide (NO). All polyphenols do that one way or another, promoting the formation of NO by blood vessel endothelium and heart endocardium (Loke et al. 2008; Schmitt and Dirsch 2009).

While it is clear that antioxidants protect cells, the contribution of enhanced NO formation to the cardiovascular system and the heart, not to mention its role in immune function, should not be underestimated. NO is so critical to cell function and immune function that Chapter 5 is devoted to it.

3.17.2 Caution about Wine As a Nutritional Source

First, it should be noted that because wine is an alcoholic beverage, it is addictive. Second, over time and depending on quantity, it can injure the liver. A study published in the journal *Alcohol and Alcoholism* in 2002, questioned the commonly held belief that all alcoholic beverages cause similar liver toxicity when drunk in high amounts as recent epidemiological surveys had suggested that drinking wine might decrease the risk of alcoholic cirrhosis in heavy drinkers. Therefore, the authors analyzed the type and intake levels of alcoholic beverages in heavy drinkers according to the severity of their liver disease. They found that the relative percentage of pure alcohol drunk in wine was significantly higher in patients with cirrhosis than in patients without cirrhosis (Pelletier et al. 2002).

Third, the extent of allergic reactions to wine is greater than generally expected. However, while the health benefits of wine are well known, this is a book about preventing accelerated aging. It would be irresponsible to recommend wine just because some of its constituents are thought to promote cardiovascular and heart health.

A study on wine allergies reported in *Deutsches Ärzteblatt International* (the official journal of the German Medical Association) in 2012, tells us that in 2010, a questionnaire-based cross-sectional study was conducted to assess the prevalence of wine intolerance among adults in Mainz, a city in the wine-cultivating region of Rhine-Hesse, Germany. Several thousand people randomly chosen from population lists were asked to fill out a questionnaire about their alcohol intake and the occurrence of various intolerance reactions and allergy-like symptoms after drinking wine.

Of the 948 persons who responded, 68 (7.2% of respondents) reported intolerance to wine and/or allergy-like symptoms after drinking wine. Self-reported wine intolerance was more prevalent in women than in men (8.9% vs. 5.2%, respectively). Wine-intolerant people also more commonly reported intolerance to beer and alcohol in general. Allergy-like symptoms were more common after the consumption of red wine.

The most commonly reported reactions to wine were skin flushing, itch, and nasal congestion.

- Flushed skin, 39 people (57.4%)
- Itching, 24 people (35.3%)
- Rhinorrhea, 22 people (32.4%)
- Diarrhea, 19 people (27.9%)
- Tachycardia, 17 people (25.0%)
- Stomach or intestinal cramps, 17 persons (25.0%)

Alcoholic drinks in general, and in particular red wine, seem to be important triggers for intolerance in some individuals. Asthma is a good example of an intolerance reaction (Vally et al. 2000).

In this study, 19 (25%) of the 68 people with wine intolerance also reported general intolerance to alcohol. This could indicate that more generalized intolerance to alcohol is one of the causes of the observed wine intolerance. Such intolerance could have several causes:

- Polar and hydrophobic ingredients in wine could be dissolved in alcohol, thereby promoting their absorption into the body.
- Alcohol promotes permeability of the intestinal mucosa, which could increase the absorption of wine ingredients.

- Alcohol-induced vasodilation could also be responsible for some symptoms of wine intolerance, such as skin flushing. Alcohol also inhibits the enzyme diaminooxidase, which degrades histamine and other biogenic amines. This would increase histamine concentrations and could lead to symptoms such as vascular dilation in the nose region (Jansen et al. 2003; Maintz and Novak 2007).

Wine intolerance was found to be more common than expected and the data were less suggestive of an immunologically mediated allergy than of intolerance to alcohol, biogenic amines, or other ingredients of wine.

The fact that only 3 out of 30 participants with self-reported wine intolerance, and 6 out of the total of 68 wine-intolerant individuals identified in the study also reported grape intolerance, supports the assumption that wine intolerance is very rarely caused by actual allergy to grapes (Wigand et al. 2012).

Wine allergies can also be linked to chemicals that enter the winemaking process including those legally permitted for use in winemaking. These include pesticides, herbicides, equipment-cleaning chemicals, sulphite preservatives, and sulfur dioxide. The extent to which chemicals are used in wine-making varies greatly between winemakers. And, if that is not enough, the *Journal of Agriculture and Food Chemistry* reported yet another wine storage-related "wine pollutant," *2,4,6-tribromoanisole* (TBA) (Chatonnet et al. 2004).

TBA is usually produced when naturally occurring airborne fungi or bacteria are exposed to certain compounds used as pesticides. TBA is used to treat wood and therefore can be found in older or used wooden barrels. Corks are also susceptible to contamination by the TBA in the winery.

3.17.3 ALCOHOL DEPLETES VITAMINS

Not only is alcohol devoid of proteins, minerals, and vitamins, but it actually also inhibits the absorption and use of vital nutrients.

3.17.3.1 Thiamin, Niacin, and Pyridoxine

Alcohol is preferentially processed in the liver by vitamin-dependent enzymes also responsible for the metabolism of other compounds, such as carbohydrates and proteins. According to Elson Haas, MD, vitamins B1 (thiamin), B3 (niacin), and B6 (pyridoxine) are directly or indirectly involved in alcohol metabolism, and are among the first nutrients to be depleted by excessive alcohol consumption.

3.17.3.2 Riboflavin and B12

The liver needs glutathione and other antioxidants to detoxify alcohol, but these compounds are not efficiently regenerated in persons who drink too much or too often. A 2011 study published in *Alcoholism: Clinical and Experimental Research* demonstrated that alcohol causes glutathione depletion which lessens the ability of the liver to metabolize alcohol. Since glutathione may also be required for optimal vitamin B12 function, heavy alcohol use creates B12 deficiency and reduced ability to store vitamin B12. Finally, vitamin B2 (riboflavin) is needed to regenerate glutathione, but this vitamin is also depleted by alcohol.

3.17.3.3 Ascorbic Acid and Fat-soluble Vitamins

These vitamins are indirectly affected by alcohol consumption because it suppresses appetite leading to poor intake of nutrient-rich foods. A lack of wholesome foods in the diet reduces the availability of the fat-soluble vitamins, A, D, E, and K, and nearly all of the B complex vitamins, including thiamin, niacin, folate, vitamin B6, biotin, and vitamin B12. Ascorbic acid (vitamin C) is also commonly depleted (Hass E., MD. http://www.livestrong.com/article/ 415965-vitamins-depleted-by-alcohol/).

3.17.4 ASTAXANTHIN

Astaxanthin is a marine carotenoid produced by a microalgae (*Haematococcus pluvialis*) to protect itself from UV radiation when its water supply dries up. It is said to be 65 times more powerful than vitamin C, 54 times more powerful than beta-carotene, and 14 times more powerful than vitamin E. It is also said to be 550 times more powerful than vitamin E and 11 times more powerful than beta-carotene at neutralizing free radicals.

The antioxidant activities of astaxanthin and related carotenoids were measured in a study published in the *Journal of Agricultural and Food Chemistry*, in 2000. Compared with alpha-tocopherol, lutein, beta-carotene, and lycopene, astaxanthin showed the highest antioxidant activity against ROS (by Trolox) (Naguib 2000).

3.18 PLANTS AS A SOURCE OF ANTIOXIDANTS

The use of natural medicinal and dietary plants as antioxidants is increasing worldwide. In large part, this is due to the observed health benefits of antioxidant-rich foods and medicinal plants. Many antioxidant compounds occurring naturally in plants, for instance, artichokes, have been identified as free radical or active oxygen scavengers (Brown and Rice-Evans 1998). A wide variety of other vegetables have also come under scrutiny including potatoes, spinach, tomatoes, and legumes, and also fruits (Furuta et al. 1997; Wan et al. 1999). Strong antioxidant activity has been found in cherries, citrus, prunes, and olives. Green and black teas have shown antioxidant properties (they contain up to 30% of their dry weight as phenolic compounds) (Lin et al. 1998).

The journal *Pharmacognosy Reviews* (2010) provided a list of Indian medicinal plants that are sources of antioxidants. Many of these plants are also commonly used in Western dietary and health-related practice. Here is a small sample from that list that would be familiar to us (the common/Ayurvedic names are in brackets):

- *Acacia catechu* (kair)
- *Allium cepa* (onion)
- *Allium sativum* (garlic, lahasuna)
- *Aloe vera* (Indian aloe, ghritkumari)
- *Camellia sinensis* (green tea)
- *Cinnamomum verum* (cinnamon)
- *Curcuma longa* (turmeric, haridra)
- *Hemidesmus indicus* (Indian sarsaparilla, anantamul),

- *Nigella sativa* (black cumin)
- *Trigonella foenum-graecum* (fenugreek)
- *Withania somnifera* (winter cherry, ashwangandha)
- *Zingiber officinale* (ginger) (Devasagayam et al. 2004; Lobo et al. 2010)

3.19   ANTIOXIDANTS PROTECT TELOMERES

The Proactive Nutrition Program is antioxidant-rich and intended to prevent the free radical and ROS damage to cells that results in abnormally rapid cycling which shortens telomeres and results in premature aging: oxidative stress shortens telomeres (von Zglinicki. 2009), but antioxidants can reduce oxidative stress (Sies 1997). The following selection of studies examines the relationship between dietary antioxidants and telomere length. These studies, accessible online in conventional medical libraries, now number in the many hundreds.

3.20   REGULAR VITAMIN CONSUMPTION PROTECTS TELOMERES

A study published in *The American Journal of Clinical Nutrition*, in 2009, aimed to determine in women whether multivitamin use results in longer telomeres. Multivitamin use and nutrient intakes were assessed with a food-frequency questionnaire, and the relative telomere length of leukocyte DNA was measured using appropriate laboratory procedures.

After age and other potential confounders were adjusted for, it was found that multivitamin use was associated with longer telomeres. Compared with non-users, the relative telomere length of leukocyte DNA was on average 5.1% longer in daily multivitamin users compared with non-users. In the analysis of micronutrients, higher intakes of vitamins C and E from foods were each associated with longer telomeres, even after adjustment for multivitamin use. The investigators concluded that multivitamin use is associated with longer telomere length in women (Xu et al. 2009).

3.20.1   DIETARY INTAKE OF ANTIOXIDANTS REDUCES THE RATE OF TELOMERES SHORTENING

A study published in the *Journal of the American Medical Association*, in 2009, aimed to determine whether the increased dietary intake of marine omega-3 fatty acids (docosahexaenoic acid [DHA] and eicosapentaenoic acid [EPA]) associated with prolonged survival in patients with coronary heart disease also impacts telomere length.

The study examined ambulatory leukocyte telomere length at baseline and again after 5 years of follow-up in outpatients in California with stable coronary artery disease. The patients were recruited from the Heart and Soul Study between September 2000 and December 2002, and followed up to January 2009.

It was reported that patients in the lowest quartile of DHA+EPA experienced the fastest rate of telomere shortening, whereas those in the highest quartile experienced the slowest rate of telomere shortening. Levels of DHA+EPA were associated with less telomere shortening before and after sequential adjustment for established risk factors and potential confounding factors. The authors concluded that in this cohort of patients with coronary artery disease, the greater the baseline blood levels of marine omega-3 fatty acids, the lesser the rate of telomere shortening over 5 years (Farzaneh-Fa et al. 2010).

3.20.2 DIETARY ANTIOXIDANT INTAKE AFFECTS BREAST CANCER RISK AND TELOMERE LENGTH IN WOMEN

A study in the *International Journal of Cancer*, in 2009, addressed the connection between white blood cell DNA telomere length and risk of breast cancer, and dietary antioxidant intake. Data were obtained from a population-based case–control study (the Long Island Breast Cancer Study Project) including control comparison individuals.

Overall, the mean level of telomere length was not significantly different between cases and controls. However, among premenopausal women only, carrying shorter telomeres as compared with the longest telomeres was associated with significantly increased breast cancer risk.

A moderate increase in breast cancer risk was observed among women with the shortest telomeres and lower dietary and supplemental intake of beta-carotene, vitamin C or E. These results provided the strongest evidence to date that breast cancer risk is associated with telomere length among premenopausal women or women with low dietary intake of antioxidants or antioxidant supplements (Shen et al. 2009).

3.21   ONE CAN'T START EARLY ENOUGH

The aim of a study conducted in Spain and published in the journal *Clinical Nutrition*, in 2015, was to evaluate the relationship between diet and leukocyte telomere length in a cross-sectional study of children and adolescents from the GENOI study. The investigators hypothesized that dietary total antioxidant capacity would be positively associated with telomere length. In fact, a positive correlation between dietary total antioxidant capacity and telomere length was found after adjustment for age and energy intake. However, higher white bread consumption was associated with shorter telomeres.

Those individuals who had both higher dietary total antioxidant capacity and lower white bread consumption significantly presented the longest telomeres. The investigators concluded that longer telomeres were associated with higher dietary total antioxidant capacity and lower white bread consumption in Spanish children and adolescents (García-Calzón et al. 2015).

3.22   THE IMPACT OF DIFFERENCES IN REGIONAL DIETARY ANTIOXIDANT INTAKE ON AGING

A study was published in the journal *Mechanisms of Ageing and Development*, in 2012. It sought to determine whether the lower level of oxidative stress and the higher antioxidant status thought to be typical in Mediterranean Southern Europe (Crete) explained the difference in incidence of diseases in Northern European (Zupthen, the Netherlands) population. The investigators compared leukocyte telomere length (LTL) in elderly men from those regions to determine whether there is a relationship between LTL and indicators of oxidative stress and antioxidant status.

It was found that the Greek men had significantly longer telomeres than the Dutch men. Endogenous antioxidants, serum albumin, and uric acid were also positively associated with LTL (de Vos-Houben et al. 2012).

The outcome of this study likely reflects not only regional but also regional/cultural differences in diet that account for the antioxidant status found in the respective samples. It is also reasonable to assume that, even as late as 2012, the dietary pattern in Crete was "Mediterranean." It should be noted that men on the Greek island of Crete live, on average, 6 years longer than their peers in Zutphen, The Netherlands (the average life expectancy in Crete is 82 years compared with 76 years in Zutphen) (http://www.sevencountriesstudy.com/about-the-study/).

3.23 WHY IT IS WISE TO CONSIDER THE MEDITERRANEAN DIET

In a report published in the journal *Metabolism*, in 2016, the authors tell us that the fact that variability in telomere shortening is independent of chronological age suggests that it is a modifiable factor. This, perhaps, can be explained at least in part by lifestyle variables such as smoking, adiposity, physical exercise, and diet. In this report, they summarize data from published studies on nutrition (nutrients, foods, and dietary patterns) and telomere length.

The investigators found that consistent with evidence of benefit or harm from chronic age-related diseases, dietary antioxidants and consumption of antioxidant-rich, plant-derived foods are thought to help maintain telomere length. In contrast, total and saturated fat intake and consumption of refined flour cereals, meat and meat products, and sugar-sweetened beverages relate to shorter telomeres. They also found evidence that adherence to the Mediterranean diet is associated with longer telomeres (Freitas-Simoes et al. 2016).

3.24 TEA IS THE BEVERAGE OF CHOICE WITH THE MEDITERRANEAN DIET

The *British Journal of Nutrition* reported in 2010 on the association between food groups and telomere length (TL) in elderly Chinese. In a sample of about 1000 men and about the same number of women aged 65 years and over, TL was measured and daily intake of food groups was assessed with a validated food questionnaire.

In men, only Chinese tea consumption was significantly associated with TL after adjustment for demographics and lifestyle factors. Mean difference in TL between those in the highest quartile of Chinese tea consumption compared with those in the lowest quartile of tea consumption corresponded to a difference of approximately 5 years of life. In women, intake of fats and oils was borderline and inversely related to TL after adjustment for demographic and lifestyle factors. It was concluded that consumption of Chinese tea protects telomere length as evidenced in elderly men (Chan et al. 2010).

3.25   AGING IS AN EQUAL OPPORTUNITY ISSUE

It had been thought that socioeconomically deprived individuals age faster and, thus, must have shorter telomeres than their more affluent counterparts. However, only a weak association between white blood cell telomere length and socioeconomic status was observed in a large heterogeneous sample of women (Adams et al. 2006).

3.26   CONSUMING VEGETABLES PROTECTS TELOMERES

Peripheral leukocyte (white immune system blood cell) telomere length (TL) was measured in hypertensive patients and normotensive control individuals aged 40–70 years, in Yinzhou, Zhejiang Province, China. Dietary intake was assessed with a brief semi-quantitative food frequency questionnaire.

Among control individuals, longer age-adjusted TL was associated with higher vegetable intake. Those with longer age-adjusted TL were 30% less likely to have hypertension. The observed TL–hypertension relationship appeared to be modified by vegetable intake: longer TL was significantly associated with lower hypertension risk only in those with greater vegetable consumption and not in those with lower vegetable intake. The report of this study appeared in *BMJ Open* in 2015 (Lian et al. 2015).

Because of the nutritional value and antioxidant capacity of foods included in the Proactive Nutrition Program, which is based on an enhanced Mediterranean diet, there may be no basis for recommending supplementation with commercial exogenous antioxidants. In addition, it should be noted that supplementation with anything may or may not be safe for any given individual and should be undertaken only under the supervision of a physician or an otherwise qualified healthcare provider.

3.27   IF "SOME ANTIOXIDANTS" ARE GOOD, ARE "MORE" BETTER

Many health authorities extol the virtue of food-derived antioxidants. However, supplements with very high antioxidant capacity may exceed safe limits, and it is not known what constitutes excess antioxidants, nor whether overdosing could be harmful. There is good reason for caution.

A report published in the *International Journal of Biochemistry & Cell Biology*, in 2007, states that ROS and reactive nitrogen species (RNS, e.g., nitric oxide) are well known to play a "dual role" as both beneficial and harmful species. Whereas overproduction of ROS results in oxidative stress, potentially damaging cell structures, ROS/RNS (e.g., superoxide radical and nitric oxide) at moderate to low concentrations have beneficial effects. Ironically, various ROS-mediated actions in fact protect cells against ROS-induced oxidative stress and re-establish or maintain oxidative free radical/antioxidant balance (Valko et al. 2007).

A report in the journal *Oxidative Medicine and Cellular Longevity*, in 2010, cautioned that the balance between oxidation and antioxidation is critical in maintaining a healthy biological system. Whereas physiologic doses of exogenous antioxidants may be required to maintain or re-establish that balance (Ratnam et al. 2006), high doses of exogenous antioxidants may disrupt it.

The authors hold that the health benefits of phytochemicals and nutrients were observed predominantly when being consumed in natural foods such as fruits, vegetables, and grain. They report that:

> Considering epidemiological studies and trials on humans taking antioxidant compounds, it is evident that the health benefits of phytochemicals and nutrients were observed predominantly when being consumed within their natural food matrices (fruits, vegetables, grain, etc.). Compounds within plant foods may therefore be considered as being more safe and healthy compared with isolated, high doses, such as present in supplements. Two main factors seem to be predisposing for the beneficial activities of plant foods: (1) the general low concentration of nutrients and non-nutrients in these natural food matrices and (2) the additive or synergistic actions of complex mixture profiles of phytochemicals and nutrients. Supplementation approaches do generally not take into account both aspects, which could explain the controversial results observed in supplementation studies. (Bouayed and Bohn 2010)

Free radicals and ROS are sometimes also called "oxidants."

There are other concerns about whether more is better. Researchers from the International Antioxidant Research Centre, Guy's Hospital, London, UK, questioned the scientific basis for supporting the argument that oxidative damage is a significant causative factor in the development of human diseases and that antioxidants are capable of preventing or ameliorating these disease processes, in a report published in the *British Journal of Nutrition*, in 1998.

Their concerns center on a number of technical factors, not least of which is that it is difficult to conduct non-invasive study of cells:

> Experimental data obtained in vivo provide evidence that antioxidants function in systems that scavenge reactive oxygen species and that these are relevant to what occurs in vivo. The relevance in vivo of these observations depends [among other things], on knowledge of the uptake and distribution of the antioxidant within the human body, and on what tissue levels of the antioxidant may be expected in relation to dietary levels. There is some way to go until validated precise methods are available for measuring biomarkers of oxidative damage in human subjects in vivo under minimally invasive conditions. (Diplock et al. 1998)

There was also a round-table discussion on the potential hazards of polyphenol consumption at the 1st International Conference on Polyphenols and Health, held in Vichy, France, in November 2003. It was reported in *The American Journal of Clinical Nutrition*, in January 2005. The authors state that:

> It is known, for example, that certain polyphenols may have carcinogenic/genotoxic effects or may interfere with thyroid hormone biosynthesis. Isoflavones are of particular interest because of their estrogenic activity, for which beneficial as well as detrimental effects have been observed. Furthermore, consumption of polyphenols inhibits nonheme iron absorption and may lead to iron depletion in populations with marginal iron stores. Finally, polyphenols may interact with certain pharmaceutical agents and enhance their biologic effects. It is important to consider the doses at which these effects occur, in relation to the concentrations that naturally occur in the human body. Future studies evaluating either beneficial or adverse effects should therefore include

relevant forms and doses of polyphenols and, before the development of fortified foods or supplements with pharmacologic doses, safety assessments of the applied doses should be performed. (Mennen et al. 2005)

Note: The authors of this book have the following concerns with supplements and nutraceuticals that directly or indirectly claim health benefits:

- Dosage: A dose that produces a beneficial effect in cell cultures may be toxic when applied in a human setting; a dose used in an experimental study may never apply in a human setting, because consumption never reaches the same level, or because the bioavailability is very low, or because the appropriate dose never reaches the target site.
- Form of administration: The form of the phenolic compound is also important. Phenolic compounds occur in food mainly as united compounds and the substances occurring in plasma and tissues are mainly mammalian forms, with some exceptions.
- Exposure levels: The risk of consuming high doses of polyphenols from naturally polyphenol-rich foods is low, but the adverse effects of other constituents in these foods, such as cholesterol-increasing fats in coffee, alcohol in wine, and fat in chocolate, must be considered. Foods can be fortified with polyphenols, but care must be taken to ensure that they are consumed by the intended target populations, and not by others who may be at risk (children, pregnant women).

Dietary supplements that contain high (i.e., pharmacologic) doses of polyphenols can be developed. The intake of polyphenols may then easily reach very high levels; in such cases, toxicologic testing may be required to ensure safe levels of intake. In this respect, a recent report on assessment of the safety of botanicals and botanical preparations for use in food and food supplements might very well apply to the field of polyphenols.

3.28   FOOD SOURCES VERSUS SUPPLEMENTS

This book is not intended to substitute for or replace medical nutrition recommendations. There are commercial antioxidant supplements available on the market. We may cite and document supplementation dosages that have been examined in medical studies, but this is only to serve as a guideline. We do not suggest following those dosage or product recommendations without first consulting a healthcare or nutrition professional.

For additional information on supplement formulations, see Schilter et al. (2003) and Kroes and Walker (2004).

REFERENCES

Adaikalakoteswari, A., M. Balasubramanyam, R. Ravikumar, et al. 2007. Association of telomere shortening with impaired glucose tolerance and diabetic macroangiopathy. *Atherosclerosis*, 195(1):83–89.

Adams, J., C. Martin-Ruiz, M. S. Pearce, et al. 2006. No association between socio-economic status and white blood cell telomere length. *Aging Cell*, 6(1):125–128.

Adiga, U., and S. Adiga. 2008. Total antioxidant activity in old age. *Biomedical Research*, 19(3):185–186.

Aguirre, J. D., H. M. Clark, M. McIlvin, et al. 2013. A manganese-rich environment supports superoxide dismutase activity in a Lyme disease pathogen, Borrelia burgdorferi. *Journal of Biological Chemistry*, 288(12):8468–8478.

Akila, V. P., H. Harishchandra, V. D'souza, et al. 2007. Changes in lipid peroxidation and antioxidant in edlerly people. *Indian Journal of Clinical Biochemistry*, 22(1):131–134.

Belinha, I., M. A. Amorim, P. Rodrigues, et al. 2007. Quercetin increases oxidative stress resistance and longevity in Saccharomyces cerevisiae. *Journal of Agricultural and Food Chemistry*, 55:2446–2451.

Benzie, I. F. 2003. Evolution of dietary antioxidants. *Comparative Biochemistry and Physiology. Part A, Molecular & Integrative Physiology*, 136(1):113–126.

Bliss RM. 2007. *Data on antioxidant food supplements aid research.* United States Department of Agriculture. http://www.ars.usda.gov/is/pr/2007/ 071106.htm, Accessed June 16, 2012.

Block, K. I., A. C. Koch, M. N. Mead, et al. 2008. Impact of antioxidant supplementation on chemotherapeutic toxicity: A systematic review of the evidence from randomized controlled trials. *International Journal of Cancer*, 123(6):1227–1239.

Booth, S. L., I. Golly, J. M. Sacheck, et al. 2004. Effect of vitamin E supplementation on vitamin K status in adults with normal coagulation status. *American Journal of Clinical Nutrition*, 80(1):143–148.

Borrá, C., J. M. Esteve, J. R. Viña, et al. 2004. Glutathione regulates telomerase activity in 3T3 fibroblasts. *Journal of Biological Chemistry*, 279(33):34332–34335.

Bouayed, J., and T. Bohn. 2010. Exogenous antioxidants—Double-edged swords in cellular redox state. Health beneficial effects at physiologic doses versus deleterious effects at high doses. *Oxidative Medicine & Cellular Longevity*, 3(4):228–237.

Brown, J. E., and C. A. Rice-Evans. 1998. Luteolin-rich artichoke extract protects low density lipoprotein from oxidation in vitro. *Free Radical Research*, 29(3):247–255.

Cannell, J. J., R. Vieth, W. Willett, et al. 2008. Cod liver oil, vitamin A toxicity, frequent respiratory infections, and the vitamin D deficiency epidemic. *Annals of Otolaringology, Rhinology, & Laryngology*, 117(11):864–870.

Cao, G., H. M. Alessio, and R. G. Cutler. 1993. Oxygen-radical absorbance capacity assay for antioxidants. *Free Radical Biology & Medicine*, 14(3):303–311.

Cao, G., S. L. Booth, J. A. Sadowsky, et al. 1998. Increases in human plasma antioxidant capacity after consumption of controlled diets high in fruit and vegetables. *American Journal of Clinical Nutrition*, 68:1081–1087.

Chan, R., J. Woo, E. Suen, et al. 2010. Chinese tea consumption is associated with longer telomere length in elderly Chinese men. *British Journal of Nutrition*, 103(1):107–113.

Chatonnet, P., S. Bonnet, S. Boutou, et al. 2004. Identification and responsibility of 2,4,6-tribromoanisole in musty, corked odors in wine. *Journal of Agriculture and Food Chemistry*, 52(5):1255–1262.

Corrêa, T. A. F., M. P. Monteiro, T. M. Mendes, et al. 2012. Medium light and medium roast paper-filtered coffee increased antioxidant capacity in healthy volunteers: Results of a randomized trial. *Plant Foods for Human Nutrition*, 67(3): 277–282.

Crozier, A., M. E. J. Lean, M. S. McDonald, et al. 1997. Quantitative analysis of the flavonoid content of commercial tomatoes, onions, lettuce, and celery. *Journal of Agricultural & Food Chemistry*, 45:590–595.

Daglia, M., M. Racchi, A. Papetti, et al. 2004. In vitro and ex vivo antihydroxyl radical activity of green and roasted coffee. *Journal of Agricultural & Food Chemistry*, 52(6):1700–1704.

De la Torre, M. R., A. Casado, and M. E. López-Fernández. 1990. Superoxide dismutase activity in the Spanish population. *Experientia*, 46(8):854–856.

de Vos-Houben, J. M., N. R. Ottenheim, A. Kafatos, et al. 2012. Telomere length, oxidative stress, and antioxidant status in elderly men in Zutphen and Crete. *Mechanisms of Ageing & Development*, 133(6):373–377.

Deichmann, R., C. Lavie, and S. Andrews. 2010. Coenzyme Q10 and statin-induced mitochondrial dysfunction. *The Ochsner Journal*, 10(1):16–21.

Deruy, E., K. Gosselin, C. Vercamer, et al. 2010. MnSOD upregulation induces autophagic programmed cell death in senescent keratinocytes. *PLoS One*, 5(9): e12712. doi: 10.1371/journal.pone. 0012712.

Devasagayam, T. P., J. C. Tilak, K. K. Boloor, et al. 2004. Free radicals and antioxidants in human health: Current status and future prospects. *The Journal of the Association of Physicians of India*, 52:794–804.

Diplock, A. T., J. L. Charleux, G. Crozier-Willi, et al. 1998. Functional food science and defence (ibid.) against reactive oxidative species. *British Journal of Nutrition*, 80 Suppl 1:S77–S112.

Dutton, P. L., T. Ohnishi, E. Darrouzet, et al. 2000. 4 Coenzyme Q oxidation reduction reactions in mitochondrial electron transport. In Kagan, V. E., and P. J. Quinn. eds. *Coenzyme Q: Molecular mechanisms in health and disease*. Boca Raton, FL: CRC Press. pp. 65–82.

Ernster, L., and G. Dallner. 1995. Biochemical, physiological and medical aspects of ubiquinone function. *Biochimica et Biophysica Acta*, 1271(1):195–204.

Espinoza, S. E., H. Guo, N. Fedarko, et al. 2008. Glutathione peroxidase enzyme activity in aging. *Journal of Gerontology Series A: Biological Sciences and Medical Sciences*, 63(5):505–509.

Essential Nutraceuticals™. 2012. *What is glutathione?* http://www.essentialgsh.com/glutathione. html.

Farzaneh-Fa, R., J. Lin, E. S. Epel, et al. 2010. Association of marine omega-3 fatty acid levels with telomeric aging in patients with coronary heart disease. *Journal of the American Medical Association*, 303(3):250–257.

Feldman, M. D., P. H. Pak, C. C. Wu, et al. 1996. Acute cardiovascular effects of OPC-18790 in patients with congestive heart failure time- and dose-dependence analysis based on pressure-volume relations. *Circulation*, 93(3):474–483.

Freitas-Simoes, T. M., E. Ros, and A. Sala-Vila. 2016. Nutrients, foods, dietary patterns and telomere length: Update of epidemiological studies and randomized trials. *Metabolism*, 65(4):406–415.

Frie, B., R. Stocke, and B. N. Ames. 1988. Antioxidant defences [ibid.] and lipid peroxidation in human blood plasma. *Proceedings of the National Academy of Sciences*, 37:569–571.

Furuta, S., Y. Nishiba, and I. Suda. 1997. Fluorometric assay for screening antioxidative activities of vegetables. *Journal of Food Science*, 62:526–528.

Gaetani, G. F., A. M. Ferraris, M. Rolfo, et al. 1996. Predominant role of catalase in the disposal of hydrogen peroxide within human erythrocytes. *Blood*, 87(4):1595–1599.

García-Calzón, S., A. Moleres, M. A. Martínez-González, et al. 2015. Dietary total antioxidant capacity is associated with leukocyte telomere length in a children and adolescent population. *Clinical Nutrition*, 34(4):694–699.

Ghirlanda, G., A. Oradei, A. Manto, S. Lippa, et al. 1993. Evidence of plasma CoQ10-lowering effect by HMG-CoA reductase inhibitors: A double-blind, placebo-controlled study. *The Journal of Clinical Pharmacology*, 33(3):226–229.

Grotto, D., L. D. Santa Maria, S. Boeira, et al. 2007. Rapid quantification of malondialdehyde in plasma by high performance liquid chromatography-visible detection. *Journal of Pharmaceutical and Biomedical Analysis*, 43(2):619–624.

Guemuri, L., Y. Artur, B. Herbeth, et al. 1991. Biological variability of superoxide dismutase, glutathione peroxidase, and catalase in blood. *Clinical Chemistry*, 37(11):1932–1937.

Halliwell, B. 1995. How to characterize an antioxidant: An update. *Biochemical Society Symposium*, 61:73–101.

Handler, J. A., and R. G. Thurman. 1990. Redox interactions between catalase and alcohol dehydrogenase pathways of ethanol metabolism in the perfused rat liver. *Journal of Biological Chemistry*, 265:1510–1515.

Handy, D. E., E. Lubos, Y. Yang, et al. 2009. Glutathione peroxidase-1 regulates mitochondrial function to modulate redox-dependent cellular responses. *Journal of Biological Chemistry*, 284(18):11913–11921.

Harikumar, K. B., and B. B. Aggarwal. 2008. Resveratrol: A multitargeted agent for age-associated chronic diseases. *Cell Cycle*, 7:1020–1035.

Hayes, J. D., J. U. Flanagan, and I. R. Jowsey. 2005. Glutathione transferases. *Annual Review of Pharmacology & Toxicology*, 45:51–88.

Jansen, S. C., M. van Dusseldorp, K. C. Bottema, et al. 2003. Intolerance to dietary biogenic amines: A review. *Annals of Allergy, Asthma Immunology*, 91:233–240.

Joseph, J. A., B. Shukitt-Hale, and G. Casadesus. 2005. Reversing the deleterious effects of aging on neuronal communication and behavior: Beneficial properties of fruit polyphenolic compounds. *American Journal of Clinical Nutrition*, 81:313–316.

Kalen, A., E. L. Appelkvist, and G. Daliner. 1989. Age-related changes in the lipid composition of rat and human tissues. *Lipids*, 24:579–584.

Kishi, T., T. Watanabe, and K. Folkers. 1977. Bioenergetics in clinical medicine XV. Inhibition of coenzyme Q10-enzymes by clinically used adrenergic blockers of beta-receptors. *Research Communications in Chemical Pathology and Pharmacology*, 17(1):157–164.

Kobayashi, S., K. Murakami, S. Sasaki, et al. 2012. Dietary total antioxidant capacity from different assays in relation to serum C-reactive protein among young Japanese women. *Nutrition Journal*, 11:91.

Kroes, R., and R. Walker. 2004. Safety issues of botanicals and botanical preparations in functional foods. *Toxicology*, 198(1–3):213–220.

Langley-Evans, S. C. 2000. Antioxidant potential of green and black tea determined using the ferric reducing power (FRAP) assay. *International Journal of Food Science & Nutrition*, 51(3):181–188.

Langsjoen, P. H. 2002. The clinical use of HMG CoA-reductase inhibitors (statins) and the associated depletion of the essential co-factor coenzyme Qlo; a review of pertinent human and animal data. http://www.fda.gov/ohrms/dockets/dailys/02/May02/052902/02p-0244-cp00001-02-Exhibit_A-vol1.pdf.

Lee, K. W., Y. J. Kim, H. J. Lee, et al. 2003. Cocoa has more phenolic phytochemicals and a higher antioxidant capacity than teas and red wine. *Journal of Agricultural & Food Chemistry*, 51(25):7292–7295.

Lian, F., J. Wang, X. Huang, et al. 2015. Effect of vegetable consumption on the association between peripheral leucocyte telomere length and hypertension: A case-control study. *British Medical Journal Open*, 5(11):e009305.

Lin, J. K., C. H. Lin, Y. C. Lin, et al. 1998. Survey of catechins, gallic acid and methylxantines in green, oolong, puerh and black teas. *Journal of Agriculture & Food Chemistry*, 46:3635–3642.

Lobo, V., A. Patil, A. Phatak, et al. 2010. Free radicals, antioxidants and functional foods: Impact on human health. *Pharmacognosy Reviews*, 4(8):118–126.

Loke. W. M., J. M. Hodgson, J. M. Proudfoot, et al. 2008. Pure dietary flavonoids quercetin and (-)-epicatechin augment nitric oxide products and reduce endothelin-1 acutely in healthy men. *American Journal of Clinical Nutrition*, 88(4):1018–1025.

Lotito, S. B., and B. Frei. 2006. Consumption of flavonoid-rich foods and increased plasma antioxidant capacity in humans: Cause, consequence, or epiphenomenon? *Free Radical Biology & Medicine*, 41(12):1727–1746.

Lu, C. Y., H. C. Lee, H. J. Fahn, et al. 1999. Oxidative damage elicited by imbalance of free radical scavenging enzymes is associated with large-scale mtDNA deletions in aging human skin. *Mutation Research*, 423(1–2):11–21.

Lushchak, V. I. 2012. Glutathione homeostasis and functions: Potential targets for medical interventions. *Journal of Amino Acids*, 2012:736837.

Maintz, L., and N. Novak. 2007. Histamine and histamine intolerance. *American Journal of Clinical Nutrition*, 85:1185–1196.

Markus, M. A., and B. J. Morris. 2008. Resveratrol in prevention and treatment of common clinical conditions of aging. *Clinical Interventions in Aging*, 3:331–339.

Maurya, P. K., and S. I. Rizvi. 2008. Protective role of tea catechins on erythrocytes subjected to oxidative stress during human aging. *Natural Product Research*, 23(12):1072–1079.

McBride, J., 1999. *High-ORAC Foods May Slow Aging*. United States Department of Agriculture. Agricultural Research Service. http://www.ars.usda.gov/is/pr/1999/990208.htm.

Mennen, L. I., R. Walker, R., C. Bennetau-Pelissero, et al. 2005. Risks and safety of polyphenol consumption. *American Journal of Clinical Nutrition*, 81(1 Suppl): 326S–329S.

Misra, U. K., B. U. Bradford, J. A. Handler, et al. 1992. Chronic ethanol treatment induces H_2O_2 production selectively in pericentral regions of the liver lobule. *Alcoholism: Clinical & Experimental Research*, 16:839–842.

Monickaraj, F., S. Aravind, K. Gokulakrishnan, et al. 2012. Accelerated aging as evidenced by increased telomere shortening and mitochondrial DNA depletion in patients with type 2 diabetes. *Molecular & Cell Biochemistry*, 365:343–350.

Mortensen, S. A., A. E. Leth, Agner, et al. 1997. Dose-related decrease of serum coenzyme Q10 during treatment with HMG-CoA reductase inhibitors. *Molecular Aspects of Medicine*, 18(Suppl): S137–S144.

Moselhy, H. F., R. G. Reid, S. Yousef, et al. 2013. A specific, accurate, and sensitive measure of total plasma malondialdehyde by HPLC. *Journal of Lipid Research*, 54(3):852–858.

Naguib, Y. M. 2000. Antioxidant activities of astaxanthin and related carotenoids. *Journal of Agricultural and Food Chemistry*, 48(4):1150–1154.

Nguyen, T., P. J. Sherratt, and C. B. Pickett. 2003. Regulatory mechanisms controlling gene expression mediated by the antioxidant response element. *Annual Review of Pharmacology & Toxicology*, 43:233–260.

Niki, E. 1993. Antioxidant defenses in eukaryotic cells. In Poli, G., E. Albano, and M. U. Dianzani, eds. *Free radicals: From Basic Science to Medicine*. Basel, Switzerland: Birkhauser Verlag. pp. 365–373.

Pandey, K. B., and S. I. Rizvi. 2009. Plant polyphenols as dietary antioxidants in human health and disease. *Oxidative Medicine & Cellular Longevity*, 2(5):270–278.

Pastori, D., R. Carnevale, R. Cangemi, et al. 2013. Vitamin E serum levels and bleeding risk in patients receiving oral anticoagulant therapy: A retrospective cohort study. *Journal of the American Heart Association*, 2(6):e000364.

Pelletier, S., E. Vaucher, R. Aider, et al. 2002. Wine consumption is not associated with a decreased risk of alcoholic cirrhosis in heavy drinkers. *Alcohol & Alcoholism*, 37(6):618–621.

Pergola, C., A. Rossi, P. Dugo, et al. 2006. Inhibition of nitric oxide biosynthesis by anthocyanin fraction of blackberry extract. *Nitric Oxide*, 15(1):30–39.

Prashan, A. V., H. Harishchandra, V. D'souza, et al. 2007. Age related changes in lipid peroxidation and antioxidants in elderly people. *Indian Journal of Clinical Biochemistry*, 22(1):131–134.

Ratnam, D. V., D. D. Ankola, V. Bhardwaj, et al. 2006. Role of antioxidants in prophylaxis and therapy: A pharmaceutical perspective. *Journal of Controlled Release*, 113(3):189–207.

Re, R., N. Pellegrini, A. Proteggente, A. Pannala, M. Yang, and C. Rice-Evans. 1999. Antioxidant activity applying an improved ABTS radical cation decolorization assay. *Free Radical Biology and Medicine*, 6(9-10):1231–1237. PMID: 10381194.

Rice-Evans, C. A., and A. T. Diplock. 1993. Current status of antioxidant therapy. *Free Radical Biology & Medicine*, 15(1):77–96.

Richelle, M., I. Tavazzi, and E. Offord. 2001. Comparison of the antioxidant activity of commonly consumed polyphenolic beverages (coffee, cocoa, and tea) prepared per cup serving. *Journal of Agricultural & Food Chemistry*, 49(7):3438–3442.

Rizvi, S. I., and P. K. Maurya. 2007a. Alterations in antioxidant enzymes during aging in humans. *Molecular Biotechnology*, 37:58–61.

Rizvi, S. I., and P. K. Maurya. 2007b. Markers of oxidative stress in erythrocytes during aging in human. *Annals of the New York Academy of Sciences*, 1100:373–382.

Schilter, B., C. Andersson, C. Anton et al. 2003. Guidance for the safety assessment of botanicals and botanical preparations for use in food and food supplements. *Food & Chemical Toxicolology*, 41:1625–1649.

Schmitt, C. A., and V. M. Dirsch. 2009. Modulation of endothelial nitric oxide by plant-derived products. *Nitric Oxide*, 21(2):77–91.

Schürks, M., R. J. Glynn, P. M. Rist, et al. 2010. Effects of vitamin E on stroke subtypes: Meta-analysis of randomised controlled trials. *British Medical Journal*, 341:c5702.

Sedighi, O., A. Makhlough, M. Shokrzadeh, et al. 2014. Association between plasma selenium and glutathione peroxidase levels and severity of diabetic nephropathy in patients with type two diabetes mellitus. *Nephro-Urology Monthly*, 6(5):e21355.

Serra, V., T. von Zglinicki, M. Lorenz, et al. 2003. Extracellular superoxide dismutase is a major antioxidant in human fibroblasts and slows telomere shortening. *Journal of Biological Chemistry*, 278(9): 6824–6830.

Setchell, K. D., M. S. Faughnan, T. Avades, et al. 2003. Comparing the pharmacokinetics of daidzein and genistein with the use of 13C-labeled tracers in premenopausal women. *American Journal of Clinical Nutrition*, 77:411–419.

Shen, J., M. D. Gammon, M. B. Terry, et al. 2009. Telomere length, oxidative damage, antioxidants and breast cancer risk. *International Journal of Cancer*, 124(7):1637–1643.

Shi, H. L., N. Noguchi, and N. Niki. 1999. Comparative study on dynamics of antioxidative action of α- tocopheryl hydroquinone, ubiquinol and α- tocopherol, against lipid peroxidation. *Free Radical Biology & Medicine*, 27:334–346.

Sies, H. 1997. Oxidative stress: Oxidants and antioxidants. *Experimental Physiology*, 82(2):291–295.

Spence, J. P., M. M. Abd El Mohsen, A. M. Minihane, et al. 2008. Biomarkers of the intake of dietary polyphenols: Strengths, limitations and application in nutrition research. *British Journal of Nutrition*, 99(1):12–22.

Sullivan-Gunn, M. J., and P. A. Lewandowski. 2013. Elevated hydrogen peroxide and decreased catalase and glutathione peroxidase protection are associated with aging sarcopenia. *BMC Geriatrics*, 13:104. doi:10.1186/1471-2318-13-104.

Tarry-Adkins, J. L., S. E. Ozanne, A. Norden, et al. 2006. Lower antioxidant capacity and elevated p53 and p21 may be a link between gender disparity in renal telomere shortening, albuminuria, and longevity. *American Journal of Physiology. Renal Physiology*, 290: F509 –F516.

Trpkovic, A., I. Resanovic,J. Stanimirovic, et al. 2015. Oxidized low-density lipoprotein as a biomarker of cardiovascular diseases. *Critical Review in Clinical Laboratory Sciences*, 52(2):70–85.

Valko, M., D. Leibfritz, J. Moncol, et al. 2007. Free radicals and antioxidants in normal physiological functions and human disease. *International Journal of Biochemistry & Cell Biology*, 39(1):44–84.

Vally, H., N. de Klerk, and P. J. Thompson. 2000. Alcoholic drinks: Important triggers for asthma. *Journal of Allergy & Clinical Immunology*, 105(3):462–467.

von Zglinicki, T. 2009. Oxidative stress shortens telomeres. *Trends in Biochemical Sciences*, 27(7):339–344.

Wan, H., G. Cao, and R. L. Prior. 1999. Total antioxidant capacity of fruits. *Journal of Agriculture & Food Chemistry*, 44:701–705.

Wang, C. C, C. Y. Chu, K. O. Chu, et al. 2004. Trolox-equivalent antioxidant capacity assay versus oxygen radical absorbance capacity assay in plasma. *Clinical Chemistry*, 50(5): 952–954.

Wang, J., and G. Mazza. 2002. Inhibitory effects of anthocyanins and other phenolic compounds on nitric oxide production in LPS/IFN-γ-activated RAW 264.7 macrophages. *Journal of Agricultural & Food Chemistry*, 50(4):850–857.

Wigand, P., M. Blettner, J. Saloga, et al. 2012. Prevalence of wine intolerance. Results of a survey from Mainz, Germany. *Deutsches Ärzteblatt International*, 109(25):437–444.

Xu, Q., C. G. Parks, L. A. DeRoo, et al. 2009. Multivitamin use and telomere length in women. *American Journal of Clinical Nutrition*, 89(6):1857–1863.

Yashin, A., Y. Yashin, J. Y. Wang, et al. 2013. Antioxidant and antiradical activity of coffee. *Antioxidants*, 2(4):230–245.

Zulueta, A., M. J. Esteve, and A. Frígola. 2009. ORAC and TEAC assays comparison to measure the antioxidant capacity of food products. *Food Chemistry*, 114:310–316.

4 Preventing Premature Cell Cycling

4.1 INTRODUCTION

Progressive age-related changes are natural and the decline of function is, for the most part, normal and inevitable. What is *not* normal is premature acceleration of the decline of function in otherwise healthy people. It helps to understand how this happens and how it can be prevented by looking at some aspects of life at the cellular level, how cells duplicate in cycles, how cells age, and why cells die. The biological life cycle of cells also helps in understanding how premature aging can be averted at the cellular level. Averting it at the cellular level is the key to averting premature aging.

The way to avoiding premature aging is to employ strategies designed to reduce oxidative stress. Oxidative stress accelerates cell division. With each division, the cells in the body are one step closer to dying as telomeres shorten. When there are none left, the cell dies. The number of cellular replications, or lives, of each cell is limited. The key to beating the cellular clock is to spread the replications out over as long a time span as possible.

Oxygen free radicals and reactive oxygen species (ROS) damage the DNA both in the mitochondria that power the cell and in the chromosomes in the nucleus of the cells. They also damage other structures in the cells, especially the membrane that is exceptionally susceptible to oxidation damage due to its high concentration of lipids. Accumulated debris in the cell is a message to the cell to speed up duplication, or to self-destruct. This chapter will explain how the rate of destruction of the mitochondria and the accumulation of debris in the cell speeds up cell reproduction that leads to premature aging.

A diet to avoid premature aging is different from a diet intended to avoid weight gain. For one thing, weight gain is reversible, while aging is not. One can apply cosmetics and one can diet; the body can reshape with exercise and surgery, but age is inscribed in every cell in the body. That inscription will fulfill its destiny. One cannot prolong the path to that destiny, but it can definitely be shortened at least by the choice of the foods in the daily diet.

There is one technical qualification to "you cannot reverse aging." At the moment, we can say that there is no practical, safe way to do that. However, scientists have found that embryonic cells as well as certain other cells can produce an enzyme that works sort of backwards: telomerase, an enzyme that can actually lengthen telomeres. The catch is that this ability also seems to confer eternal life on cancer cells. In fact, scientists are looking at ways to inhibit the production of telomerase in cancer cells so that they will die on schedule, as they should (Blackburn 2005; Shay and Wright 2011).

4.2 BODY WEIGHT MAY BE AN UNRELIABLE CLUE TO CELL AGING

It is generally held that overweight is unhealthy and the trend in increasing body weight in Western society is a concern to many individuals, as well as to health authorities. For most people, it is tied to worsening self-image over time. However, in terms of overall health, a recent analysis revealed some very interesting data.

A study published in the *Journal of the American Medical Association* in 2013 examined published analyses of body mass index (BMI) and all-cause mortality in almost 3 million individuals, and 300,000 deaths. The investigators concluded that relative to normal weight, grade 1 obesity (BMI of 30.0–34.9) overall was not associated with higher mortality. To everyone's surprise, it was associated with significantly lower all-cause mortality (Flegal et al. 2013). This is not to suggest that abandoning efforts to maintain a healthy weight has merit, but it indicates a greater concern with appearance than with what happens to the body that cannot be seen. And, that is really what matters most.

Appearance is generally accepted as a hallmark of aging, but aging is really about what happens over time inside cells in the body, in fact, inside the nucleus and especially in mitochondria. One cannot see or otherwise experience any of this, yet what happens there over time is not reversible.

4.3 CELL DIVISION: MITOSIS

We live from the top-down, and we die from the bottom-up. What does this mean? At any moment, the cells in all the body organs are newborn "daughters" of a previous cell that has just "died," perhaps "ceased to exist" might be a more apt description. This reproductive cycle is called *mitosis*. It is the point where cells divide. This process is repeated fairly quickly for a fixed number of such new generations—approximately 50–70 times (Hayflick 1965). That is the *Hayflick limit*. Parenthetically, it may be appropriate to talk about "daughter cells" because it is a reminder that mitochondria are passed on to us only by our mothers. Fathers play no role in this.

The biologist Dr. Leonard Hayflick noticed that cells reproducing in cultures do so only a finite number of times before the process stops for good and the cells die. What is more, cells frozen during their lifetimes and later returned to an active state, had a kind of *cellular memory*: the frozen cells picked up right where they left off. In other words, interrupting the cell lifespan did nothing to lengthen it.

Hayflick found that cells go through a number of phases, but once a cell reaches the end of its lifespan, it undergoes programmed cellular death, *apoptosis*. The implications of the *Hayflick limit* are not appealing: there is a molecular clock that inexorably winds down from the moment of conception (Hayflick 1965; Hayflick and Moorhead 1961).

So the body is constantly replacing old cells with new ones at the rate of millions per second and by the time one finishes reading this sentence, about 50 million of the cells will have died and been replaced by others. Some are lost through *wear and tear*, some reach the end of their life, and others *deliberately* self-destruct. It is said to be "deliberately" because there is no other rational explanation for their action, but that is not to say that in the sense in which it would apply to our voluntary actions as commonly understood. There is no explanation, nor is there a vocabulary to explain what cells do other than common terms.

The more quickly cells divide, the sooner they will die. Avoiding premature aging requires the rate of cell division to be slowed because each time they divide, they are just one step closer to dying, causing accelerated and, therefore, premature aging.

4.4 CELL SUICIDE: APOPTOSIS

The number and kind of cells in the body is closely regulated in three ways: first, by controlling the rate of cell division; second, by senescence, or aging, of the cell (when cells become dysfunctional due to age, they become debris excreted by the body); and third, when a cell is no longer needed, an enzyme is activated that begins cell death. Cells undergo *apoptosis,* or self-destruction. Apoptosis is a genetically pre-programmed process initiated within the cell DNA that directs it to self-destruct when certain internal conditions have been met. Here again, scientists use the term "cell suicide," implying volition but with no basis for such a concept other than observing what a cell does.

The extent of apoptosis that takes place is staggering. In a healthy adult human, billions of cells die in the intestine every hour. It seems remarkably wasteful for so many cells to die, especially as the vast majority may be perfectly healthy at the time they self-destruct. However, there are several reasons why a cell should be programmed to die after a certain point. In the developmental stages, for example, human fetuses have tissues that create some webbing between the fingers. As the fetus develops in the uterus, these tissues undergo apoptosis that ultimately allows the fingers to form. Shedding the lining of the uterus in menstruation also occurs as apoptosis.

4.5 THE CELL-OWNER'S MANUAL

There are many kinds of cells in the body and some, including nerve cells, do not divide at all. However, they share some common elements. Cells that have a membrane that encloses them, and a nucleus and *organelles* inside that make them work and replicate, are called *eukaryotes.*

Most cells that make up the body are eukaryotes, but not all of them. There are many types of cells that have no nucleus or any kind of organelles, and a fair number of those also live inside us.

Figure 4.1 depicts a simplified *slice-through* model of a eukaryote cell showing only a very small number of the organelles that are ordinarily found in such cells. Selected structures and organelles feature prominently in concerns about premature aging: these include the double-walled membrane that surrounds the cell, the *smooth endoplasmic reticulum*, the mitochondria, and the nucleus holding DNA in chromosomes. Each organelle is responsible for a specific function needed by the cell and also by the tissues or organ of which it is a part.

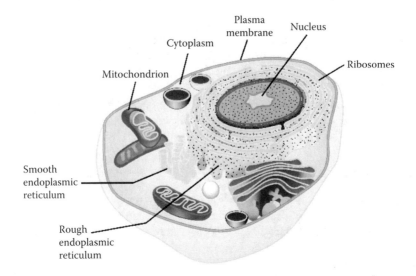

FIGURE 4.1   **(See color insert.)** The eukaryote cell. (From Stuart Nezin. With permission.)

4.5.1   THE MEMBRANE

The plasma membrane that surrounds the cell is two layered, flexible, and selectively permeable. It encloses *cytoplasm*, a jelly-like substance made mostly of water and salt. The membrane is made primarily of phospholipids in a bilayer with embedded proteins that separate the internal contents of the cell from the surrounding environment. The plasma membrane controls the movement of organic molecules, ions, water, and oxygen in and out of the cell. In addition, wastes including carbon dioxide and ammonia also pass out of the cell through the plasma membrane.

Figure 4.2 represents a section of cell membrane showing that its structure depends largely on proteins and various kinds of lipids including sugar-containing lipid molecules (glycolipids).

The membrane is not just an envelope or wall enclosing a cell but a very complex biological entity performing a multitude of its own separate actions, as well as those integral to cell function. The membrane encloses the cytoplasm that contains all the organelles. In a sense, in addition to enclosing the cell and maintaining its shape, the wall also has *valve* functions which permit various molecules to enter the cell and other to exit in accordance with the metabolic and defense functions of the cell (Tillman and Cascio 2003).

It is important to note also that these functions are highly dependent on the availability of lipids integrated into the membrane wall structure. Cholesterol is an important element of membrane structure and function. More than 90% of cellular cholesterol is located in the plasma membrane and in fact, cells falter without an adequate supply. Membrane functions also falter when lipids oxidize and therefore cells form antioxidants to prevent that from happening. Chapter 3 detailed these endogenous antioxidants.

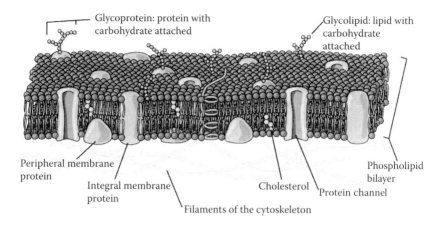

FIGURE 4.2 **(See color insert.)** Section of the membrane of a eukaryote cell. (From Nickels, J.D., et al. *Chem. Phys. Lipids*, 192, 87–99, 2015. With permission.)

The crucial role of cholesterol in cell membrane function is often undervalued in connection with the clinical effort to reduce serum lipids in the treatment of cardiovascular and heart disease. Furthermore, the age-associated decline in endogenous antioxidants, also described in Chapter 3, jeopardizes the membrane, and therefore, cell functions (Goluszko and Nowic 2005).

Material entering the cells starts with the process (endocytosis) whereby cells take up macromolecules, microscopic substances and, in specialized cases, even other cells. The material to be ingested is encapsulated in a small portion of the plasma membrane that forms an *endocytic vesicle* containing it.

There are two main types of endocytosis: "cellular eating" (*phagocytosis*) involves the ingestion of large particles, such as microorganisms or dead cells, via large vesicles called phagosomes, while "cellular drinking" (*pinocytosis*) is the ingestion of fluid and solutes via small pinocytic vesicles. Most eukaryote cells are continually ingesting fluid and solutes by pinocytosis, while large particles are most efficiently ingested by specialized phagocytic cells (Alberts et al. 2002).

Membranes are a dynamic environment that permits bi directional exchange of substances with their surroundings (Tillman and Cascio 2003). This allows the condition inside the cell to be very different from that outside. For example, nerve cells will maintain a high concentration of potassium inside, whereas outside there is very little of it, and lots of sodium. Such concentration differences functionally "tolerated" by the cell membrane are absolutely necessary for its function.

4.5.1.1 Reactive Oxygen Species (ROS): Cell Killers

Because the membrane holds cholesterol, a vital component of cell membrane structure, it is an easy target for free radicals that can oxidize it. Free radicals, a natural by-product of normal metabolism, form *lipid peroxide* that "steals" electrons from the cholesterol in cell membranes. This process causes a free radical chain reaction that jeopardizes cell function.

As noted in Chapter 3, there are different substances in the body, usually lipids but also proteins, that are oxidized by free radicals to form different "species" of reactive molecules. They are called "reactive oxygen species" (ROS). Some are reactive nitrogen species (RNS). ROS are the prime suspects in cell damage, setting the stage for apoptosis and premature aging.

Lipid peroxidation causes changes in membrane fluidity, a very important physical feature known to affect protein formation by the cell. The resulting disturbance of the bilayer structure alters the physiological functions of the membranes and contributes to cell membrane damage. Oxidative stress and damage to the membrane could then lead the cell down one of two paths, survival or apoptosis (de la Haba et al. 2013).

4.5.2   THE NUCLEUS

The nucleus, typically the most prominent organelle in a cell, contains the DNA. It stores chromatin (DNA plus proteins) in a gel-like substance called the nucleoplasm. The nucleolus is the condensed region of chromatin where ribosome synthesis occurs. The ribosomes synthesize proteins that are needed in some organelles.

The nuclear envelope forms the boundary of the nucleus. It consists of an outer membrane and an inner membrane continuous with the endoplasmic reticulum. Nuclear pores allow substances to enter and exit the nucleus.

The nuclear envelope is perforated with pores that control the passage of ions, molecules, and RNA between the nucleoplasm and the cytoplasm. The nucleoplasm is the semi-solid fluid inside the nucleus. It contains the chromatin and the nucleolus.

4.5.2.1   Chromosomes

Chromosomes are structures within the nucleus that hold DNA, the material that confers heredity. There are 23 pairs of chromosomes, DNA strands containing genes, in the nucleus of human eukaryote cells. Two pairs determine gender: XX in women and XY in men.

Every eukaryote cell-type has a specific number of chromosomes in the nucleus. Chromosomes are only visible and individually distinguishable just before cell division. When the cell is in the growth and maintenance phases of its life cycle, proteins are attached to chromosomes, making them appear to be unwound disorganized threads. In that state, they are called chromatin.

Both exogenous and endogenous free radicals as well as ROS are known to damage DNA (Dizdaroglu and Jaruga 2012). On the bright side, a study by Lobo et al. (2010) titled "Free radicals, antioxidants and functional foods: impact on human health," published in the journal *Pharmacognosy Reviews*, reports that while free radicals adversely alter lipids, proteins, and DNA and trigger a number of human diseases, application of external source of antioxidants can assist in coping with this oxidative stress. The authors propose relying on effective, non-toxic natural compounds with antioxidative activity and dietary antioxidants as functional foods (Dizdaroglu and Jaruga 2012). This book likewise proposes this strategy in Chapter 8.

The Proactive Nutrition Program was developed to help avoid accelerated aging because nutrition can be shown to directly affect the chromosomes and, therefore, lifespan; the rate of cell reproduction appears geared to cellular ability to weather the continuous free radical storm which is mostly created by metabolism within the cells. However, countering free radical damage with optimal antioxidant-enhanced nutrition can change the rate at which cells cycle/duplicate or die.

4.5.3 ENDOPLASMIC RETICULUM

The endoplasmic reticulum consisting of folded membranes, channels, and flattened sacs in cell cytoplasm forms, stores, and transports various substances necessary to cell function. Principal among those functions is calcium storage and protein formation (called "folding"). Protein formation results in free radicals in the endoplasmic reticulum just as might any metabolic function involving oxygen. Persistent oxidative stress can initiate a cascade of cell apoptosis that is now linked to many human diseases including diabetes, atherosclerosis, and neurodegenerative conditions (Malhotra and Kaufman 2007).

The adverse effects of the free radicals generated by the endoplasmic reticulum affect its function in ways that can translate into many common diseases such as diabetes and liver and kidney disease. In some instances, there are errors in the production of proteins (protein *misfolding*) that ultimately cascade into organ malfunction. Researchers reported in 2006, in *The International Journal of Biochemistry & Cell Biology*, that, given type 2 diabetic conditions, oxidative stress can cause the endoplasmic reticulum to activate an enzyme that further suppresses insulin production and insulin action.

The good news is that antioxidants reduce stress in the endoplasmic reticulum and improve protein formation/folding. It seems that free radicals are profusely generated when the endoplasmic reticulum makes errors in protein synthesis, apparently not a rare occurrence. However, evidence points to a reduction of free radicals by antioxidants (Malhotra et al. 2008), and antioxidants can be supplied through "proactive" nutrition.

4.5.4 THE MITOCHONDRIA

Mitochondria, as can be seen in their DNA, are much like parasitic bacteria now living in and off most of our body cells. They are double membrane–bound organelles found in most eukaryote cells. Their number in a cell can vary widely within and among different organism, tissue, and cell types. For instance, red blood cells have no mitochondria, while liver cells can have more than 2000 (Bruce et al. 1994). A mitochondrion is depicted in Figure 1.1, Chapter 1, and their place in a typical cell is shown in Figure 4.1.

Mitochondria manage and transport most of the cell's source of chemical energy in adenosine triphosphate (ATP). They control cell metabolism (aerobic "respiration"), waste disposal, growth, cycle, and apoptosis.

Although most of a cell's DNA is contained in the cell nucleus, the mitochondria have their own independent complete set of DNA, including all of its genes (genome) that, as previously noted, show substantial similarity to bacterial genomes.

Mitochondria are very much involved in cell self-destruction. Scientists writing in the *Annual Review of Pharmacology and Toxicology*, in 2007, reported that the regulation of cell death (apoptosis), a second major function of these organelles, appears to be closely linked to their generation of ROS (Orrenius et al. 2007).

Reporting in the *Proceedings of the National Academy of Sciences* in 2001, investigators described a study intended to determine the importance of free radicals formed by mitochondria in aging and senescence. They analyzed changes in mitochondrial function with age in mice with partial or complete deficiencies in the antioxidant enzyme manganese superoxide dismutase (MnSOD, commonly termed SOD).

Liver mitochondria in mice with complete deficiency in MnSOD exhibited substantially slower metabolism. Mice with normal MnSOD levels showed the same age-related mitochondrial decline, but it occurred later in life. The investigators concluded that mitochondrial free radical production leading to oxidative stress causes functional decline and the initiation of apoptosis, and this process appears to be a central component of aging (Kokoszka et al. 2001).

In addition to the well-established role of the mitochondria in energy metabolism, regulation of cell death is emerging as the second major function of mitochondria because their metabolism (respiration) is the principal source of free radicals in cells.

Free radicals destroy, whereas antioxidants protect, albeit not invariably. Excessive free radical production has been implicated in mitochondrial DNA mutations, aging, and cell death. Conversely, mitochondrial antioxidant enzymes protect against apoptosis and it seems that there may be a direct link between mitochondria, oxidative stress, and cell death (Ott et al. 2007). How can that be prevented?

It has been shown that the source of free radicals does not matter when it comes to oxidative stress damage to our body. In one study, oxidative stress was induced in red blood cells (erythrocytes) by low doses of gamma radiation. An imbalance between the radiation-mediated oxidative damage and the antioxidant capacity of the erythrocytes was observed in the hours after radiation exposure. Antioxidant enzyme activities, mainly catalase and glutathione peroxidase, were found to decrease after irradiation (Benderitter et al. 2003).

4.5.4.1 The Mitochondrial Theory of Aging

The "mitochondrial theory of aging" (Harman) is that mitochondria are both the primary sources of free radicals and the primary targets of those same free radicals. In addition to effects on lifespan and aging, mitochondrial free radicals have been shown to play a central role in the healthspan of many vital organ systems. In the following article, the authors review the evidence supporting the role of mitochondrial oxidative stress, damage, and dysfunction in aging and healthspan, including cardiac aging, age-dependent cardiovascular diseases, skeletal muscle aging, neurodegenerative diseases, insulin resistance and diabetes as well as age-related cancers.

Potential treatment strategies to improve mitochondrial function in aging and healthspan are reviewed, with a focus on protective drugs, such as the mitochondrial antioxidants *MitoQ*, *SkQl*, and the protective peptide *SS-31* (Cui et al. 2012; Dai et al. 2014).

Note:

- MitoQ is a mitochondria-targeted antioxidant designed to protect against oxidative damage. It is the first substance specifically designed to decrease mitochondrial oxidative damage to have undergone clinical trials in humans specifically in connection with liver damage (Gane et al. 2010) and Parkinson's disease (Snow et al. 2010).
- SkQ1, designed to penetrate cell membranes, has antioxidant properties and has been found to improve skin wound healing (Demyanenko et al. 2015).
- SS-31, targeted at mitochondrial oxidative stress, protects the kidneys (Birk et al. 2013).

These studies, and many others, conclude that the oxidative metabolism of mitochondria generates free radicals in quantity. These result in ROS that attack the mitochondria that gave rise to them. It seems equally clear that in many cases, the antioxidant protective enzyme systems of the cell, SOD, catalase, etc., may not be sufficient to neutralize them. As a consequence, the resulting debris that accumulates in the cell ages it, and the age of the cell and proximity to self-destruction depend on the degree of that accumulation.

4.6   FREE RADICALS: INSIDE AND OUTSIDE THE CELL

Science is now revising our knowledge of the principal causes of oxidative stress. It is known that plasma membranes and mitochondria are a major source of free radicals. Protein production generates free radicals and therefore, free radicals cannot be perceived anymore as a mere consequence of external factors, or by-products of altered cellular metabolism as was commonly thought. This may explain why the indiscriminate use of antioxidants has not produced beneficial results in many popular or medical applications so far. There is still a lack of deeper understanding of the biological roles of free radicals, particularly in organelles (Moldovan and Moldovan 2004).

4.7   WHAT TRIGGERS MITOSIS?

Mitosis is the process of cell division. The nucleus first splits into two, then follows division of the parent cell components into two daughter cells. Parenthetically, injecting cytoplasm from a cell undergoing mitosis into another cell in other stages of the cell cycle can induce the non-dividing cells to start mitosis. This suggested that there is a chemical signal in the cytoplasm of dividing cells that "tells" the cells to divide. By analyzing the cytoplasm into its components, scientists were able to find small proteins that trigger mitosis (CDKs).

Each time a cell divides into two daughter cells, the resultant telomeres at the end of the chromosomes become shorter. The life of the cell hangs in balance when there is not enough telomere left to protect the end of the chromosome.

Figure 4.3 depicts the resulting shortening of the *telomeres*, the caps at the end of the chromosomes, with each subsequent cell division as the cell ages. When no *telomeres* are left, the cell dies. This process affects all eukaryote cells in the body.

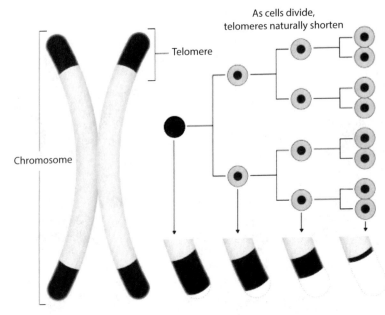

FIGURE 4.3 **(See color insert.)** Abbreviation of the telomeres with each cell cycle. (From Dr. David Eifrig Jr., Strawberry Research, http://retirementmillionairedaily.com/this-ocean-animal-could-hold-the-key-to-extending-human-life/. With permission.)

4.8 CAN TELOMERE LENGTH BE DIRECTLY CONTROLLED?

4.8.1 Telomerase

Telomerase is the enzyme that replaces short bits of DNA on telomeres that are otherwise shortened when the cell divides. But it is only present in viable quantity in embryonic stem cells and other rapidly reproducing cells such as sperm cells, and especially cancers. In ordinary cases, when low levels of telomerase are present in most cells, mitosis will reach the *Hayflick limit* and division will stop.

Telomerase seems a candidate for averting aging. Researchers are now able to extract telomerase and synthesize it. There is hope that if telomerase could be added to normal adult cells, they will continue to replicate beyond their Hayflick limit. In one study that supports this notion, researchers found that cells to which they had introduced telomerase replicated 20 times more often than their normal expected lifespan and they were still dividing at the time of the report (Cherfas 2000).

4.8.1.1 Meditation and Telomeres

Researchers at the University of California, Davis Center for Mind and Brain, recently reported investigating the effects of a 3-month meditation retreat on telomerase activity and two major contributors to the experience of stress: perceived control (associated with decreased stress) and neuroticism (associated with increased subjective distress). They also tried to determine whether two aspects of meditative practice, increased mindfulness and purpose in life, accounted for retreat-related changes in the two stress-related variables and in telomerase activity.

It was reported that telomerase activity was significantly greater in retreat participants than in control comparison participants at the end of the retreat (Jacobs et al. 2011). What this study seems to point out is that perhaps any behavior that results in reducing oxidative stress, including life stress, will contribute to slowing telomere shortening. It turns out that stress/distress is not telomere friendly.

4.9 THE PROACTIVE NUTRITION PROGRAM

The Proactive Nutrition Program is a simple, easy to implement nutritional plan designed to preserve telomere length. This plan combines a Mediterranean food pattern with "sirtfoods." Sirtfoods activate sirtuins, especially sirtuin 1. The Proactive Nutrition Program is low in sugar (both refined and from simple carbohydrates) to reduce free radicals generated by insulin dysregulation. Second, this plan is high in antioxidants and rich in nitrates and in the amino acid L-arginine, a nitric oxide (NO) donor. These foods are shown to protect telomeres (see Chapter 5 on nitric oxide).

Sirtfoods activate an ancient highly adaptive gene that controls energy (calories) storage and metabolic down-regulation. This is thought to be related to Paleolithic times when food availability was unpredictable and "feast or fast" was the common dietary principle. This gene has been called the "thrifty gene" because it helped ancestors conserve body weight between hunts. Unfortunately, as we now have almost unlimited access to food (except in cases of extreme poverty), the thrifty gene no longer serves its purpose and has been implicated in our growing rates of obesity (Neel 1962).

4.10 THE SIRTUIN FAMILY

Sirtuin activators, a "family" of seven similar neuropeptide molecules, are very new to the science of nutrition. The first sirtuin activator identified, SIRT1—and still the best known—is found in resveratrol, concentrated mostly in the skin of red grapes, pomegranates, and Japanese knotweed. Sirtuin influences the formation of DNA. DNA is encased in proteins called histones that stabilize their structure. It has been shown that calorie restriction is one way to activate sirtuin (Guarente 2013; Morselli et al. 2010). When the sirtuin gene is activated by low caloric intake or another dietary stimulus, increased activation also slows chromosome replication, thus reducing errors. Replication errors can cause cell self-destruction or, worse case, cancer.

Activation of SIRT1 affects food intake, metabolism, calories, fat storage, inflammation, circadian rhythm, and aging. Other sirtuin activators have since been discovered, such as catechins (found in green tea) and epicatechins in cocoa powder (responsible for the health benefits claimed for dark chocolate).

SIRT1 helps to promote survival by protecting cells in those times when food (and therefore energy) is scarce. Activating it regulates a number of body functions including fat storage in the body: sirtuin activation mimics low energy levels and therefore enhances fat oxidation.

Although sirtuin activators are found throughout the plant kingdom, only certain fruits, vegetables, and beverages have large enough amounts to qualify as "sirtfoods." Examples are:

- Apples
- Blackcurrants
- Blueberries
- Capers
- Citrus fruits
- Dark chocolate
- Cocoa powder
- Green tea
- Kale
- Extra-virgin olive oil
- Onions
- Parsley
- Red wine
- Tofu and other soy products
- Turmeric

These foods are incorporated in the Proactive Nutrition Program detailed in Chapter 7.

Most importantly, SIRT1 activation is strongly associated with longevity and is said to turn on a "fountain of youth" in cells. Although this is an age of plenty, the biological mechanisms that evolved in hunter-gatherers from prehistoric times promoted eating everything in sight, and storing as much fat as possible for later. These mechanisms are still alive and well in modern times, but they clash with the wish to remain trim and "fit."

Efforts to reduce calorie consumption and reduce fat storage are at odds with firmly entrenched biological dictates to *pig-out* whenever possible: the modern Western diet now largely dictates that with simple carbohydrates, especially refined sugar, foods that were not readily available in ancient times.

The Proactive Nutrition Program prevents accelerated aging by appropriately restricting overall calories and adding sirtfoods to promote the expression of the all-important SIRT1 gene. Although this type of food plan has been shown to promote moderate weight loss, the emphasis here is on preventing accelerated aging by protecting cells from accelerated aging. As documented earlier, body weight, except in the extreme, is not a reliable index of longevity, whereas slowing cell cycling is.

4.10.1 Sirtfoods Protect the Cell Membrane, Organelles, and Telomeres

The sirtuins are a multifunction family. Among the many benefits of sirtuin activation are:

- Promoting longevity and the integrity of plasma membrane function (Crane et al. 2013)
- Supporting glucose metabolism and heart action (Pillai et al. 2014)

- Reducing oxidative stress-induced apoptosis, thus increasing the lifespan of the cell (Shoba et al. 2009)
- Protecting mitochondria from ROS (Verma et al. 2013)

Recent studies in animal models have shown impressive benefits with activating SIRT1. L.P. Guarente (Massachusetts Institute of Technology [MIT], Cambridge, MA) showed that SIRT1 promotes the formation of new mitochondria in the cell. This is called mitochondrial *biogenesis*. It is strongly suspected that the SIRT1 activator resveratrol stimulates mitochondrial biogenesis and delivers health benefits in treated mice. Dr. Guarente believes that mitochondrial biogenesis may have beneficial effects on aging and, perhaps, diseases of aging. Furthermore, he believes that SIRT1-mediated mitochondrial rejuvenation may reduce the production of the ROS that may accelerate aging (Guarente 2007).

Other investigators, using mouse models, reported in *The Journal of Cell Biology* in 2010 that SIRT1 appears to promote telomere length in vivo (in live beings) and attenuates telomere shortening associated with aging, an effect dependent on telomerase activity. In short, SIRT1 averts DNA damage (Palacios et al. 2010).

Mice over-producing SIRT1 have an increased lifespan, remaining healthy for longer than their littermates. SIRT1-deficient mice have shorter telomeres, whereas SIRT1 over production boosts telomere length, preventing them from shortening as the mice grow older.

SIRT1 may also influence a second maintenance pathway called "alternative lengthening of telomeres" (ALT): SIRT1 over production promoted chromosome end DNA repair. Conversely, SIRT1-deficient cells showed increased damage at their chromosome ends. SIRT1 therefore maintained telomere length and integrity, which may explain why SIRT1-overexpressing mice stay healthier for longer (Short 2010).

4.10.2 Sirtuin and Cancer: The Possible Dark Side of SIRT1

Hepatocellular carcinoma (HCC) is a form of liver cancer that most commonly occurs in people with chronic hepatitis B or C. The treatment for HCC, a highly malignant tumor with a poor prognosis, is complicated because it is often diagnosed at an advanced stage when it may no longer respond to chemotherapy or to surgery.

A study, published in the journal *Cancer Research* in 2011, reported that SIRT1, essential for the transformation of normal cells into HCC cancer cells, occurs at very low levels in normal livers, but was over-produced in HCC cell lines and in a subset of HCC. Furthermore, tissue analysis of HCC, and adjacent non-tumor liver tissues, revealed a positive correlation between the production levels of SIRT1 and advancement in tumor grades. On the other hand, down-regulation of SIRT1 consistently suppressed the proliferation of HCC cells by induction of cellular senescence or apoptosis.

The authors reported that these findings reveal a novel function for SIRT1 in telomere maintenance of HCC and suggested that inhibition of SIRT1 might prove helpful in treating HCC (Chen et al. 2011).

4.10.3 Sirtuin and Cancer: The Possible Bright Side of SIRT1

Recent studies have identified small chemical compounds that modulate sirtuins, and these modulators have enabled a greater understanding of the biological function and molecular mechanisms of sirtuins. A review in the journal *Molecule*, in 2014, highlights the possibility of using sirtuins, especially SIRT1 and SIRT2, for cancer therapy, and focuses on the therapeutic potential of sirtuin modulators in both cancer prevention and treatment (Kozako et al. 2014).

4.11 20:20 HINDSIGHT

It seems, in retrospect, that nature endowed Paleolithic ancestors with a metabolic adjustment of caloric need mechanism, sirtuin1, for surviving during times of food shortage when there was no agriculture to produce and guarantee a consistent food supply. But it seems ironic that this mechanism that actually averts premature aging by protecting telomeres came at a time in prehistory when premature aging could hardly have been a serious problem.

Now that, on average, a longer lifespan can be expected, it is more important than ever to consider the Proactive Nutrition Program to help avoid telomere shortening that could promote premature aging. The Proactive Nutrition Program is also designed to help provide better overall health outcomes.

The typical Western diet (see Chapter 6) supplies the metabolic furnace with an almost unending supply of sugars for fuel. Why is overconsumption of sugar not a good idea? Among other things, sugar causes dental cavities; it contributes to obesity, type 2 diabetes, and cancer; and, most important, it also shortens telomeres to cause premature aging.

A cooperative study published in the *American Journal of Public Health*, in 2014, involved investigators from the Center for Health and Community, School of Medicine, University of California, San Francisco, as well as many other clinical and research centers. The aim of the study was to determine whether leukocyte telomere length maintenance, which underlies healthy cellular aging, provides a link between sugar-sweetened beverage (SSB) consumption and the risk of cardio-metabolic disease.

The investigators examined cross-sectional associations between the consumption of SSBs, diet soda, and fruit juice and telomere length in a nationally representative sample of healthy adults. The study population included more than 5000 American adults, aged 20–65 years, with no history of diabetes or cardiovascular disease, from the 1999 to 2002 National Health and Nutrition Examination Surveys (NHANES).

Leukocyte telomere length was determined from DNA specimens. Diet was assessed using 24-hour dietary recalls. After the usual adjustments for sociodemographic and health-related characteristics, sugar-sweetened soda consumption was associated with significantly shorter telomeres.

Consumption of 100% fruit juice was marginally associated with longer telomeres, and no significant associations were observed between consumption of diet sodas or non-carbonated SSBs and telomere length. The authors concluded that regular consumption of sugar-sweetened sodas might influence metabolic disease development through accelerated cell aging (Leung et al. 2014).

The average daily sugar-sweetened soda consumption for all survey participants in this study was 12 oz. About 21% in this nationally representative sample reported drinking at least 20 oz of sugar-sweetened soda a day.

The researchers also found that each daily 8 oz serving of sugar-sweetened sodas was directly related to shorter telomeres, roughly equivalent to 1.9 additional years of aging, independent of sociodemographic and health-related variables. For a daily 20 oz serving, the current standard serving size, this translates into approximately 4.6 additional years of aging. More than 20% of adults in the study population reported at least 20 oz of sugar-sweetened soda consumption per day.

Although these are modest associations, the magnitude of the association for consuming 20 oz of sugar-sweetened soda is comparable to observed associations between telomere length and moderate/vigorous levels of physical activity (4.4 years) and smoking (4.6 years, in the opposite direction).

This study is one of many establishing the association of telomere length with dietary patterns and supports the logic behind the Proactive Nutrition Program.

REFERENCES

Alberts, B., A. Johnson, J. Lewis, et al. 2002. *Molecular Biology of the Cell*, 4th edition. New York: Garland Science.

Benderitter, M., L. Vincent-Genod, J. P. Pouget, et al. 2003. The cell membrane as a biosensor of oxidative stress induced by radiation exposure: A multiparameter investigation. *Radiation Research*, 159(4):471–483.

Birk, A. V., S. Liu, Y. Soong, et al. 2013. The mitochondrial-targeted compound SS-31 re-energizes ischemic mitochondria by interacting with cardiolipin. *Journal of the American Society of Nephrology*, 24(8):125012–125061.

Blackburn, E. H. 2005. Telomerase and cancer: Kirk A. Landon—AACR prize for basic cancer research lecture. *Molecular Cancer Research*, 3:477. doi: 10.1158/1541-7786. MCR-05-0147.

Bruce. A., A. Johnson, J. Lewis, et al. 1994. *Biology of the Cell*. New York: Garland Publishing. ISBN 0-8153-3218-1.

Chen, J., B. Zhang, N. Wong, et al. 2011. Sirtuin 1 is upregulated in a subset of hepatocellular carcinomas where it is essential for telomere maintenance and tumor cell growth. *Cancer Research*, 71(12):4138–4149.

Cherfas, J. 2000. Hayflick licked: Telomerase lengthens life of normal human cells. *Science Watch*, May/June 2000. http://archive.sciencewatch.com/may-june2000/sw_may-june2000_page8.htm.

Crane, F. L., P. Navas, H. L. Low, et al. 2013. Sirtuin activation: A role for plasma membrane in the cell growth puzzle. *Journals of Gerontology Series A: Biological Sciences & Medical Sciences*, 68(4):368–370.

Cui, H., Y. Kong, and H. Zhang. 2012. Oxidative stress, mitochondrial dysfunction, and aging. *Journal of Signal Transduction*, 2012:646354.

Dai, D-F., Y. A. Chiao, D. J. Marcinek, et al. 2014. Mitochondrial oxidative stress in aging and healthspan. *Longevity & Healthspan*, 3:6. doi:10.1186/ 2046-2395-3-6.

de la Haba, C., J. R. Palacio, P. Martínez, et al. 2013. Effect of oxidative stress on plasma membrane fluidity of THP-1 induced macrophages. *Biochimica et Biophysica Acta*, 1828(2):357–364.

Demyanenko, I. A., E. N. Popova, V. V. Zakharova, et al. 2015. Mitochondria-targeted antioxi-
    dant SkQ1 improves impaired dermal wound healing in old mice. *Aging*, 7(7):475–485.
Dizdaroglu, M., and P. Jaruga. 2012. Mechanisms of free radical-induced damage to DNA.
    Free Radical Research, 46(4):382–419.
Flegal, K. M., B. K. Kit, H. Orpana, et al. 2013. Association of all-cause mortality with over-
    weight and obesity using standard body mass index categories: A systematic review and
    meta-analysis. *Journal of the American Medical Association*, 309(1):71–82.
Gane, E. J., F. Weilert, D. W. Or, et al. 2010. The mitochondria-targeted anti-oxidant mito-
    quinone decreases liver damage in a phase II study of hepatitis C patients. *Liver
    International*, 30:1019–1026.
Goluszko, P., and B. Nowic. 2005. Membrane cholesterol: A crucial molecule affecting
    interactions of microbial pathogens with mammalian cells. *Infection and Immunity*,
    73(12):7791–7796.
Guarente, L. 2007. Sirtuins in aging and disease. *Cold Spring Harbor Symposia on Quantitative
    Biology*, 72:48348–4838.
Guarente, L. 2013. Calorie restriction and sirtuins revisited. *Genes & Development*,
    27(19):2072–2085.
Hayflick, L. 1965. The limited in vitro lifetime of human diploid cell strains. *Experimental
    Cell Research*, 37(3):614–636.
Hayflick, L., and P. S. Moorhead. 1961. The serial cultivation of human diploid cell strains.
    Experimental Cell Research, 25(3):585–621.
Jacobs. T. L., E. S. Epel, J. Lin, et al. 2011. Intensive meditation training, immune cell telomer-
    ase activity, and psychological mediators. *Psychoneuroendocrinology*, 36(5):664–681.
Kokoszka, J. E., P. Coskun, L. A. Esposito, et al. 2001. Increased mitochondrial oxidative
    stress in the Sod2 (+/−) mouse results in the age-related decline of mitochondrial
    function culminating in increased apoptosis. *Proceedings of the National Academy of
    Sciences*, 98(5):2278–2283.
Kozako, T., T. Suzuki, M. Yoshimitsu, et al. 2014. Anticancer agents targeted to sirtuins.
    Molecules, 19(12):20295–20313.
Leung. C. W., B. A. Laraia, B. L. Needham, et al. 2014. Soda and cell aging: Associations
    between sugar-sweetened beverage consumption and leukocyte telomere length in
    healthy adults from the National Health and Nutrition Examination Survey. *American
    Journal of Public Health*, 104(12):2425–2431.
Lobo,V., A. Patil, A. Phatak, et al. 2010. Free radicals, antioxidants and functional foods:
    Impact on human health. *Pharmacognosy Review*, 4(8):118–126.
Malhotra, J. D., H. Miaob, K. Zhanga, et al. 2008. Antioxidants reduce endoplasmic reticulum
    stress and improve protein secretion. *Proceedings of the National Academy of Sciences*,
    105(47):18525–18530.
Malhotra, J. D., and R. J. Kaufman. 2007. Endoplasmic reticulum stress and oxidative
    stress: A vicious cycle or a double-edged sword? *Antioxidants & Redox Signaling*,
    9(12):2277–2293.
Moldovan, L., and N. I. Moldovan. 2004. Oxygen free radicals and redox biology of organ-
    elles. *Histochemistry & Cell Biology*, 122(4):395–412.
Morselli. E., M. C. Maiuri, M. Markaki, et al. 2010. Caloric restriction and resveratrol pro-
    mote longevity through the Sirtuin-1-dependent induction of autophagy. *Cell Death &
    Disease*, 1:e10. doi:10.1038 /cddis.2009.8.
Neel, J. V. 1962. Diabetes mellitus: A "thrifty" genotype rendered detrimental by "progress"?
    American Journal of Human Genetics, 14(4):353–362.
Nickels, J. D., J. C. Smith, and X. Cheng. 2015. Lateral organization, bilayer asymmetry,
    and inter-leaflet coupling of biological membranes. *Chemistry and Physics of Lipids*,
    192:87–99.

Orrenius, S., V. Gogvadze, and B. Zhivotovsky. 2007. Mitochondrial oxidative stress: Implications for cell death. *Annual Review of Pharmacology & Toxicology*, 47:143–183.

Ott, M., V. Gogvadze, S. Orrenius, et al. 2007. Mitochondria, oxidative stress and cell death. *Apoptosis*, 12(5):913–922.

Palacios, J. A., D. Herranz, M. L. De Bonis, et al. 2010. SIRT1 contributes to telomere maintenance and augments global homologous recombination. *Journal of Cell Biology*, 191(7):1299–1313.

Pillai, V. B., N. R. Sundaresan, and M. P. Gupta. 2014. Regulation of Akt signaling by sirtuins. Its implication in cardiac hypertrophy and aging. *Circulation Research*, 114:368–378.

Shay, J. W., and W. E. Wright. 2011. Role of telomeres and telomerase in cancer. *Seminars in Cancer Biology*, 21(6):349–353.

Shoba, B., Z. M. Lwin, L. S. Ling, et al. 2009. Function of sirtuins in biological tissues. *The Anatomical Record*, 292:536–543.

Short, B. 2010. Telomeres get SIRT-ified. *Journal of Cell Biology*, 191(7):1299–1313.

Snow, B. J., F. L. Rolfe, M. M. Lockhart, et al. 2010. A double-blind, placebo-controlled study to assess the mitochondria-targeted antioxidant MitoQ as a disease-modifying therapy in Parkinson's disease. *Movement Disorders*, 25:1670–1674.

Tillman, T. S., and M. Cascio. 2003. Effects of membrane lipids on ion channel structure and function. *Cell Biochemistry & Biophysics* 38(2):161–190.

Verma, M., N. Shulga, and J. G. Pastorino. 2013. Sirtuin-4 modulates sensitivity to induction of the mitochondrial permeability transition pore. *Biochimica et Biophysica Acta*, 1827(1):38–49.

5 Nitric Oxide Is Said to Be the "Miracle Molecule" That "Reverses Aging"

5.1 INTRODUCTION

Science tells us that when cells come under attack by oxygen free radicals, they do the best they can to protect themselves by drawing on endogenous antioxidants to prevent the formation of damaging reactive oxygen species (ROS) that are formed by these free radicals. We also know that we can help our cells extend their life, preventing accelerated cycling that contributes to premature aging, by adopting the antioxidant-rich Proactive Nutrition Program.

This chapter focuses on a curious molecule, a gas actually, nitric oxide (NO), made by the cells in the inner lining of our blood vessels, the *endothelium*. The cells use an enzyme, nitric oxide synthase (NOS), to derive NO from the amino acid L-arginine, a component of protein in foods in the diet. There is also another source of NO: it can be derived directly from nitrates found mostly in common vegetables consumed regularly. This is detailed in Chapter 7.

5.2 HOW THE BODY FORMS NITRIC OXIDE

The demands of increased physical activity cause the brain to release a molecule, acetylcholine (ACh), that starts a chain of events resulting in increasing blood flow to the appropriate muscles. Acetylcholine stimulates the endothelium, the inner lining of arterial blood vessels, to form NO to relax the blood vessel. This results in the vessel dilating, which allows the volume of blood flowing through it to increase. So, NO is both made by the endothelium and used by the endothelium to control the volume of blood flowing through the vessel at any given time in response to the needs of the body.

Why the quotation marks in the title of this chapter? They actually represent quotes from scientists writing in conventional medical journals. For instance, "reverses aging" comes from the title of the report "Aging-associated endothelial dysfunction in humans is reversed by L-arginine" published in the *Journal of the American College of Cardiology* in 1996. The authors concluded that:

> aging selectively impairs endothelium-dependent coronary microvascular function and… this impairment can be restored by administration of L-arginine, a precursor of nitric oxide. (Chauhan et al. 1996)

Their conclusion in common terms is that the endothelium deteriorates with age. But—good news—it can be rejuvenated with nitric oxide (NO) that we can get from the amino acid L-arginine (Fried and Merrell 1999). The authors suggest "administration," which is ambiguous medical jargon. However, L-arginine from which the "miracle molecule" is derived is actually plentiful in many of the foods commonly consumed, so it is just a matter of picking the right ones. Chapter 7 explains all that.

After the publication of this discovery, doctors might immediately have given all their cardiovascular and heart patients a list of foods high in L-arginine, such as nuts, beans, and salmon, with the instruction to be sure to include these in the daily diet. However, the advice was not widely adopted, and the scientific revelation sank without making much of a ripple in the medical community.

Quotes such as that above are rare in science because scientists pride themselves on calm objectivity and are seldom given to exaggeration. In fact, it is likely that a scientist suspended in mid-air by no visible means, being interviewed by the media following his claim to have discovered *antigravity*, is likely to be quoted as saying, "Early trials are encouraging but we need further research...."

Be assured, however, that enthusiasm about the discovery of the biological role of nitric oxide (NO), a gas that was thought to be little more than an air pollutant until the early 1980s, is well earned. And in fact, like so many scientific discoveries, it was found by accident to be a "miracle molecule" that "reverses aging."

5.3 THE LABORATORY OVERSIGHT THAT LED TO THE NOBEL PRIZE

In the early 1900s, the Austrian pharmacologist Otto Loewi discovered a substance made by cells in the nervous system that he termed "*vagus material.*" Some years later, Sir Henry Dale, with whom Loewi came to collaborate at the University of London, and with whom he shared the 1936 Nobel Prize in Medicine, named it "acetylcholine" (ACh).

This was the beginning of modern neuropharmacology based on the new knowledge of *neurotransmitters*, chemical signals by which cells in the nervous system and brain communicate with each other, and turn things ON and OFF. Acetylcholine was found to relax arterial smooth muscles by turning ON blood vessel relaxation and this seemed a promising road to lower blood pressure to treat hypertension. However, it did so unreliably and unpredictably. No one knew why.

In 1980, Dr. Robert F. Furchgott, professor of pharmacology at SUNY Downstate Medical Center in Brooklyn, NY, published his findings in the journal *Nature* that ACh relaxation of arterial smooth muscle depended on the simultaneous presence of a mysterious substance made by the endothelium, the inner lining of blood vessels. It was termed "*endothelium-derived relaxing factor*" (EDRF): acetylcholine relaxed the vessels only when EDRF was also present (Furchgott and Zawadzki 1980). The identity of EDRF was a mystery.

However, it did not take long to verify the finding. In 1993, Dr. Salvador Moncada at Wellcome Research Laboratories, UK, who had previously first identified EDRF as a gas, nitric oxide (NO), detailed its role in health and disease in *The New England Journal of Medicine* (Moncada and Higgs 1993).

At first, this news was met with disbelief, even derision. A gas, indeed! It was not known then that NO had a biological role, much less in blood vessels: as previously noted, NO is derived in the body principally from the food-borne amino acid L-arginine, and similarly from inorganic (water soluble) nitrates as well.

In 1998, Dr. Furchgott and two colleagues, Drs. Ferid Murad and Louis Ignarro, were awarded the Nobel Prize in Medicine for the discovery of the biological role of nitric oxide (NO) in blood vessels, cardiovascular and heart function, and the nervous system and brain. The immune system was soon added to the list.

One of the three recipients, Dr. Louis J. Ignarro, detailed how ACh in sexual arousal caused increased and sustained production of NO synthesized from the amino acid L-arginine by the endothelium lining the spongy chambers of the penis, the cavernosa(e). This causes them to relax (dilate), allowing increased blood inflow. This research ultimately led to the development of a class of drugs now used by millions of men for erectile dysfunction, the type 5 phosphodiesterase (PDE-5) inhibitor drugs such as VIAGRA® and Cialis®.

5.3.1 A SIMPLE ERROR

Why doesn't ACh reliably cause vasodilation in human blood circulation or in blood vessel strips in the laboratory, as it should? What Dr. Furchgott discovered in strips of swine arterial blood vessels that did not relax when exposed to ACh, is that laboratory preparation, handling the samples, had often inadvertently rubbed away the inner surface of the blood vessel, the endothelium, thereby damaging it. Damaged endothelium cannot form NO and therefore the blood vessel cannot dilate by relaxing.

The observation that damaged endothelium cannot produce NO in amounts sufficient to cause dilation and maintain adequate blood circulation now explains cardiovascular disorders such as hypertension, atherosclerosis, heart disease, and erectile dysfunction: erectile dysfunction is typically a cardiovascular impairment (Fried 2014). All these are now said to be due to, or result from, damage to the endothelium and each, in turn, causes further damage to the endothelium. But, it is understood now that the damage is not due to inept handling, but due to attack by free radicals and ROS, that is, oxidative stress.

The cardiovascular disorders mentioned above impair endothelium function as surely as if the blood vessels were mechanically damaged by mishandling in the laboratory. One prime culprit in this scenario is damage caused by free radicals formed by ordinary metabolism and compounded by the failure to "quench" those due to our antioxidant-poor Western pattern diet.

However, "handled carelessly" is not really accurate because no one had any idea then that the endothelium had any biological function, so why spare it? It was thought to be not much more than a sort of lining between the bloodstream and the blood vessel wall—something like a bedsheet—to keep undesirable stuff in blood out of the vessel walls.

But "carelessly" may now be the right word, because we allow blood vessels to be damaged by atherosclerosis. Atherosclerosis is considered the prime culprit in cardiovascular and heart disease, a product of free radicals and ROS toxic sludge circulating in blood, hardening the vessel wall, and damaging the endothelium (Singh et al. 2015). And there is a strong connection between atherosclerosis and dietary habits.

This chapter first describes the essential role of nitric oxide (NO) derived from dietary sources, the amino acid L-arginine in common foods, and dietary nitrates, in supporting major organ functions, and exposes the harm done by NO insufficiency. Then, it describes the role of NO in protecting telomeres and details the best ways of promoting an adequate supply of NO from an ample supply of dietary L-arginine and nitrate foods—"Greens, Beans and Staminators" (Fried and Nezin 2006). There is also a means to determine whether one is forming enough nitric oxide to maintain a healthy body.

5.4 NITRIC OXIDE DERIVED FROM L-ARGININE

Nitric oxide (NO) is formed in the body from the amino acid L-arginine, a constituent of proteins in common foods in our diet. How can it be determined that regular consumption of food high in L-arginine actually results in increased serum levels of NO?

A study appearing in the journal *Nutrients*, in 2016, aimed to determine whether regular dietary intake of L-arginine correlates with serum levels of nitrate+nitrite and NO. Men and women recruits in the third Tehran Lipid and Glucose Study were evaluated for demographics, anthropometrics, and biochemical variables. Dietary data were collected using a validated food item semi-quantitative food frequency questionnaire, and dietary intake of L-arginine was calculated. It was found that as intake of L-arginine rose, so did serum NO.

Further analysis, stratified by age, body mass index, and hypertension status, showed the effect to be more pronounced in middle-aged and older adults. A greater association was also observed between L-arginine intake and serum NO in non-hypertensive versus hypertensive individuals. The authors concluded that dietary L-arginine intake is associated with serum NO, but that this association can be affected by gender, age, body mass index, and blood pressure status (Mirmiran et al. 2016).

Studies such as the one cited above, and there are many, help the medical community to understand how diet translates into serum levels of NO. But they are of no help (pun unintended) to the typical consumer trying to improve his/her health. The good news is that now there is a way of estimating NO formation and availability with nitric oxide indicator strips that will be described later in this chapter (https://www.humann.com).

Nitric oxide (NO) is formed from L-arginine by nitric oxide synthase enzymes (NOS), there being three isoforms: eNOS forms NO in the endothelium to control blood flow in the vessels; nNOS forms NO in nerve and brain cells to effect their communication; and inducible iNOS forms NO in macrophages activated to combat inflammation (Alderton et al. 2001; Daff 2010). All NOS enzymes metabolize L-arginine to another amino acid, L-citrulline, and NO: L-arginine creates nitric oxide and L-citrulline inside cells. Citrulline is then recycled back into arginine, making even more nitric oxide.

In one study, it was shown that L-citrulline plus L-arginine supplementation caused a more rapid increase in plasma L-arginine levels and marked enhancement of NO bioavailability, including plasma cGMP (see below) concentrations (Morita et al. 2014).

Ample L-arginine can be found in protein-rich foods such as meat and fish, and in protein and nitrate-rich plant foods, nuts, and seed, including:

- The staminators (from animal and fish sources): pork, beef, chicken, turkey, dairy products, and seafood. The top choices for seafood are tuna, salmon, halibut, trout, and tilapia.
- Greens and beans (plant-based choices): soybeans, pumpkin seeds, sesame seeds, peanuts, and walnuts. You will also get L-arginine from sweet green peppers and the seaweed spirulina, and from grains such as quinoa, oats, and wheat germ.

This is only a partial list but extensive details can be accessed at the SELFNutrition Data website: http://nutritiondata.self.com/foods-000089000000000000000.html. The healthiest source of L-arginine are plant foods.

A Note of Caution: It has been said that a diet rich in L-arginine is contraindicated for individuals with a dormant or active herpes infection. A list of foods showing L-arginine and L-lysine content per serving, as well as the arginine/lysine ratio can be found at the website: http://www.herpes.com/Nutrition.shtml. L-lysine is reported to suppress herpes virus.

In a study published in the journal *Dermatologica*, in 1978, patients with frequently recurring herpes infection were given 312–1200 mg of lysine daily in single or multiple doses. Supplementary lysine accelerated recovery from herpes simplex infection and suppressed recurrence. Tissue culture showed an enhancing effect on viral replication when the amino acid ratio of arginine to lysine favors arginine. The opposite ratio, lysine to arginine, suppresses viral replication (Griffith et al. 1978). It is left to the reader's discretion to decide what is best.

There are other medical conditions such as sepsis when it is desirable to suppress NO formation and there are pharmaceutical drug treatments that can do that (Víteček et al. 2012).

5.5 NITRIC OXIDE DERIVED FROM NITRATES

Just as dietary L-arginine is a source of nitric oxide, so are nitrates in the foods commonly consumed. They are for the most part vegetables and legumes. Ranking high among these are arugula (known to be one of the nitrate richest-foods), spinach, beets, celery, and iceberg lettuce.

Tables 5.1 and 5.2 list food sources of nitrate and nitrite and appeared in a report published in *The American Journal of Clinical Nutrition*, in 2009, titled "Food sources of nitrates and nitrites: the physiologic context for potential health benefits" (Hord et al. 2009).

TABLE 5.1
Nitrate and Nitrite Contents of Edible Vegetables

Vegetable Types and Varieties	Nitrite mg/100 g Fresh Weight	Nitrate mg/100 g Fresh Weight
Root vegetables		
Carrot	0.002–0.023	92–195
Mustard leaf	0.012–0.064	70–95
Green vegetables		
Lettuce	0.008–0.215	12.3–267.8
Spinach	0–0.073	23.9–387.2
Cabbage		
Chinese cabbage	0–0.065	42.9–161.0
Bok choy	0.009–0.242	102.3–309.8
Cabbage	0–0.041	25.9–125.0
Cole	0.364–0.535	76.6–136.5
Melon		
Wax gourd	0.001–0.006	35.8–68.0
Cucumber	0–0.011	1.2–14.3
Nightshade		
Eggplant	0.007–0.049	25.0–42

Source: Hord, N.G., *Am. J. Clin. Nutr.*, 90(1), 1–10, 2009. With Permission.

TABLE 5.2
Classification of Vegetables According to Nitrate Content

Nitrate Content (mg/100 g Fresh Weight)	Vegetable
Very low, <20	Artichoke, asparagus, broad bean, eggplant, garlic, onion, green bean, mushroom, pea, pepper, potato, summer squash, sweet potato, tomato, watermelon
Low, 20 to <50	Broccoli, carrot, cauliflower, cucumber, pumpkin, chicory
Middle, 50 to <100	Cabbage, dill, turnip, Savoy cabbage
High, 100 to <250	Celeriac, Chinese cabbage, endive, fennel, kohlrabi, leek, parsley
Very high, >250	Celery, cress, chervil, lettuce, red beetroot, spinach, rocket (rucola)

Source: Hord, N.G., *Am. J. Clin. Nutr.*, 90(1), 1–10, 2009. With Permission.

5.5.1 The "Nitrites Cause Cancer" Controversy

Normal digestion converts nitrates to nitrites in the body and in the process, also forms NO. A study by the Cancer Research Center of Hawaii and the University of Southern California suggested there was a link between eating processed meats and cancer risk. The study followed almost 200,000 people, aged 45–75, for 7 years, and found that those who ate the most processed meats had a 67% higher risk of pancreatic cancer than those who ate the least amount.

Processed meats are manufactured using sodium nitrite. During the process of cooking certain meats, sodium nitrites combine with naturally present amines in the meat to form carcinogenic N-nitroso compounds. According to the study, when these are ingested, they can cause cancer. (Nöthlings et al. 2005)

The authors of this book are not in a position to evaluate the merits of this proposition. But it is suggested that there is likely a basic difference between nitrites derived in the body from nitrates in common food—especially plant foods—and the consequences of the addition of sodium nitrite to meats in manufacturing. Furthermore, meat consumption entails other health hazards not the least being high sodium content.

Here follow several expert opinions on the matter and it is left to the reader's discretion to decide on their merits. The journal *Nitric Oxide* reported, in 2012, on the safety controversy surrounding nitrate and nitrite in the diet. Here is the abstract of the report taken from the NCBI/PubMed website:

Nitrate and nitrite are part of the human diet as nutrients in many vegetables and part of food preservation systems. In the 1950s and 1960s the potential for formation of nitrosamines in food was discovered and it ignited a debate about the safety of ingested nitrite which ultimately focused on cured meats. Nitrate impurities in salt used in the drying of meat in ancient times resulted in improved protection from spoilage during storage. This evolved into their deliberate modern use as curing ingredient responsible for "fixing" the characteristic color associated with cured meats, creating a unique flavor profile, controlling the oxidation of lipids, and serving as an effective antimicrobial. Several critical reports and comprehensive reviews reporting weak associations and equivocal evidence of nitrite human health safety have fostered concerns and debate among scientists, regulators, press, consumer groups, and consumers. Despite periodic controversy regarding human health concerns from nitrite consumption, a building base of scientific evidence about nitrate, nitrite, heme chemistry, and the overall metabolism of nitrogen oxides in humans has and continues to affirm the general safety of nitrate/nitrite in human health. As nitrite based therapeutics emerge, it is important to consider the past controversies and also understand the beneficial role in the human diet. (Sindelar and Milkowski 2012)

And again, from the *Journal of Food Protection*, in 2002:

The literature was reviewed to determine whether ingested nitrate or nitrite may be detrimental or beneficial to human health. Nitrate is ingested when vegetables are consumed. Nitrite, nitrate's metabolite, has a long history of use as a food additive, particularly in cured meat products. Nitrite has been a valuable antibotulinal agent in cured meats and may offer some protection from other pathogens in these products as well. Nitrite's use in food has been clouded by suspicions that nitrite could react with amines in the gastric acid and form carcinogenic nitrosamines, leading to various cancers. Nitrate's safety has also been questioned, particularly with regard to several cancers. Recently, and for related reasons, nitrite became a suspected developmental toxicant. A substantial body of epidemiological evidence and evidence from chronic feeding studies conducted by the National Toxicology Program refute the suspicions of detrimental effects. Recent studies demonstrate that nitrite, upon its ingestion and mixture with gastric acid, is a potent bacteriostatic and/or bactericidal agent and that ingested nitrate is responsible for much of the ingested nitrite. Acidified nitrite has been shown to be bactericidal for gastrointestinal, oral, and skin pathogenic bacteria. Although these are in vitro studies, the possibility is raised that nitrite, in synergy with acid in the stomach, mouth, or skin, may be an element of innate immunity. (Archer 2002)

Finally, nitrite is essential for human health and food safety. It has a proven track record of preventing botulism which can cause paralysis and possible death if left untreated. The government of Canada requires that nitrite be added to cured meat products (deli meats, bacon, and more) to protect against food-borne illness. The levels of nitrate and nitrite required by the Food and Drugs Regulations are found in the Health Canada List of Permitted Preservatives (http://www.knowyournitrites. com/nitrite-nitrate-and-your-health).

5.6   HOW DOES NO CONTROL BLOOD FLOW IN BLOOD VESSELS?

Ordinarily, blood pressure, and therefore blood flow volume, is a function of the internal diameter of blood vessels, the *caliber*. The smaller the caliber, the higher will be the blood pressure; the larger the caliber, the lower the blood pressure. The inside passageway of a blood vessel through which blood flows is called the *lumen*. The diameter of the lumen varies with the caliber. The caliber of the blood vessels is determined by physiological factors that can either cause the vessel to dilate (larger caliber) or to constrict (smaller caliber).

Arterial blood vessels are never totally constricted and it would be fatal (shock) if they were to totally dilate. Thus, caliber normally remains somewhere between these extremes, plus or minus, fluctuating from moment to moment in a sort of mid-state called *tonus*.

What the 1998 Nobel Prize in Medicine described is the physiological mechanism that maintains that state of normal tonus. Figure 5.1 shows the cross-section of an arteriole, a very small blood vessel, and also shows the red blood cells in the lumen.

The fluted structure is the inner lining of the blood vessel, the *endothelium*. It is the fluting that, like an accordion, allows the vessel to dilate increasing the caliber, thus increasing blood flow on demand. It is the cells in the endothelium that form NO that causes it to relax and thus dilate. The smooth muscle cells of the artery envelop the blood vessel and have no known mechanism for changing their shape.

NO does not directly cause the blood vessel to relax (vasodilation) but, in turn, causes the formation of yet another substance by the endothelium termed cGMP which is the actual vasodilator. Before the publications of the research by Dr. Furchgott and colleagues, scientists knew only about ACh, the very first step in the process. They did not know about the role of nitric oxide or of cGMP.

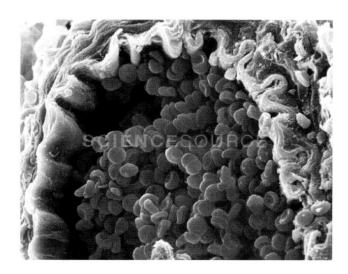

FIGURE 5.1   **(See color insert.)** Electron micrograph of a section of arterial blood vessel showing the endothelium surrounding red blood cells flowing in the bloodstream. (Courtesy of Steve Gschmeissner, Science Source, New York, NY.)

ACh signaling ends when increased formation of NO is no longer required. Endothelium then forms another enzyme, type 5 phosphodiesterase (5PDE), that disintegrates cGMP. Following that, NO production returns to a low level and the blood vessels return to their previous tonus caliber.

VIAGRA® (the first 5PDE inhibitor), and other drugs in that class, prevent the disintegration of cGMP, thus maintaining NO formation and, therefore, blood flowing into the penis to maintain erection. However, 5PDE inhibitors are not selective and affect blood flow in all the vessels in the body, which is why men are cautioned about taking VIAGRA® when they are also taking antihypertensive medications that are vasodilators like nitrate patches or nitroglycerin. These are NO donors.

5.7   THE ENDOTHELIAL FLOW-MEDIATED DILATION TEST MEASURES THE EFFECTS OF NO ON BLOOD VESSELS

There are a number of physiological factors that can affect blood flow through arterial blood vessels. This chapter focuses on blood vessel relaxation that is due to the action of NO formed by the endothelium. When the endothelium is healthy, its ability to form NO from L-arginine or from nitrates is adequate and the blood vessel relaxes to meet increased demand. However, when the endothelium is damaged, as is the case for instance in atherosclerosis, diabetes, and heart disease, its ability to form NO from L-arginine or from nitrates is impaired: vessels do not relax as they should and blood flow is likewise impaired.

In brief, the most widely used non-invasive test for assessing endothelial function in research, and now in the clinical setting, is endothelial flow-mediated dilation (FMD). A blood pressure cuff is placed over an artery, either the brachial artery in the arm or the femoral artery in the leg, and the cuff is temporarily inflated. The blood flow in the artery is observed using Doppler ultrasound. This technique measures endothelial function by first restricting circulation, and then when the pressure in the cuff has been released, measuring and timing the resultant relative increase in blood vessel diameter and flow velocity via Doppler ultrasound (Corretti et al. 2002).

Another method measures the viability of the endothelium in forming NO by "challenging" blood vessels to relax with ACh. However, FMD is the most commonly used method in both the laboratory and the clinic.

There are also immediately observable objective measures of the benefits of dietary promotion of NO formation in the body. A report titled "Effect of vegetable consumption on the association between peripheral leucocyte telomere length and hypertension: a case–control study," published in the journal *BMJ Open*, in 2015, tells us that higher vegetable intake was associated with longer telomeres, and those individuals with longer telomeres were also 30% less likely to have hypertension. The observed telomere–hypertension relationship appeared to be highly dependent on vegetable intake: the longer the telomeres, the lower also the risk of hypertension (Lian et al. 2015).

Also, according to a study titled "Dietary patterns, food groups, and telomere length in the Multi-Ethnic Study of Atherosclerosis (MESA)," reported in *The American Journal of Clinical Nutrition*, in 2008, the more meat consumed, the shorter the telomeres (Nettleton et al. 2008).

5.8 ORAL L-ARGININE VERSUS ORAL L-CITRULLINE

Oral L-arginine supplementation has been used in many studies to improve endothelium-dependent, nitric oxide (NO)-mediated vasodilation, but it is hampered by some degree of elimination in the stomach. In contrast, L-citrulline is readily absorbed and, at least in part, converted to L-arginine. The aim of the following study was to assess this metabolic conversion and its subsequent effects.

Healthy volunteers received six different doses of either comparison placebo, citrulline, or L-arginine. After 1 week of supplementation, L-citrulline increased plasma L-arginine concentration more effectively than did L-arginine. Moreover, urinary nitrate and cGMP were significantly increased. The data show for the first time that oral L-citrulline supplementation raises plasma L-arginine concentration and augments NO-dependent activity in a dose-dependent manner (Schwedhelm et al. 2008).

5.9 BLOOD PRESSURE

A number of factors can cause blood pressure to rise including strenuous exercise, but it is usually a health hazard only when that elevation is consistently present, when it is known as "essential hypertension." Essential hypertension can be caused by elevation of the "action hormone" norepinephrine which belongs to the class of hormones called catecholamines. Its function is to mobilize the brain and body for action—fight or flight.

Blood pressure also rises when the body retains water due to low sodium elimination (low diuresis). There are additional mechanisms that can come into play and thus hypertension is treated medically with a number of prescription medications that address these factors. These mechanisms are superimposed on the basic way that arterial blood vessels circulate blood throughout the body and the brain under the control of NO.

5.9.1 Blood Pressure Normally Rises Progressively with Age

Blood pressure normally rises progressively with age as the formation of nitric oxide in the body declines. A report in the *Postgraduate Medical Journal*, in 2007, tells us that data from the Framingham Heart Study which followed patients for 30 years, showed systolic blood pressure rising continuously between the ages of 30 and 84 years. Diastolic blood pressure was variable, but rising until the fifth decade and slowly decreasing from the age of 60 to at least 84 years of age.

The report in that journal might serve as an enticement to consider an antioxidant- and L-arginine- and nitrate-rich diet to avoid over-treatment of elevated blood pressure in the elderly. The authors aver that while treating the elderly hypertensive patient will reduce the risk of cardiovascular events, this may not apply to the very elderly:

> There is no evidence yet for the very elderly. This population is particularly susceptible to side effects of treatments and the reduction of blood pressure, although reducing the risk of cardiovascular events such as stroke, may result in increased mortality. (Pinto 2007)

In a study conducted on Russian medical students reported in the journal *Advances in Gerontology*, in 2012, the concentration of nitrates and nitrites, a marker of NO availability, was found to decrease with age as blood pressure rose. Because nitrate and nitrite levels corresponded to "biological age," the authors concluded that NO can be considered an "anti-aging" molecule (Barbarash et al. 2012).

The normal age-related decline in the ability of the endothelium to form NO, resulting in a progressive rise in blood pressure, may well be a window into the extent of the damage done to the endothelium by free radicals and ROS over the course of the lifespan. In this book, we recommend an antioxidant-rich Proactive Nutrition Program to support endothelium function. But, it should be noted for the record that, while no specific recommendations can be made, oral L-arginine supplementation has shown clinical value in many cases including coronary artery disease (see below) (Adams et al. 1997).

The *Journal of the Association of Physicians of India* reported in 2000 on a study of the effect of free radicals and ROS on coronary artery endothelium. Plasma levels of malonaldehyde (MDA, a byproduct of ROS encountered in a previous chapter) and nitrite, markers of oxidative stress and antioxidant activity, were measured in patients with acute myocardial infarction. Levels of superoxide dismutase (SOD) enzyme were obtained as an indicator of antioxidant activity.

It was found that the plasma levels of MDA and nitrite were significantly elevated in the acute myocardial infarction patients compared to a comparison group,

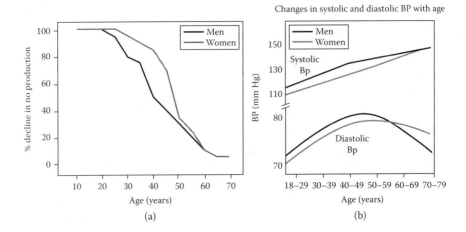

FIGURE 5.2 (See color insert.) Age-related decline in endothelial nitric oxide (NO) (a) compared to age-related rise in systolic and diastolic blood pressure in men and in women (b). (From Franklin, S.S., *Circulation*, 103, 1245–1249, 2001. With permission.)

indicating that oxygen free radicals cause endothelial damage. The SOD levels were also found to be elevated in these patients.

These results indicate that acute myocardial infarction results from advanced free radical activity causing endocardium (heart lining) damage. The elevated SOD levels reflect the attempts by the body to combat this oxidative stress by raising endogenous levels of anti-oxidants—a common form of self-defense (Jain et al. 2000).

The progressive age-related decline in NO formed by the endothelium, and the concomitant rise in blood pressure over the lifespan, are illustrated in Figure 5.2.

Endothelial NO formation declines more rapidly in men than in women over the lifespan; systolic blood pressure rises in men and women, and diastolic blood pressure rises into the middle years in both men and women. There is no evidence that, except in unusual conditions, these findings are due to the unavailability of L-arginine, which is a rare occurrence discussed in the next section. Rather, the evidence points to free radical and ROS damage to the endothelium. The message is clear: damage is avoidable by a diet that supplies adequate antioxidants.

5.9.2 Dietary L-Arginine and the Arginine Paradox

Despite saturation of the enzyme nitric oxide synthase (NOS) by L-arginine, oral and intravenous supplementation of L-arginine may actually enhance NO formation. This is known as the "L-arginine paradox." However, L-arginine is a source not only of NO but also of derivatives which inhibit the activity of the NOS. Therefore, L-arginine supplementation may not always result in enhanced NO formation (Schneider et al. 2015).

It is important to take this paradox into consideration because failure to do so may lead to the false conclusion that failure of NO to relax a blood vessel is due to L-arginine insufficiency. There is no substantiated clinical evidence of L-arginine insufficiency.

5.9.3 Nitric Oxide from Dietary L-Arginine and Nitrate Lowers Blood Pressure

A study published in the *International Journal of Angiology*, in 2008, reports that a diet rich in protein-derived L-arginine lowers blood pressure. It explains that, among other things, this may be due to arginine improving insulin resistance, increasing nitric oxide (NO) availability, and decreasing oxidative stress.

The authors also explain that the Dietary Approaches to Stop Hypertension (DASH) study demonstrated that this diet, rich in vegetables, fruits, and low-fat dairy products, low in fat, and including whole grains, poultry, fish, and nuts, lowered blood pressure even more than a typical Western diet with similar reduced sodium content (http://dashdiet.org/default.asp). As the DASH diet is rich in protein, the blood pressure-lowering effects may be due to higher L-arginine-containing protein and higher antioxidant content (and low salt content) (Vasdev and Gill 2008).

The *International Journal of Cardiology* reported, in 2002, that endothelium-dependent vasodilation and increased blood flow responding to NO formation is attenuated in patients with hypertension. However, the effects of oral L-arginine on the endothelial function of the conduit arteries, the arteries that become stiffer with age, in patients with essential hypertension have not previously been investigated.

Patients with essential hypertension received either 6 g of L-arginine or a comparison placebo. Blood flow in the arm (FMD) was tested in patients before and 1½ hours after administration of L-arginine or placebo.

The two groups of individuals who received either L-arginine or placebo were similar with regard to age, gender, level of blood lipids, smoking, presence or absence of diabetes, coronary artery disease, body mass index, blood pressure, and baseline arm (brachial) artery vasodilation measures. L-Arginine resulted in a significant increase in measures of brachial artery vasodilation (FMD). The authors concluded that oral L-arginine significantly improved the relaxation of the brachial artery and increased blood flow in patients with essential hypertension (Lekakis et al. 2002).

According to a report in the *International Journal of Hypertension*, appearing in 2016, poor eating habits are cardiovascular risk factors since a high intake of fat and saturated fatty acids contributes to elevated serum cholesterol, obesity, diabetes mellitus, and hypertension. The Dietary Approach to Stop Hypertension (DASH) plan may be an effective intervention strategy for the prevention and non-pharmacological management of hypertension. The beneficial effects of the DASH diet on blood pressure may be related to the high inorganic nitrate (water soluble) content of foods in this meal plan.

Beetroot and other food plants considered as nitrate sources account for approximately 60–80% of the daily nitrate exposure in the Western population. The increased levels of nitrite by nitrate intake may have beneficial effects in many of the physiological and clinical settings (d'El-Rei et al. 2016).

5.9.4 "Beet" the Clock

Beets (red beetroot) deliver nitrates that metabolize to nitrite that, in turn, deliver NO (Hobbs, et al. 2012; Lundberg et al. 2008). It seems pretty clear that adding beets to the diet brings cardioprotective and other benefits that are mediated by nitrate and subsequent conversion to NO. The antioxidative and anti-inflammatory effects are mediated by betalains and other phenolics.

Betalains are a new class of antioxidants. Betalains and their metabolites were found to inhibit lipid peroxidation of membranes (Kanner et al. 2001; Reddy et al. 2005). The intense red color of beets is due to high concentrations of betalains, a group of phenolic secondary plant metabolites. Betalains are used as natural colorants by the food industry, but have also received increasing attention due to possible health benefits in humans, especially because of their antioxidant and anti-inflammatory activities (Georgiev et al. 2010; Zielinska-Przyjemska et al. 2009).

Red beet products used regularly in the diet may provide protection against certain oxidative stress-related disorders. While there are currently no anticipated negative health outcomes associated with other constituents of beetroot, consumers should be aware that some supplements (i.e., juices) could have a relatively high sugar content, which might need to be taken into consideration by some individuals (i.e., those suffering from diabetes) (Clifford et al. 2015; Tesoriere et al. 2003).

5.9.4.1 The Case for Supplements versus Beets

In a study published in the journal *Nutrition Research*, in 2012, it was reported that nitrate and nitrite are increased by a high-nitrate supplement but not by high-nitrate foods in older adults. The investigators examined the effect of a 3-day control diet compared to a high-nitrate diet, with and without a high-nitrate supplement (beetroot juice), on plasma nitrate and nitrite and blood pressure. In healthy older adults only, a high-nitrate supplement consumed at breakfast elevated plasma nitrate and nitrite levels throughout the day (Miller et al. 2012).

Many beetroot supplements are commercially available, for instance, the products shown on the HumanN™ website (https://www.humann.com/products/?gclid=CIy8gs3 DqM8CFYwkhgodQVcBmw). The science supporting these products is impressive. Parenthetically, the authors have no commercial connection to the company, nor do they derive any financial benefits from the products.

5.10 FERRIC REDUCING ANTIOXIDANT POWER (FRAP) ASSAY

A number of reports on the antioxidant capacity of red beetroot as well as other foods center on the antioxidant assay termed FRAP, or *ferric reducing antioxidant power*. FRAP was developed at The Hong Kong Polytechnic University, Kowloon, Hong Kong, SAR, and reported in the *Journal of Agricultural and Food Chemistry*, in 1999 (Benzie and Strain 1996; Benzie and Zeto 1999).

The investigators developed the FRAP assay to measure the total antioxidant power of freshly prepared infusions of 25 types of teas. Their results showed that different teas had widely different antioxidant power and that the antioxidant capacity was strongly correlated with the total phenolic content of the tea. Their assay showed that one cup of usual strength tea (1–2%) can provide the same potential for improving antioxidant status as about 150 mg of pure ascorbic acid (vitamin C).

For instance, Table 5.3 is taken from an article published in the *Journal of Food Composition and Analysis*, in 2015. Note the comparison of different measures of

TABLE 5.3

Total Phenolic Content (TPC), Antioxidant Capacity (ORAC and FRAP), Pigments, and Phenolic Acid Concentration of Seven Beetroot Varieties

Variety	TPC (g/l)	ORAC (mM TE)	FRAP (mM TE)	Pigments (mg/l)			Phenolic acids (mg/l)			
				Betalain Total	Betacyanins	Betaxanthins	Gallic Acid	Syringic Acid	Caffeic Acid	Ferulic Acid
Mona Lisa	1.28 ± 0.223	37.9 ± 2.82	37.1 ± 6.21	1309 ± 140	807 ± 99.3	501 ± 46.7	27.7	2.02	10.3	1.24
Moronia	1.29 ± 0.175	24.0 ± 1.71	23.3 ± 2.88	1135 ± 127	633 ± 75.6	501 ± 53.9	17.8	0.865	3.14	0.335
Redval	0.85 ± 0.146	19.7 ± 6.56	17.8 ± 3.16	853 ± 80.1	466 ± 41.7	387 ± 38.6	14.4	1.34	3.03	0.751
Ägyptische Plattrunde	1.01 ± 0.271	25.7 ± 0.78	22.6 ± 4.05	933 ± 147	576 ± 87.9	357 ± 61.9	30.2	0.674	5.78	0.399
Robuschka	0.885 ± 0.136	28.5 ± 2.93	23.2 ± 2.94	767 ± 101	465 ± 69.5	301 ± 32.6	10.8	2.91	4.46	0.764
Forono	0.984 ± 0.214	23.7 ± 0.73	17.4 ± 4.03	826 ± 197	515 ± 135	311 ± 62.8	21.3	1.63	3.74	0.246
Bolivar	1.10 ± 0.257	28.0 ± 3.86	19.4 ± 4.77	789 ± 177	487 ± 86.3	301 ± 93.3	30.4	3.54	3.32	0.854
Mean	1.06	26.8	23	1103	705	397	21.8	1.85	4.82	0.651
SD	0.209	5.75	6.73	253	156	100	7.95	1.15	2.62	0.335
%CV	17.4%	21.4%	17.4%	23.0%	22.2%	25.2%	36.1%	58.1%	54.6%	58.0%

Source: Wruss, J., et al. *J. Food Comp. Anal.*, 42, 46–55, 2015. With Permission.

Note: "±" indicates SD from three individual measurements.

antioxidant content or capacity including total phenolic content (TPC), and ORAC and FRAP values, in different varieties of beetroot (Wruss et al. 2015).

The problem is that data such as this, while they show that science can develop measures of antioxidant capacity, are not presented in a form that is helpful to the health-conscious consumer in selecting foods for a balanced antioxidant diet. To be fair, it is still not known how to measure individual needs for antioxidants at any given moment, nor has science any way to help determine how much or what kind of antioxidants are best suited to individual needs at any given time. However, there is a scientific basis for the Proactive Nutrition Program because it relies on analysis of the scientific evidence connecting foods to antioxidants and preventing premature aging.

The nitrate–nitrite–nitric oxide (NO) association with important vascular effects has only recently been recognized. Dietary nitrate has a range of beneficial cardiovascular effects, including reducing blood pressure and improving endothelial function. Clinical studies with nitrate or nitrite also show evidence that suggests a reduction in cardiovascular risk with diets high in nitrate-rich vegetables (such as the Mediterranean diet). Interactions with other nutrients, such as vitamin C, polyphenols, and fatty acids, may enhance or inhibit these effects.

A report in the *British Journal of Clinical Pharmacology*, in 2013, provided simple guidance on nitrate intake from different vegetables in the form of a "Nitrate 'Veg-Table'" and listed the nitrate units, each one equal to 62 mg of nitrate, required to achieve a nitrate intake that is likely to be high enough to provide benefits (Lidder and Webb 2013).

The discovery that dietary (inorganic) nitrate has important vascular effects came from the relatively recent realization of the 'nitrate-nitrite-nitric oxide (NO) pathway'. Dietary nitrate has been demonstrated to have a range of beneficial vascular effects, including reducing blood pressure, inhibiting platelet aggregation, preserving or improving endothelial dysfunction, enhancing exercise performance in healthy individuals and patients with peripheral arterial disease. Pre-clinical studies with nitrate or nitrite also show the potential to protect against ischaemia-reperfusion injury and reduce arterial stiffness, inflammation and intimal thickness. However, there is a need for good evidence for hard endpoints beyond epidemiological studies. Whilst these suggest reduction in cardiovascular risk with diets high in nitrate-rich vegetables (such as a Mediterranean diet), others have suggested possible small positive and negative associations with dietary nitrate and cancer, but these remain unproven. Interactions with other nutrients, such as vitamin C, polyphenols and fatty acids may enhance or inhibit these effects. In order to provide simple guidance on nitrate intake from different vegetables, we have developed the Nitrate 'Veg-Table' with 'Nitrate Units' [each unit being 1 mmol of nitrate (62 mg)] to achieve a nitrate intake that is likely to be sufficient to derive benefit, but also to minimize the risk of potential side effects from excessive ingestion, given the current available evidence. The lack of data concerning the long term effects of dietary nitrate is a limitation, and this will need to be addressed in future trials.

The aim of a report in the journal *Hypertension*, appearing in 2015, was to assess whether dietary nitrate might sustain lower blood pressure in patients with hypertension. Patients with hypertension received daily dietary supplementation with either dietary nitrate (250 ml daily, as beetroot juice) or a nitrate comparison placebo for 4 weeks.

Daily supplementation with dietary nitrate was associated with a reduction in blood pressure. Endothelial function improved, arterial stiffness was reduced and 24-hour ambulatory blood pressure was significantly lowered after dietary nitrate consumption with no change after comparison placebo. The intervention was well tolerated.

This was the first evidence of durable blood pressure reduction with dietary nitrate supplementation in a relevant patient group. It was suggested that there may be a role for dietary nitrate as an affordable, readily available, and tasty adjunctive treatment in the management of patients with hypertension (the study was funded by The British Heart Foundation) (Kapil et al. 2015).

This is only a small sample of the medical reports on the benefit of dietary nitrates for clinical disorders. These reports all document clinical response to increasing the formation of NO from dietary nitrates. What is learned from these studies is that NO helps "repair" the damage done to blood vessel endothelium by free radicals. This is certainly an example of age reversal. The enhanced antioxidant-rich Mediterranean diet, like the Proactive Nutrition Program, is designed to prevent damage and even repair of basic body structures and functions damaged by free radicals and ROS. This is key to the goal of preventing accelerated aging.

5.11 ATHEROSCLEROSIS

Atherosclerosis is a disorder of blood vessels where an artery wall is thickened by an invasion of white blood cells, actually in the form of "foam cells," containing peroxidized cholesterol. These cells enter a particular layer of the artery wall, the intima, where a cascade of events causes them to form an accumulation of blood platelet cell detritus plastered over by calcium that hardens as *plaque*. The wall stiffening may eventually encroach inward (remodeling), narrowing the lumen, which impairs blood flow and raises blood pressure. This process also has the potential to breach the endothelium and cause a blood clot (embolism) to form in the *lumen*, raising the real prospect of stroke.

Atherosclerosis is considered a chronic inflammatory response to the combination of white blood cells and other hardened debris and sludge in the artery wall. Inflammation is known to be related to free radical activity (see Chapter 8).

Because atherosclerosis is usually the prime reason for impaired blood flow in an artery, the conventional test of any treatment is to measure blood flow before and after treatment. Measuring blood flow in the brachial artery (FMD) in the arm is one way to do this. Further details about the procedure(s) can also be found in Chapter 2, Measuring and evaluating function, impairment and change with intervention, in the book *Erectile Dysfunction as a Cardiovascular Impairment* (Fried 2014).

5.11.1 Preventing, Even Reducing, Atherosclerosis with Dietary L-Arginine and Nitrate

The journal *Integrative Medicine Alert* reported, in 1999, that a diet rich in the amino acid L-arginine may help patients with clinically elevated serum cholesterol (hypercholesterolemia) and patients with atherosclerosis-related disease.

Because hypercholesterolemia can impair vascular function, the protein foods rich in L-arginine should not be red meats but seafood, poultry, nuts, and beans. The diet can supply an adequate amount of L-arginine and is the recommended method of supplementation (Sorrentin 1999).

The objective of a study published in 2005 in the *Proceedings of the National Academy of Sciences* was to evaluate the influence of dietary L-arginine, L-citrulline, and antioxidants (vitamins C and E) on the progression of atherosclerosis in rabbits fed a high-cholesterol diet.

It is often not feasible to conduct long-term studies of the effects of a treatment on humans which is one reason why animal models may be used. Curiously, rabbits have a cardiovascular system that responds to a high-cholesterol and saturated fats diet very much as people do: they rapidly develop atherosclerosis and heart disease. For that reason, they are usually chosen as the animal model in many nutrition studies.

The fatty diet caused a marked impairment in the blood flow that should have been controlled by NO in isolated thoracic (chest, or its equivalent in a rabbit) aorta, and the blood flow in a live rabbit ear artery. The rabbits developed atherosclerotic plaque (atheroma) and lesions and there were indications of ROS-related blood vessel damage.

The rabbits were then treated for 12 weeks with oral L-arginine, L-citrulline, and/or antioxidants. L-arginine plus L-citrulline, either alone or in combination with antioxidants, caused a marked improvement in blood vessel relaxation response and blood flow, a dramatic regression in plaque, and a decrease in ROS.

The investigators further report that these therapeutic effects followed increases in markers of NO formation and in particular, cGMP levels. This means that consuming NO-donor foods including L-arginine and L-citrulline, plus antioxidants, can overturn oxidative stress and reverse the progression of atherosclerosis. They conclude that "This approach may have clinical utility in the treatment of atherosclerosis in humans" (Hayashi et al. 2005).

"Inorganic nitrite supplementation for healthy arterial aging" is the title of a report published in the *Journal of Applied Physiology*, in 2014. The authors tell us that aging is the major risk factor for cardiovascular diseases and that it is due to adverse changes in arteries and impairment of the endothelium in forming NO. This results in oxidative stress.

Inorganic nitrite is a promising way to augment NO bioavailability and nitrite may be effective in the treatment of vascular aging: in old mice, short-term oral sodium nitrite supplementation reduced large elastic artery stiffness and ameliorated endothelial dysfunction. These improvements in age-related vascular dysfunction with nitrite are mediated by reductions in oxidative stress and inflammation, and may be linked to increases in mitochondrial rejuvenation (biogenesis) and health. Increasing nitrite levels, via dietary intake of nitrate, appears to have similarly beneficial effects in many of the same physiological and clinical settings.

In summary, dietary nitrate supplementation is said to be a promising therapy for the treatment of arterial aging and prevention of age-associated cardiovascular disease in humans (Sindler et al. 2014).

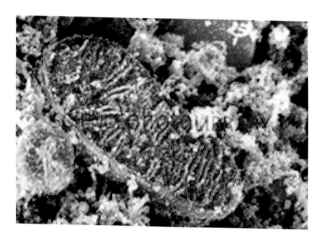

FIGURE 1.1 Mitochondrion. Colored scanning electron micrograph (SEM) of a mitochondrion in a nerve cell. (Courtesy of Furness, D., Keele University/Science Photo Library, http://www.sciencephoto.com/media/77027/view.)

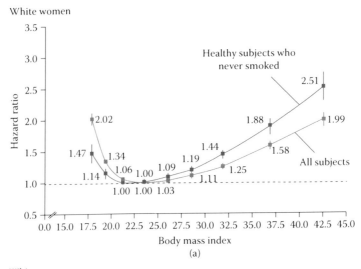

White women

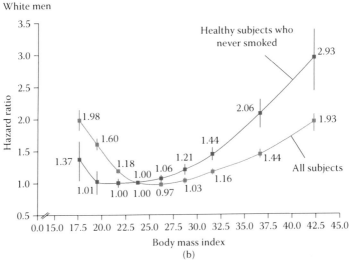

White men

FIGURE 1.2 Estimated hazard ratios for death from any cause according to body mass index (BMI) for all study participants and for healthy subjects who never smoked. Hazard ratios and 95% confidence intervals are shown for white women (a) and white men (b). The hazard ratios were adjusted for alcohol intake (grams per day), educational level, marital status, and overall physical activity. (From Berrington de Gonzalez, A., et al., *N. Engl. J. Med.*, 363, 2211–2219, 2010. With permission.)

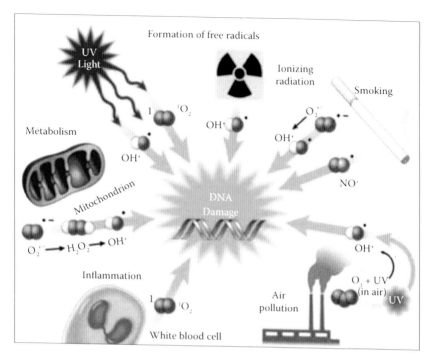

FIGURE 2.1 Environmental and metabolic sources of free radicals. (From Pendyala et al., *J. Indian Soc. Periodontol.*, 12, 3, 79–83, 2008. With permission.)

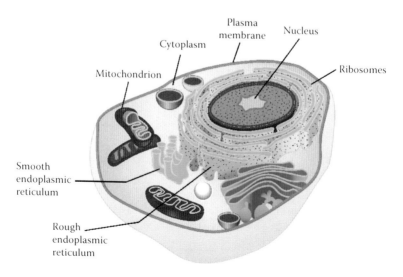

FIGURE 4.1 The eukaryote cell. (From Stuart Nezin. With permission.)

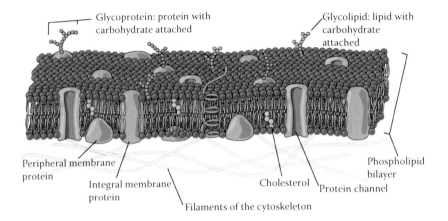

FIGURE 4.2   Section of the membrane of a eukaryote cell. (From Nickels, J.D., et al. *Chem. Phys. Lipids*, 192, 87–99, 2015. With permission.)

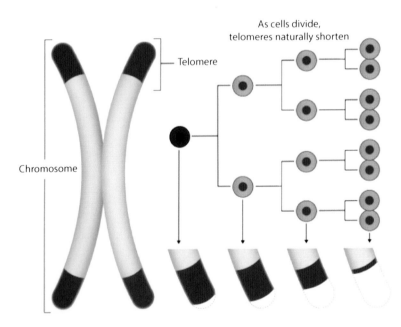

FIGURE 4.3   Abbreviation of the telomeres with each cell cycle. (From Dr. David Eifrig Jr., Strawberry Research, http://retirementmillionairedaily.com/this-ocean-animal-could-hold-the-key-to-extending-human-life/. With permission.)

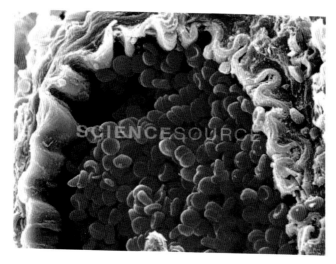

FIGURE 5.1 Electron micrograph of a section of arterial blood vessel showing the endothelium surrounding red blood cells flowing in the bloodstream. (Courtesy of Steve Gschmeissner, Science Source, New York, NY.)

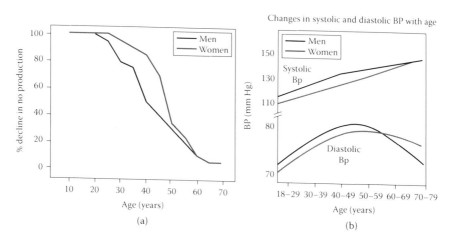

(a)

(b)

FIGURE 5.2 Age-related decline in endothelial nitric oxide (NO) (a) compared to age-related rise in systolic and diastolic blood pressure in men and in women (b). (From Franklin, S.S., *Circulation*, 103, 1245–1249, 2001. With permission.)

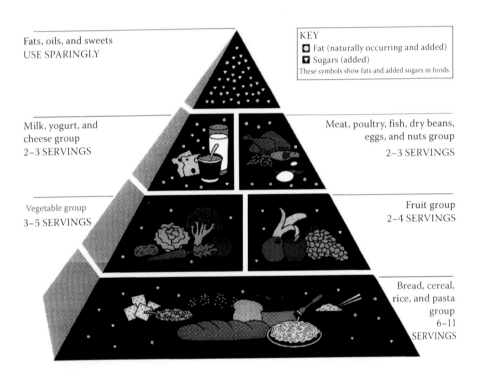

FIGURE 6.1 The 1992 Food Guide Pyramid. (Courtesy of USDA, Washington, DC.)

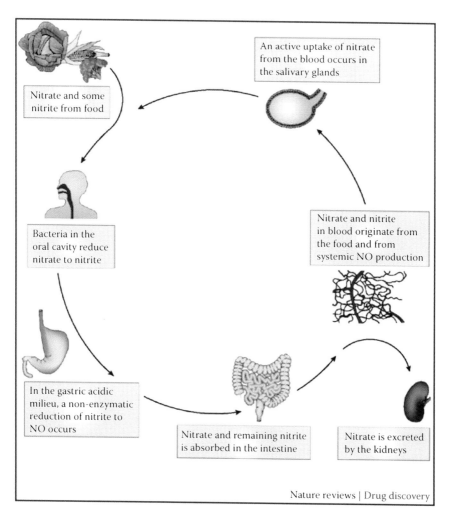

FIGURE 7.2 The entero-salivary circulation of nitrate in humans. (From Lundberg, J.O., *Nat. Rev. Drug Discov.*, 7, 156–167, 2009. With permission.)

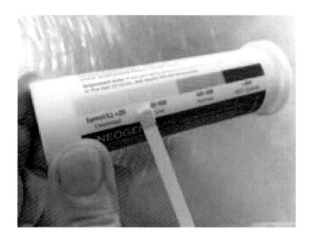

FIGURE 7.3 N-O indicator strips. HumanN® N-O indicator strips are used to assess nitrite levels in saliva as an index of NOx availability. (With permission.)

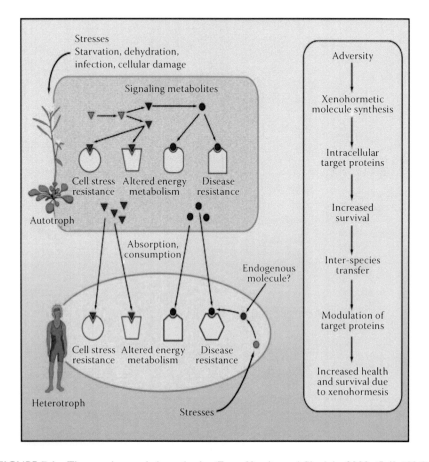

FIGURE 7.4 The xenohormesis hypothesis. (From Howitz and Sinclair, 2008. *Cell*, 133(3), 387–391, 2008. With permission.)

Another study published in the journal *Experimental Gerontology*, in 2012, is titled "Sodium nitrite de-stiffening of large elastic arteries with aging." This translates to sodium nitrite "de-stiffens" large arteries that stiffen with age. Nitrite derived in the body from dietary nitrates helps reverse atherosclerosis and *voilá*—anti-aging (Fleenor et al. 2012).

5.11.2 DIETARY NITRATE IMPROVES BLOOD CIRCULATION IN ATHEROSCLEROSIS

A study published in *The American Journal of Clinical Nutrition*, in 2015, examined the effects Go to: of 6-week, once-daily, intake of dietary nitrate (nitrate-rich beetroot juice) compared with a placebo consisting of nitrate-depleted beetroot juice on markers of elevated serum cholesterol. Dietary nitrate resulted in an absolute increase in measures of blood flow, while the placebo group experienced worsening. Dietary nitrate also caused a small but significant reduction in platelet aggregation. No adverse effects of dietary nitrate were detected.

The conclusions were that sustained dietary nitrate ingestion improves blood vessel function in hypercholesterolemic patients, providing additional support for the assessment of the potential of dietary nitrate as a preventative strategy against the development of atherosclerosis. This trial was registered at clinicaltrials.gov as NCT01493752 (Velmurugan et al. 2016).

5.12 HEART DISEASE

There are many forms of heart disease including:

- *Congestive heart failure*: Congestive heart failure is a condition where the heart pumping function is inadequate to meet body needs.
- *Coronary heart disease*: Coronary heart disease, also known as coronary artery disease, is due to narrowing of the small arterial blood vessels that supply blood and oxygen to the heart. This is usually, although not invariably, due to atherosclerosis. It is the leading cause of death in the United States for both men and women. This condition is also known as ischemic heart disease due to the impaired blood flow to the heart.

There is extensive documentation of the benefits of dietary L-arginine and dietary nitrates in the treatment of various aspects of heart disease. In 2001, the *Annual Review of Pharmacology & Toxicology* published a review of the clinical pharmacology of L-arginine. There are multiple studies showing positive results for L-arginine in the prevention and improvement of cardiovascular disease including:

- Oral administration of 6.6 g/day in patients with peripheral arterial disease. After 2 weeks, there was increased pain-free total walking distance and increased quality of life (by 66% and 23%, respectively).
- Oral administration of 15 g/day in patients with congestive heart failure. After 5 days there was also improved kidney function.

- Oral administration of 2×3.3 g/day in a type I diabetic patient with debilitating angina pectoris on exertion. After 7 days, the angina resolved and the patient was able to exercise to capacity.
- Oral administration of 8.4 g/day in hypercholesterolemic patients. After 2 weeks, platelet aggregation had normalized.
- Oral administration of 17 g/day oral in a healthy smoking elderly population. After 14 days, subjects showed decreased serum total cholesterol and decreased low-density lipoprotein cholesterol, but not decreased high-density lipoproteins cholesterol (Böger and Bode-Böger 2001).

Furthermore,

- Patients with peripheral artery disease improved their walking distances after L-arginine supplementation with 16 g daily for 14 days (Böger et al. 1998).
- L-arginine improved heart function in patients with severe congestive heart failure (Bednarz et al. 2004; Wascher et al. 1997).
- L-arginine reduced heart rate and improved hemodynamics in severe congestive heart failure (Bocch et al. 2000).

5.12.1 Heart Disease Patients Improve with Dietary Nitrate or L-Arginine

A report in the journal *Cardiovascular Research*, in 2010, supported the role of inorganic nitrate in cardiovascular health and disease. The authors held that dietary inorganic nitrates are now better known for their role in forming nitric oxide (NO). As shown earlier in this chapter, NO reduces blood pressure, inhibits platelet aggregation, and protects arterial blood vessels. Importantly, all the effects of nitrate are achievable with amounts corresponding to a rich intake of vegetables. A theory is now emerging suggesting nitrate is the active constituent of vegetables which contributes to the beneficial health effects of this food group, including protection against cardiovascular disease and type 2 diabetes (Lundberg et al. 2010).

A study reported in *Nature Reviews Drug Discovery*, in 2015, investigated the association between regular dietary intake of L-arginine and the incidence of coronary heart disease and changes in blood pressure. Eligible adults who participated in the Tehran Lipid and Glucose Study were followed for a mean of 4.7 years. Dietary intake of L-arginine was assessed at baseline, and clinical laboratory variables were evaluated at baseline and at the follow-up examination.

During a mean of follow-up of 4.7±1.4 years, 57 participants experienced "events." A significant inverse relationship was observed between plant-derived L-arginine intake and changes in both systolic and diastolic blood pressure, while animal-derived L-arginine intake was related to increased levels of diastolic blood pressure. The risk of cardiovascular heart disease declined with increasing plant-derived L-arginine intake.

It was concluded that a higher intake of plant-derived L-arginine may be protective, while animal-derived L-arginine may be a risk factor for the development of hypertension and cardiovascular and heart events (Bahadoran et al. 2016; see also Lundberg et al. 2015; Thadani 1997).

In another study, patients with angina showed improved exercise tolerance after L-arginine supplementation. Two 1 g capsules of L-arginine given three times per day significantly lengthened mean exercise time (Ceremuzyński et al. 1997; see also Schwartz 2003).

5.12.2 CONGESTIVE HEART FAILURE REDUCED BY DIETARY L-ARGININE OR NITRATE

A study conducted in Poland, published in *Kardiologia Polska* (Polish Cardiology) in 2004, investigated the effect of oral supplementation with L-arginine on exercise capacity and looked at markers of oxidative stress in patients with mild to moderate congestive heart failure.

Patients with stable congestive heart failure underwent three exercise tests after oral administration of either 9 g/day of L-arginine for 7 days, or comparison placebo. Blood samples were collected before each test for plasma lipid peroxides and other free radical markers. The L-arginine group showed prolongation of exercise duration time, while the comparison group did not (Bednarz et al. 2004).

In a study published in the *Journal of Hypertension*, patients with chronic congestive heart failure received oral L-arginine (15 g/day) or placebo, or placebo and arginine sequentially for 5 days each. The 24-hour excretion level was higher and plasma endothelin level was lower with L-arginine treatment compared to placebo treatment.

Endothelins are very potent vasoconstrictors. In any healthy individual, there must be a delicate balance between vasoconstriction and vasodilation which is maintained by endothelin and other vasoconstrictors on the one hand, and nitric oxide and other vasodilators on the other. Thus, endothelin and nitric oxide are antagonist. The authors concluded that oral administration of L-arginine has beneficial effects on kidney filtration rate and kidney sodium excretion, and on plasma endothelin level in patients with chronic congestive heart failure (Watanabe et al. 2000).

5.12.3 AN IMPORTANT CONSIDERATION

In a study designed to evaluate the effects of L-arginine (9 g/day) supplementation for 6 months following myocardial infarction, no significant change in vascular stiffness or left ejection fraction was shown. However, 8.6% of the patients died in the L-arginine group, while no deaths occurred in the comparison control group, so the trial was terminated. Researchers concluded that L-arginine should not be given to patients following an acute myocardial infarction and suggested that diffuse atherosclerosis in older patients may worsen the clinical outcome (Schulman et al. 2006).

5.13 PERIPHERAL ARTERY DISEASE

Peripheral artery disease (PAD) is a narrowing of the arteries in the legs, and sometimes in the stomach, arms, and head, but most commonly in the legs. PAD is similar to coronary artery disease because both are caused by atherosclerosis that narrows and blocks arteries in various critical regions of the body. The most common symptoms of PAD involving the lower extremities are cramping, pain, or tiredness in the leg or hip muscles while walking or climbing stairs. Typically, this pain goes away with rest and returns again with walking (http://www.heart.org/HEARTORG/Conditions/More/PeripheralArteryDisease/About-Peripheral-Artery-Disease-PAD_UCM_301301_Article.jsp#.V2rUTPkrLcs).

A study appearing in the *Journal of the American College of Cardiology*, in 1998, looked at whether prolonged intermittent intravenous therapy with L-arginine improves the clinical symptoms of intermittent claudication, common in PAD. Intermittent claudication features cramping and pain in the legs induced by exercise, and is typically caused by obstruction in the arteries.

Patients with intermittent claudication received 8 g of L-arginine twice a day, or 40 μg of prostaglandin E1 (PGE1) twice a day for comparison, or no active treatment for 3 weeks. The pain-free and absolute walking distances were assessed on a walking treadmill at 3 km/hour, on a 12% slope. Nitric oxide-mediated blood flow measures in the femoral artery were assessed at 1, 2, and 3 weeks of therapy, and 6 weeks after the end of treatment. Urinary nitrate and cGMP were assessed as indices of NO production.

It was found that L-arginine significantly improved the pain-free walking and the absolute walking distance compared with control patients who experienced no significant change. L-arginine therapy improved blood flow in the femoral artery, and increased urinary nitrate and cyclic GMP excretion rates, indicating normalized NO formation. The authors concluded that restoring NO formation and endothelium-dependent vasodilation by L-arginine improves the clinical symptoms of intermittent claudication in patients with peripheral arterial occlusive disease (Böger et al. 1998).

5.13.1 THE ANKLE-BRACHIAL INDEX

The ankle-brachial index (ABI) test is a quick, non-invasive test for peripheral artery disease (PAD). The test is valuable because people with PAD are at increased risk of heart attack and stroke. The test compares the blood pressure measured at the ankle with the blood pressure measured at the arm. A low ABI score can indicate narrowing or blockage of the arteries in the legs, indicating increased risk of cardiovascular disease.

The ABI is done 10 minutes after lying down. The systolic blood pressure is measured at both the right and left brachial arteries and both the right and left dorsalis pedis and posterior tibial arteries. Typically, the systolic pressures are recorded with a handheld 5 or 10 mHz Doppler instrument. However, this can also be done with a standard blood pressure cuff.

The procedure is as follows. An ABI is calculated for each leg: the ABI is the higher pressure of the two arteries at the ankle, divided by higher systolic brachial arterial pressure. ABI values should be calculated to two decimal places:

ABI = Highest pressure in right or left foot/highest pressure in both arms.

Normal ABI ranges from 1.0 to 1.4. An ABI below 0.9 is considered diagnostic of PAD.

Additional detail may be obtained online including from the following web pages:

- https://www.nhlbi.nih.gov/health/health-topics/topics/pad/diagnosis
- http://circ.ahajournals.org/content/126/24/2890
- http://stanfordmedicine25.stanford.edu/the25/ankle.html
- http://emedicine.medscape.com/article/1839449-overview

5.14   METABOLIC SYNDROME AND TYPE 2 DIABETES

Metabolic syndrome is a group of risk factors that raises the risk of coronary heart disease and other health problems, such as diabetes and stroke. Metabolic risk factors include:

- A large waistline. This also is called abdominal obesity or "having an apple shape." Excess fat in the stomach area is a greater risk factor for heart disease than excess fat in other parts of the body, such as on the hips.
- A high triglyceride level (or being on medicine to treat high triglycerides).
- A low HDL cholesterol level (or being on medicine to treat low HDL cholesterol).
- High blood pressure (or being on medicine to treat high blood pressure).
- High fasting blood sugar (or being on medicine to treat high blood sugar).

One can have any of these risk factors by itself, but they tend to occur together. At least three metabolic risk factors are required for a diagnosis of metabolic syndrome (http://www.nhlbi.nih.gov/health/health-topics/topics/ms).

5.14.1   THE ROLE OF MITOCHONDRIA IN METABOLIC SYNDROME

The main components of metabolic syndrome, especially visceral obesity, insulin resistance, and type 2 diabetes, are now thought to be related to changes in mitochondrial metabolism in different tissues. The main mechanisms implicated in the development of metabolic syndrome include increased generation of mitochondrial ROS (Litvinova et al. 2015).

5.14.2   DIETARY L-ARGININE AND NITRATE IN THE TREATMENT OF METABOLIC SYNDROME AND TYPE 2 DIABETES

Type 2 diabetes mellitus is a long-term metabolic disorder that is characterized by high blood sugar, insulin resistance, and relatively low insulin production. A study conducted in Greece, appearing in the *Journal of the American Dietetic Association*, in 2007, reported on the relationship between foods or food patterns and the characteristics of the metabolic syndrome. Dietary habits were evaluated using a semi-quantitative food frequency questionnaire. The characteristics of the metabolic syndrome (i.e., blood pressure, waist circumference, glucose, triglycerides, and high-density lipoprotein cholesterol) were also recorded in the volunteers.

Six clinical components were found. Component 1 was the consumption of cereals, fish, legumes, vegetables, and fruits; component 2 was the intake of potatoes and meat; component 6 was characterized by alcohol intake. The other components were mainly related to consumption of dairy and sweets.

Component 1 was inversely associated with waist circumference, systolic blood pressure, triglycerides, positively associated with high-density lipoprotein cholesterol levels, and inversely related to the likelihood of having metabolic syndrome. Components 2 and 6 were positively correlated with the previous indices, and the likelihood of having metabolic syndrome.

It was concluded that a dietary pattern that includes cereals, fish, legumes, vegetables, and fruits was independently associated with reduced levels of clinical and biological markers of metabolic syndrome, whereas meat and alcohol intake had opposite effects (Panagiotakos et al. 2007).

A report in the *Asia Pacific Journal of Clinical Nutrition* in 2006 reviewed original research papers from the Medline database for dietary patterns that may be associated with metabolic syndrome. Three large-scale epidemiological studies were found fitting the authors criteria. Dietary patterns high in fruit and vegetable content were generally found to be associated with a lower prevalence of metabolic syndrome, while those with high meat intake were frequently associated with a high prevalence of metabolic syndrome, especially impaired glucose tolerance.

High dairy intake was generally associated with a reduced risk of metabolic syndrome, with some inconsistency in the literature regarding risk of obesity. Minimally processed cereals appeared to be associated with decreased risk, while highly processed cereals with a high glycemic index were found to be associated with higher risk. Fried foods were noticeably absent from any dietary pattern associated with a decreased prevalence of metabolic syndrome.

The conclusion from this review is that no individual dietary component could be considered wholly responsible for any association between diet and metabolic syndrome, rather it is the overall quality of the diet that appears to offer protection against lifestyle disease such as metabolic syndrome (Baxter et al. 2006).

5.14.3 L-ARGININE AND GLUCOSE TOLERANCE

L-arginine stimulates insulin secretion and enhances insulin-mediated glucose disposal. A long-term study of L-arginine supplementation in patients with type 2 diabetes (9 g/day for 1 month) showed improved peripheral and hepatic insulin sensitivity. No changes in body weight, glycated hemoglobin, serum potassium, diastolic blood pressure, or heart rate were demonstrated, although systolic blood pressure decreased in the L-arginine group compared to a control comparison group (Piatti et al. 2001).

5.15 DIETARY L-ARGININE AND NITRATE IN KIDNEY DYSFUNCTION

Medical research on the benefits or adverse effects of L-arginine as a treatment or as a dietary supplement in kidney disease is equivocal. There are many different forms of kidney disease and L-arginine has been found to be beneficial in some types and detrimental in others (Carlström et al. 2010; Peters and Noble 1996; Reyes et al. 1994).

5.16 NO PROTECTS TELOMERES

Two articles propose that NO can directly protect telomeres. The first, appearing in the journal *Circulation Research*, in 2000, makes the tantalizing suggestion that "shortening of telomeres is not strictly a function of the number of cellular divisions but can be modulated." According to the investigators looking at endothelial cell (EC) telomeres, NO interferes with telomerase activity thereby inhibiting telomere shortening. It is thought that NO may react with tissue-derived oxygen radicals, thereby reducing oxidative stress which has been shown to accelerate the senescence of endothelial cells.

Regardless of the molecular mechanisms involved in the modulation of telomerase activity, the demonstration that NO affects telomerase activity and delays EC senescence suggests NO has a novel endothelial protective function (Vasa et al. 2000).

In most cancer cells, the length of telomeres is maintained by telomerase. Heat shock protein 90 (Hsp90) stabilizes proteins against heat stress and aids in protein degradation. It also stabilizes a number of proteins required for tumor growth, which is why it is under consideration as an anti-cancer drug. Hsp90 facilitates the assembly of telomerase and is thought to have a direct involvement in telomere length regulation.

A study appearing in the journal *Molecular and Cell Biology*, in 2006, concerned an effort to detect the effects of inhibiting the action of Hsp90 on the function and viability of human prostate cancer cells. Both pharmacological and other approaches to target Hsp90 were used. Depletion of Hsp90 caused dramatic telomere shortening followed by apoptosis. It is particularly significant that these cells exhibit a high level of nitric oxide synthase (NOS)-dependent free radical production, and simultaneous treatment of cells with an NOS inhibitor (L-NAME) resulted in telomere elongation and prevention of apoptosis (Compton et al. 2006).

5.17 NITRIC OXIDE CONCENTRATION IS USUALLY MEASURED INDIRECTLY (NOx), BUT CAN IT BE MEASURE DIRECTLY?

The clinical studies that were cited above in connection with the biological activity of nitric oxide (NO) concerned mostly cardiovascular and related disorders. These assumed endothelial impairment and some sort of enhancement of NO by supplementing its sources, that is, a regimen of clinically supervised dosage of L-arginine or dietary L-arginine and/or nitrate. But reported clinical measures rarely consist of direct measurement of concentration of NO, those being usually inferred from serum or plasma levels of nitrate or by change in some clinical signs. To avoid confusion, outcome measures of NO derived from nitrate/nitrite assay should really be noted as NOx. That is not often the case.

Why are so few instances of direct measurement of NO concentration cited in clinical studies? For one thing, they are fairly difficult to execute.

There are a number of scientifically validated techniques for measuring NO directly. The earliest methods measured concentration in the breath because it was shown that in ordinary circumstances, and in ordinary healthy people, L-arginine measurably increases exhaled NO (Kharitonov et al. 1994). Nitric oxide is produced by various cells in the lower respiratory tract, including inflamed epithelial cells, and is detectable in normal exhaled air. In 1994, a study in *The Lancet* reported that NO was measured reproducibly using a chemiluminescence analyzer in patients with asthma (Kharitonov et al. 1995).

NO formation is, of course, also associated with an increased concentration of nitrite in plasma. However, it does not invariably prove readily feasible to disentangle the proportion of NO produced in the lungs in various types of pulmonary infections from the proportion produced by the immune system and the endothelium elsewhere in the body.

5.18　MEASURING NO IN CLINICAL OUTCOME

There are two kinds of clinical outcome measures: (a) those that measure change in the type or the severity of the symptoms, and (b) those that measure change in serum, plasma, or other established "lab" markers. Ideally, these two types of measures correspond to indicate either success or failure of the treatment. A few select articles on laboratory-type assessment of nitric oxide levels either as indices of severity of the disorder or as indices of the success of treatment are listed below:

- Measurement of nitric oxide in biological models (Archer 1993). Assay by ozone chemiluminescence.
- Different plasma levels of nitric oxide in arterial and venous blood (Cicinelli, E, Ignarro, L. J., L. M. Schonauer et al. 1999). Endothelium derived NO (eNO) comes primarily from arteries and not from veins.
- Measuring nitric oxide production in human clinical studies (Granger, D. L., Anstey, N. M., W. C. Miller et al. 1999).
- L-arginine increases exhaled nitric oxide in normal human subjects (Kharitonov, S. A., Lubec, G., B. Lubec et al. 1995).

If successful treatment of cardiovascular and heart disease were aimed at restoring endothelium function, and if restored endothelium function can be expected to result in increased NO formation, and if NO is detectable in breath, then it stands to reason that a breath test for change in exhaled NO concentration should indicate the success or failure of treatment even before any change in signs or symptoms is detected. Something to that effect can be read into the report by Cikach and Dweik, titled "Cardiovascular biomarkers in exhaled breath," which appeared in the journal *Progress in Cardiovascular Diseases*, in 2012 (Cikach and Dweik 2012).

There are disadvantages to the most common indirect techniques used to assess NO. The methods largely rely on the fact that NO is rapidly metabolized to nitrite in the body, and further converted to nitrate in body fluids. The nitrate is then converted to nitrite because the conventional method of assay can only detect nitrite. Nitrate/nitrite appears as a marker of inflammation in fluid such as urine, saliva, etc.

The interpretation of results from such tests can be unclear due to complications. For instance, an article in *Circulation*, the journal of the American Heart Association (AHA), cites a few examples. Diet is a potential source of nitrate and nitrite and patients need to consume a diet low in green leafy vegetables for several days before measurements. Intestinal bacteria can be a source of plasma nitrate, plasma NO in the blood can result from the activity of three different NO synthase enzymes, and there are a number of other caveats concerning "markers" (Dzau 2004). Nevertheless, many authorities recognize the value of assessing endothelial NO formation and especially its impact and conveyance in blood (Lauer et al. 2002).

5.18.1 Measuring NO in Exhaled Air

Investigators from the Department of Internal Medicine, Tokyo University aimed to evaluate NO production in patients with end-stage chronic renal failure using an ozone chemiluminescence method and measuring plasma nitrate and nitrite levels by the Griess method (which detects the presence of nitrite ion in solution). They found that patients with chronic renal failure had higher exhaled nitric oxide concentrations, greater nitric oxide output, and higher plasma nitrate/nitrite concentrations than comparison controls (Matsumoto et al. 1999).

The aim of one study was to measure NO in the exhaled air of patients with chronic rheumatic heart disease with and without pulmonary hypertension. The NO concentration in exhaled air was determined with a chemiluminescence analyzer. Echocardiography was performed in all patients to assess the severity of valve disease and for the measurement of pulmonary artery pressure. The level of exhaled NO was found to be significantly greater in patients with rheumatic heart disease than in comparison control patients. NO concentration in exhaled air was significantly increased in patients with pulmonary hypertension as compared with patients who had normal pulmonary artery systolic pressure (Gölbaşi et al. 2001).

The purpose of another study was to evaluate the relationship between body mass index (BMI), asthma, and fractional exhaled nitric oxide (FeNO) in a sample of US adults using data from the National Health and Nutrition Examination Surveys (NHANES) for 2007–2010. Adjusted asthma prevalence was positively associated with BMI, and subjects with asthma had higher adjusted FeNO levels than subjects without asthma (Singleton et al. 2014).

5.18.2 Measuring NO in Serum or Plasma

The Lancet reported in 1994 that plasma nitrate, the stable end-product of NO production, was significantly increased in patients with heart failure compared with normal comparison controls (Winlaw et al. 1994).

A study published in the journal *Vascular Medicine*, in 1999, aimed to evaluate fluctuations in plasma concentrations of L-arginine over the day depending on diet. Plasma L-arginine concentrations were found to change during the day and to be influenced by dietary intake (Tangphao et al. 1999).

Another study published in the *Journal of the Medical Association of Thailand*, in 2001, aimed to determine whether serum NO, as shown by nitrate and nitrite levels, was elevated in patients with coronary artery disease (CAD). A number of blood components including cholesterol, triglyceride, LDL-C, HDL-C and blood sugar were compared to serum NO.

It was found that serum NOx (nitrate and nitrite) levels in the CAD groups were significantly higher in a group with abnormal lipid profiles (cholesterol, triglyceride, LDL-C) and blood sugar than in a group with normal profiles. The results suggested that there was an increased NOx level in patients with CAD and much higher in patients with multiple underlying conditions such as hyperlipidemia and hyperglycemia. Measurement of NOx levels at different times was suggested to help monitor CAD (Akarasereenont et al. 2001).

Researchers reported in 2011, in the *International Journal of Applied & Basic Medical Research*, that serum NOx was observed to be significantly low in diabetic participants as compared to comparison control participants along with differences in other biochemical parameters. The Griess reaction was used for indirect assay of stable decomposition products in serum (serum nitrite and nitrate levels) as an index of NO generation (Ghosh et al. 2011).

5.19 NOx SELF-TEST

By adhering to the Proactive Nutrition Program, one can make sure that it provides ample antioxidants, mostly from plant-derived L-arginine and nitrates. Now, the HumanN™ (Formerly Neogenis Labs®) N-O Indicator Strips provide a simple way to measure levels of nitric oxide in the body (see https://www.humann.com/products/).

Dr. N. S. Bryan (adjunct assistant professor at Baylor College of Medicine in the Department of Molecular and Human Genetics) pioneered the use of salivary nitrite as a marker of human NO status. He proposes sampling of salivary nitrite as an accurate representation of total body NO production/availability, as up to now

> there have not been any new developments in the use of NO biomarkers in the clinical setting for diagnostic or prognostic utility. In fact, NO status is still not part of the standard blood chemistry routinely used for diagnostic purposes. This is simply unacceptable given the critical nature of NO in many disease processes and new technologies should be developed in Humans. (Personal communication)

HumanN™ (formerly Neogenis Labs®) is a leader in nitric oxide research and invented the world's first standard non-invasive salivary nitric oxide test strip that can be used to measure nitric oxide levels at home. Using one's own saliva, it is quick and easy to conduct the test: saliva is applied to a strip whose coloration is then compared to a color code on the side of the strip container.

The test strip measures salivary nitrite which indicates total body NO availability. If one consumes a nitrate-rich diet (containing green leafy vegetables), but lacks the proper oral nitrate-reducing bacteria, then there may be no increase in salivary nitrite, resulting in NO deficiency. If on the other hand, one has the right oral nitrate-reducing bacteria but does not eat sufficient nitrate-rich vegetables, then the test strip will also reflect low NO availability because the body is not getting enough nitrate from the diet to convert to nitrite. Only 5% of the nitrate is reduced to nitrite in saliva.

The use of such a test strip provides *"feedback"*—knowledge of results—insofar as it may help to determine sooner the positive outcome of one's attention to daily nutrition. This test is further detailed in Chapter 7.

Because of the implications for health risks, hypertension, atherosclerosis, cardiovascular and heart disease (CVHD), and diabetes, the value of discovering that one has a LOW NO reading cannot be underestimated. Such a reading may be interpreted to mean that one's diet may be low in the foodstuffs that are used in the body to form NO.

The Proactive Nutrition Program is based on the most recent science concerning the impact of nutrition on telomere length. This approach to eating can reduce free radical damage to the cells in the body. The logic is that reducing free radical damage can prevent accelerated cell cycling and premature aging. Using the N-O Indicator Strips is the easiest way to track the availability of nitric oxide in the body and can help in making food choices to maintain desirable levels. As this chapter has shown, adequate NO formation is very important for lowering the free radical and ROS load. Reducing this load is the key to improving and maintaining cardiovascular and metabolic health.

REFERENCES

Adams, M. R., R. McCredie, W. Jessup, et al. 1997. Oral L-arginine improves endothelium-dependent dilatation and reduces monocyte adhesion to endothelial cells in young men with coronary artery disease. *Atherosclerosis*, 129(2):261–269.

Akarasereenont, P., T. Nuamchit, A. Thaworn, et al. 2001. Serum nitric oxide levels in patients with coronary artery disease. *Medical Association of Thailand*, 84 Suppl 3:S730–S739.

Alderton, W. K., C. E. Cooper, and R. G. Knowles. 2001. Nitric oxide synthases: Structure, function and inhibition. *Biochemical Journal*, 357(3):593–615.

Archer, D. L. 2002. Evidence that ingested nitrate and nitrite are beneficial to health. *Journal of Food Protection*, 65(5):872–875.

Archer, S. 1993. Measurement of nitric oxide in biological models. *FASEB J*, 7(2):349–360.

Bahadoran, Z., P. Mirmiran, Z. Tahmasebinejad, et al. 2016. Dietary L-arginine intake and the incidence of coronary heart disease: Tehran lipid and glucose study. *Nutrition & Metabolism Open Access*, 201613:23. doi: 10.1186/s12986-016-0084-z.

Barbarash, N. A., D. Y. Kuvshinov, M. V. Chichilenko, et al. 2012. Nitric oxide and human aging. *Advances in Gerontology*, 2(1):71–74.

Baxter, A. J., T. Coyne, and C. McClintock. 2006. Dietary patterns and metabolic syndrome—A review of epidemiologic evidence. *Asia Pacific Journal of Clinical Nutrition*, 15(2):134–142.

Bednarz, B., T. Jaxa-Chamiec, J. Gebalska, et al. 2004. L-arginine supplementation prolongs exercise capacity in congestive heart failure [in English, Polish]. *Kardiologia Polska*, 60(4):348–353.

Benzie, I. F. F, and J. J. Strain. 1996. Reducing ability of plasma (FRAP) as a measure of "Antioxidant Power": The FRAP. *Analytical Biochemistry*, 239:70–76.

Benzie, I. F. F, and Y. T. Zeto. 1999. Total antioxidant capacity of teas by the ferric reducing/antioxidant power assay. *Journal of Agricultural & Food Chemistry*, 47(2):633–636.

Bocch, E. A., A. V. Vilella de Moraes, A. Esteves-Filho, et al. 2000. L-arginine reduces heart rate and improves hemodynamics in severe congestive heart failure. *Clinical Cardiology*, 23(3):205–210.

Böger, R. H., and S. M. Bode-Böger. 2001. The clinical pharmacology of L-arginine. *Annual Review of Pharmacology & Toxicology*, 41:79–99.

Böger, R. H., S. M. Bode-Böger, W. Thicle, et al. 1998. Restoring vascular nitric oxide formation by L-arginine improves the symptoms of intermittent claudication in patients with peripheral arterial occlusive disease. *Journal of the American College of Cardiology*, 32(5):1336–1344.

Carlström, M., A. E. G. Persson, E. Larsson, et al. 2010. Dietary nitrate attenuates oxidative stress, prevents cardiac and renal injuries, and reduces blood pressure in salt-induced hypertension. *Cardiovascular Research*, 89(3):574–585. doi: doi.org/10.1093/cvr/cvq366 574-585.

Ceremuzyński, L., T. Chamiec, and K. Herbaczyńska-Cedro. 1997. Effect of supplemental oral L-arginine on exercise capacity in patients with stable angina pectoris. *American Journal of Cardiology*, 80(3):331–333.

Chauhan, A., R. S. More, P. A. Mullins, et al. 1996. Aging-associated endothelial dysfunction in humans is reversed by L-Arginine. *Journal of the American College of Cardiology*, 28(7):1796–1804.

Cikach, F. S., Jr, and R. A. Dweik. 2012. Cardiovascular biomarkers in exhaled breath. *Progress in Cardiovascular Diseases*, 55(1):34–43.

Cicinelli, E, L. J. Ignarro, L. M. Schonauer, et al. 1999. Different plasma levels of nitric oxide in arterial and venous blood. *Clinical Physiology*, 19:440–442.

Clifford, T., G. Howatson, D. J. West, et al. 2015. The potential benefits of red beetroot supplementation in health and disease. *Nutrients*, 7(4):2801–2822.

Compton, S. A., L. W. Elmore, K. Haydu, et al. 2006. Induction of nitric oxide synthase-dependent telomere shortening after functional inhibition of Hsp90 in human tumor cells. *Molecular & Cell Biology*, 26(4):1452–1462.

Corretti, M. C., T. J. Anderson, E. G. Benjamin, et al. 2002. Guidelines for the ultrasound assessment of endothelial-dependent flow-mediated vasodilation of the brachial artery. A report of the International Brachial Artery Reactivity Task Force. *Journal of the American College of Cardiology*, 39(2):257–265.

d'El-Rei, J., A. R. Cunha, M. Trindade, et al. 2016. Beneficial effects of dietary nitrate on endothelial function and blood pressure levels. *International Journal of Hypertension*, 2016: 6791519.

Daff, S. 2010. NO synthase: Structures and mechanisms. *Nitric Oxide*, 23(1):1–11.

Dzau, V. J. 2004. Markers of malign across the cardiovascular continuum: Interpretation and application. *Circulation*, 109(25 Suppl 1):IV1–2.

Fleenor, B. S., A. L. Sindler, J. S. Eng, et al. 2012. Sodium nitrite de-stiffening of large elastic arteries with aging: Role of normalization of advanced glycation end-products. *Experimental Gerontology*, 47(8):588–594.

Franklin, S. S., M. G. Larson, S. A. Khan, et al. 2001. Does the relation of blood pressure to coronary heart disease risk change with aging? The Framingham Heart Study. *Circulation*, 103:1245–1249.

Fried R. 2014. *Erectile Dysfunction as a Cardiovascular Impairment*. Boston, MA: Academic Press/Elsevier.

Fried, R., and W. C. Merrell. 1999. *The Arginine Solution*. New York: Warner Books.

Fried, R., and L. Nezin. 2006. *Great Food, Great Sex*. New York: Ballantine Books.

Furchgott, R. F., and J. V. Zawadzki. 1980. The obligatory role of endothelial cells in the relaxation of arterial smooth muscle by acetylcholine. *Nature*, 288:373–376.

Georgiev, V. G., J. Weber, E. M. Kneschke, et al. 2010. Antioxidant activity and phenolic content of betalain extracts from intact plants and hairy root cultures of the red beetroot Beta vulgaris cv. *Detroit dark red*. *Plant Foods for Human Nutrition*, 65(2):105–111.

Ghosh, A., M. L. Sherpa, Y. Bhutia, et al. 2011. Serum nitric oxide status in patients with type 2 diabetes mellitus in Sikkim. *International Journal of Applied & Basic Medical Research*, 1(1):31–35.

Gölbaşi, Z., S. Dinçer, H. Bayol, et al. 2001. Increased nitric oxide in exhaled air in patients with rheumatic heart disease. *European Journal of Heart Failure*, 3(1):27–32.

Granger, D. L., N. M. Anstey, W. C. Miller et al. 1999. Measuring nitric oxide production in human clinical studies. *Methods in Enzymology*, 301:49–61.

Griffith, R. S., A. L. Norins, and C. Kagan. 1978. A multicentered study of lysine therapy in Herpes simplex infection. *Dermatologica*, 156(5):257–267.

Hayashi, T., P. A. R. Juliet, H, Matsui-Hirai, et al. 2005. L-citrulline and L-arginine supplementation retards the progression of high-cholesterol-diet-induced atherosclerosis in rabbits. *Proceedings of the National Academy of Sciences, USA*, 102(38):13681–13686.

Hobbs, D. A., N. Kaffa, T. W. George, et al. 2012. Blood pressure-lowering effects of beetroot juice and novel beetroot-enriched bread products in normotensive male subjects. *British Journal of Nutrition*, 108(11):2066–2074.

Hord, N. G., Y. Tang, and N. S. Bryan. 2009. Food sources of nitrates and nitrites: The physiologic context for potential health benefits. *American Journal of Clinical Nutrition*, 90(1):1–10.

Jain, A. P., A. Mohan, O. P. Gupta, et al. 2000. Role of oxygen free radicals in causing endothelial damage in acute myocardial infarction. *Journal of the Association of Physicians of India*, 48(5):478–480.

Kanner, J., S. Harel, and R. Granit R. 2001. Betalains—A new class of dietary cationized antioxidants. *Journal of Agricultural and Food Chemistry*, 49(11):5178–5185.

Kapil, V., R. S. Khambata, A. Robertson, et al. 2015. Dietary nitrate provides sustained blood pressure lowering in hypertensive patients: A randomized, phase 2, double-blind, placebo-controlled study. *Hypertension*, 65(2):320–327.

Kharitonov, S. A., G. Lubec, B. Lubec, et al. 1995. L-arginine increases exhaled nitric oxide in normal human subjects. *Clinical Science*, 88:135–139.

Kharitonov, S. A., D. Yates, R. A. Robbins, et al. 1994. Increased nitric oxide in exhaled air of asthmatic patients. *Lancet*, 343(8890):133–135.

Lauer, T., P. Kleinbongard, and M. Kelm. 2002. Indexes of NO bioavailability in human blood. *News in Physiological Sciences*, 17:251–255.

Lekakis, J. P., S. Papathanassiou, T. G. Papaioannou, et al. 2002. Oral L-arginine improves endothelial dysfunction in patients with essential hypertension. *International Journal of Cardiology*, 86(2–3):317–323.

Lian, F., J. Wang, and X. Huang, et al. 2015. Effect of vegetable consumption on the association between peripheral leucocyte telomere length and hypertension: A case-control study. *British Medical Journal Open*, 5(11):e009305.

Lidder, S., and A. J. Webb. 2013. Vascular effects of dietary nitrate (as found in green leafy vegetables and beetroot) via the nitrate-nitrite-nitric oxide pathway. *British Journal of Clinical Pharmacology*, 75(3):677–696.

Litvinova, L., D. N. Atochin, N. Fattakhov, et al. 2015. Nitric oxide and mitochondria in metabolic syndrome. *Frontiers in Physiology*, 6:20.

Lundberg, J. O., M. Carlström, F. J. Larsen, et al. 2010. Roles of dietary inorganic nitrate in cardiovascular health and disease. *Cardiovascular Research*, 89(3):525–532.

Lundberg, J. O., M. T. Gladwin, and E. Weitzberg. 2015. Strategies to increase nitric oxide signalling in cardiovascular disease. *Nature Reviews Drug Discovery*, 14:623–641.

Lundberg, J. O., E. Weitzberg, and M. T. Gladwin MT. 2008. The nitrate-nitrite-nitric oxide pathway in physiology and therapeutics. *Nature Reviews Drug Discovery*, 7(2):156–167.

Matsumoto, A., Y. Hirata, M. Kakoki, et al. 1999. Increased excretion of nitric oxide in exhaled air of patients with chronic renal failure. *Clinical Science (London)*, 96(1):67–74.

Miller, G. D., A. P. Marsh, R. W. Dove, et al. 2012. Plasma nitrate and nitrite are increased by a high-nitrate supplement but not by high-nitrate foods in older adults. *Nutrition Research*, 32(3):160–168.

Mirmiran, P. Z. Bahadoran, A. Ghasemi, et al. 2016. The association of dietary L-arginine intake and serum nitric oxide metabolites in adults: A population-based study. *Nutrients*, 8(5) pii: E311.

Moncada, S., and A. Higgs. 1993. The L-arginine-nitric oxide pathway. *New England Journal of Medicine*, 329(27):2002–2012.

Morita, M., T. Hayashi, M. Ochiai. 2014. Oral supplementation with a combination of L-citrulline and L-arginine rapidly increases plasma L-arginine concentration and enhances NO bioavailability. *Biochemical & Biophysical Research Communications*, 454(1):53–57.

Nettleton, J. A., A. Diez-Roux, N. S. Jenny, et al. 2008. Processed meat intake showed an expected inverse association with telomere length. Dietary patterns, food groups, and telomere length in the Multi-Ethnic Study of Atherosclerosis (MESA). *American Journal of Clinical Nutrition*, 88(5):1405–1412.

Nöthlings, U., L. R. Wilkens, S. P. Murphy, et al. 2005. Meat and fat intake as risk factors for pancreatic cancer: The multiethnic cohort study. *Journal of the National Cancer Institute*, 97:1458–1465.

Panagiotakos, D. B., C. Pitsavos, Y. Skoumas, et al. 2007. The association between food patterns and the metabolic syndrome using principal components analysis: The ATTICA Study. *Journal of the American Dietetic Association*, 107(6):979–987; quiz 997.

Peters, H., and N. A. Noble. 1996. Dietary L-arginine in renal disease. *Seminars in Nephrolology*, 16(6):567–575.

Piatti, P. M., L. D. Monti, G. Valsecchi, et al. 2001. Long-term oral L-arginine administration improves peripheral and hepatic insulin sensitivity in type 2 diabetic patients. *Diabetes Care*, 24(5):875–880.

Pinto, E. 2007. Blood pressure and ageing. *Postgraduate Medical Journal*, 83(976):109–114.

Reddy, M. K., R. K. Alexander-Lindo, and M. G. Nair. 2005. Relative inhibition of lipid peroxidation, cyclooxygenase enzymes, and human tumor cell proliferation by natural food colors. *Journal of Agricultural and Food Chemistry*, 53(23):9268–9273.

Reyes, A. A., I. E. Karl, and S. Klahr S. 1994. Role of arginine in health and in renal disease. *American Journal of Physiology*, 267(3 Pt 2):F331–F346.

Schneider, J. Y., S. Rothmann, F. Schröder, et al. 2015. Effects of chronic oral L-arginine administration on the L-arginine/NO pathway in patients with peripheral arterial occlusive disease or coronary artery disease: L-Arginine prevents renal loss of nitrite, the major NO reservoir. *Amino Acids*, 47(9):1961–1974.

Schulman, S. P., L. C. Becker, D. A. Kass, et al. 2006. L-arginine therapy in acute myocardial infarction: The Vascular Interaction With Age in Myocardial Infarction (VINTAGE MI) randomized clinical trial. *Journal of the American Medical Association*, 295(1):58–64.

Schwartz, L. 2003. Amelioration of microvascular angina with arginine supplementation. *Annals of Internal Medicine*, 138(2):160.

Schwedhelm, E., R. Maas, R. Freese, et al. 2008. Pharmacokinetic and pharmacodynamic properties of oral L-citrulline and L-arginine: Impact on nitric oxide metabolism. *British Journal of Clinical Pharmacology*, 65(1):51–59.

Sindelar, J. J., and A. L. Milkowski. 2012. Human safety controversies surrounding nitrate and nitrite in the diet. *Nitric Oxide*, 26(4):259–266.

Sindler, A. L., A. E. Devan, B. S. Fleenor, et al. 2014. Inorganic nitrite supplementation for healthy arterial aging. *Journal of Applied Physiology*, 116(5):463–477.

Singh, R., S. Devi, and R. Gollen. 2015. Role of free radical in atherosclerosis, diabetes and dyslipidaemia: larger-than-life. *Diabetes/Metabolism Research & Reviews*, 31(2):113–126.

Singleton, M. D., W. T. Sanderson, and D. M. Mannino. 2014. Body mass index, asthma and exhaled nitric oxide in U.S. adults, 2007–2010. *Journal of Asthma*, 51(7):756–761.

Sorrentin, M. J. 1999. Oral L-arginine for improving vascular function in hypercholesterolemia, PVD, and atherosclerotic heart disease. *Integrative Medicine Alert*, 2:121–124.

Tangphao, O., S. Chalon, A. M. Coulston, et al. 1999. L-arginine and nitric oxide-related compounds in plasma: Comparison of normal and arginine-free diets in a 24-h crossover study. *Vascular Medicine*, 4:27–32.

Tesoriere, L., D. Butera, D. D'Arpa, et al. 2003. Increased resistance to oxidation of betalain-enriched human low-density lipoproteins. *Free Radical Research*, 37(6):689–696.

Thadani, U. 1997. Oral nitrates: More than symptomatic therapy in coronary artery disease? *Cardiovascular Drugs & Therapy*, 11 Suppl 1:213–218.

Vasa, M., K. Breitschopf, A. M. Zeiher, et al. 2000. Nitric oxide activates telomerase and delays endothelial cell senescence. *Circulation Research*, 87:540–542.

Vasdev. S., and V. Gill. 2008. The antihypertensive effect of arginine. *International Journal of Angiology*, 17(1):7–22.

Velmurugan, S., J. M. Gan, K. S. Rathod, et al. 2016. Dietary nitrate improves vascular function in patients with hypercholesterolemia: A randomized, double-blind, placebo-controlled study. *American Journal of Clinical Nutrition*, 103(1):25–38.

Víteček, J., A. Lojek, and G. Valacchi, et al. 2012. Arginine-based inhibitors of nitric oxide synthase: Therapeutic potential and challenges. *Mediators of Inflammation*, 2012:318087.

Wascher, T. C., K. Posch, S. Wallner, et al. 1997. Vascular effects of L-arginine: Anything beyond a substrate for the NO-synthase? *Biochemistry & Biophysics Research Communication*, 234(1):35–38.

Watanabe, G., H. Tomiyama, and N. Doba. 2000. Effects of oral administration of L-arginine on renal function in patients with heart failure. *Journal of Hypertension*, 18(2):229–234.

Winlaw, D. S., G. A. Smythe, A. M. Keogh, et al. 1994. Increased nitric oxide production in heart failure. *Lancet*, 344:373–374.

Wruss, J., G. Waldenberger, S. Huemer, et al. 2015. Compositional characteristics of commercial beetroot products and beetroot juice prepared from seven beetroot varieties grown in Upper Austria. *Journal of Food Composition and Analysis*, 42:46–55.

Zielinska-Przyjemska, M., A. Olejni, A. Dobrowolska-Zachwieja, et al. 2009. In vitro effects of beetroot juice and chips on oxidative metabolism and apoptosis in neutrophils from obese individuals. *Phytotherapy Research*, 23(1):49–55.

6 Three Common Diets Compared for Their Effects on Cell Aging

6.1 INTRODUCTION

Premature aging can be averted by neutralizing free radicals formed by metabolism and physical activity, and by reducing their accumulation in the body. This will slow cell recycling and protect telomeres. This can be accomplished with a diet that centers on foods that minimize free radical formation, supply adequate antioxidants to avoid their accumulation, and activate longevity-promoting *sirtuins*. The choice of the right diet plan, the Proactive Nutrition Program, is therefore at the core of preventing the free radical damage that shortens telomeres and, therefore, shortens lifespan.

Diet is also about what fuels metabolism, the process of energy formation. Here follows a comparison of three well-known diets, the Western/Standard American Diet (SAD), the Heart-Healthy/Prudent diet, and the Mediterranean diet, with respect to their potential for minimal or maximal reduction of free radical damage to telomeres. In addition, it will be shown that a Mediterranean diet, the best way we know to reduce telomere damage, can be enhanced with foods that activate Sirtuin 1, a protein that regulates telomere length by its ability to trigger genes that can signal cells to slow down recycling in response to free radical oxidative stress.

6.2 OXIDATIVE METABOLISM

But first, here is how MedlinePlus (US National Library of Medicine[*]) defines metabolism:

> Metabolism refers to all the physical and chemical processes in the body that convert or use energy, such as:
>
> - Breathing
> - Circulating blood
> - Controlling body temperature
> - Contracting muscles
> - Digesting food and nutrients
> - Eliminating waste through urine and feces
> - Functioning of the brain and nerves

---

[*] National Institutes of Health (NIH). https://www.nlm.nih.gov/medlineplus/ency/article/002257.htm

What's wrong with this definition? Actually, everything—nothing is right: If one picks up a rock from the ground, that is a *physical process that converts energy* from that stored in muscles to that used to lift the rock against the opposing force of gravity. For instance, "breathing" is not metabolism, "contracting muscles" is not metabolism, "functioning of the brain and nerves" is not metabolism. Metabolism is none of the above.

Metabolism is the chemical combination of oxygen with consumed foods. When something combines with oxygen it is said to *oxidize*. Oxidation creates energy often in the form of heat, and it usually creates water, "waste," and other by-products. Therefore, "metabolism" is only one-half of the correct term—*oxidative metabolism*. The distinction is an important reminder because, bottom line, oxidation results in oxygen free radicals. Hence, metabolism results in oxygen free radicals.

Oxidative metabolism "burns calories." Well, one does not actually "burn calories": a calorie is a unit of measurement—not height or weight, but *energy*. Something containing 100 calories describes how much energy the body could get from eating or drinking it. How are calories measured?

The calories indicated on a food package label is actually a *kilocalorie* (kcal) or 1000 calories. A kcal is the amount of energy needed to raise the temperature of 1 kilogram of water by 1°C. So, calorie is really a measure of how much heat is produced by oxidation.

In normal circumstances, we—all of different body heights and weights—each oxidize a sufficient amount of food/fuel to provide the energy required by the physiological body processes that maintain life and activate motion, all the while maintaining body temperature at about 98.6°F. That is quite a juggling act. An average person needs about 2400 calories per day to do that and still maintain body weight.

And now, to the point, to avert premature aging, oxidative metabolism needs to be fine-tuned so as to maximize energy production—calories—and energy storage as fat in the body, all the while minimizing free radical formation and accumulation. Anybody can maximize energy production and storage, but it takes knowledge and determination to minimize free radical formation.

It is feasible to practically maximize energy production and storage and minimize free radical formation by the choice of foods/fuel in a nutrition plan such as the one proposed in this book. Such a plan both eliminates foods that maximize free radical formation and accumulation—like "burning sugar" versus "burning fat"—and simultaneously supplies antioxidants to reduce both the formation and accumulation of free radicals.

American health authorities have agonized for more than a century over what are the best ways that nutrition can make us healthy and thrive. Their efforts, numerous and varied, have met with relatively little success: their criteria for success were limited early on to observing physical development by age, and identifying the absence of the few known vitamins and other deficiencies (iodine, for instance) that, with some notable exceptions like scurvy and beriberi, likewise mostly impeded physical development.

In fact, grandmother's pediatrician evaluated the general health of a baby by its weight for its age. Presumably, there were no unhealthy fat babies as birth weight was a relatively successful predictor of baby survival.

It took a long time for the connection between diet and longevity in the seemingly healthy person to be made. The focus became preventing death from dread diseases.

It stands to reason that were an effective diet for health ever devised, there would be no need for the countless reappraisals and revisions that mark the field of public health nutrition guidelines and advice.

This chapter reviews the evolution of dietary guidelines—mostly from the US Department of Agriculture (USDA)—that show its focus on grouping various foods in keeping with the Victorian idea that "moderation in all things is best," a popular notion in those days. The USDA was far more successful in producing useful nutrition guidelines for cattle, pigs, and other farm animals than for humans.

Ultimately, the American Heart Association (AHA) developed updated versions of USDA nutrition guidelines into the so-called Heart-Healthy and Prudent diets to reduce consumption of animal fat considered to cause cardiovascular and heart disease via cholesterol-driven atherosclerosis. Mention of the hazard of excessive dietary sodium, carbohydrates, and sugar came late in the game, especially sugar and carbohydrates, as metabolic syndrome and type 2 diabetes rose in popularity as diagnostic categories.

The Mediterranean diet gained popularity with early studies that reported that those who adhered to it in various regions of the world had a lower incidence of the cardiovascular, heart, and metabolic diseases that plague us here. At about the same time, rising insight into the role of antioxidants and the Mediterranean diet, which is rich in antioxidants, was credited with success in promoting cardiovascular and heart health.

The USDA jumped on the bandwagon, with one of its laboratories devising a means of measuring antioxidant food capacity, the *oxygen radical absorbance capacity* (ORAC). But it suddenly leaped off the bandwagon, repudiating ORAC as a meaningful measure of anything other than how many trillions of free radicals a given food could neutralize, and it removed the ORAC values tables from its website, making them inaccessible to the general consumer public.

Finally, it will become clear that the best diet approach to health and longevity is the Proactive Nutrition Program because of the antioxidant capacity of the Mediterranean diet to protect telomeres, boosted with the "sirtfoods" that activate sirtuin1 that likewise protects telomeres.

6.3 HOW AND WHY NUTRITION GUIDELINES CHANGE OVER TIME

Despite overwhelming evidence that diet influences lifespan, and with seeming determination, most Americans are now still eating themselves into an early grave. Health authorities tell us that epidemic "preventable" catastrophes such as cardiovascular and heart disease, metabolic syndrome, type 2 diabetes, etc., even cancer, are related to "poor diet."

It is clearly our fault, of course, because we do not watch what we eat. To help us watch what we eat, health authorities, especially the USDA, periodically issued dietary guidelines intended to provide us with "healthy" nutrition.

These guidelines changes are apparently driven by two main forces. First, there are periodic changes in the foods that are promoted as being vital to health by the special interests of the corporate dairy, beef, and processed foods industry. Second, it becomes periodically known that, for one reason or another, some foods, or food constituents, are in fact, inadequate if not outright harmful.

Many changes are crisis-driven. There are also many instances where the outcome of a given diet was supported by reputable establishment research. One example is the *low saturated fat-diet reduces coronary heart disease*, which appeared in 1972 (Miettinen et al. 1972), a conclusion that was overturned by equally reputable conventional establishment research in 2004 (Knopp and Retzlaff 2004).

6.4 EARLY FOOD GUIDANCE: 1900s–1940s

Here is an abridged history. The US Department of Agriculture (USDA) has issued well-intentioned dietary recommendations for over 100 years. Yet, despite changing patterns of nutrition, many current guidelines are quite similar to the earliest ones. When it published the first dietary recommendations in 1894, some vitamins and minerals were not yet known. Food policies including iodine fortification of salt, and the enrichment of flour products with B vitamins and milk with vitamin D, together with consumer education, have lessened some nutritional deficiencies in the United States.

The first published dietary guidance by the USDA was a *Farmers' Bulletin* written in 1894 by Wilbur O. Atwater, the first director of the Office of Experiment Stations in the USDA. It suggested diets for American men based on the content of protein, carbohydrate, fat, and mineral matter ("ash"). Atwater initiated the scientific basis for connecting food composition, dietary intake, and health, and emphasized the importance of *variety, proportionality*, and *moderation* in healthful eating (Atwater 1894). His research on food composition and nutritional needs set the stage for the development of a food guide for selecting the kinds and amounts of foods that provide a nutritionally sound diet.

The first USDA food guide, *Food for Young Children*, by the nutritionist Caroline Hunt, appeared in 1916 (Hunt 1916). It classified foods into five groups:

- Milk and meat
- Cereals
- Vegetables and fruits
- Fats and fatty foods
- Sugars and sugary foods

This food guide was followed in 1917 by dietary recommendations likewise based on these five food groups, but targeted to the general public in *How to Select Foods* (Hunt and Atwater 1917) and later adapted for the average family (Hunt 1921).

Early in the Depression years of the 1930s, a USDA food economist proposed plans consisting of 12 major food groups to buy and use in a week at four cost levels to help people shop for food (Cleveland et al. 1983; Stiebeling and Ward 1933).

6.5 DIETARY GUIDANCE: 1940s TO 1970s

In 1941, President Franklin D. Roosevelt called for a National Nutrition Conference for Defense (Anonymous 1941). It provided the first set of Recommended Dietary

Allowances (RDAs) by the Food and Nutrition Board of the National Academy of Sciences, recommending intakes for calories and nine essential nutrients:

- Protein
- Iron
- Calcium
- Vitamin A
- Vitamin D
- Thiamin
- Riboflavin
- Niacin
- Ascorbic acid (vitamin C)

This was followed in 1943 by the USDA *National Wartime Nutrition Guide* (revised in 1946 as the *National Food Guide*) promoting the "Basic 7" food groups. It specified a basic diet to provide a major share of the RDAs for nutrients but only a portion of caloric needs. The 1946 version suggested numbers of food group servings and was widely used for over a decade (Anonymous 1946). However, its complexity and lack of specifics regarding serving sizes led in 1956 to a new food guide popularly known as the *Basic Four*, which recommended a minimum number of foods from each of four food groups: milk, meat, fruits and vegetables, and grain products (Page and Phipard 1956).

6.6 THE EARLY 1970s TO THE 1990s

In 1977, the report *Dietary Goals for the United States* by the Senate Select Committee on Nutrition and Human Needs shifted the focus from obtaining adequate nutrients to avoiding excessive intakes of food constituents linked to chronic diseases. It followed the 1979 USDA publication *Food* with a new guide to the role of fats, sugars, and sodium in risks for chronic diseases and modified the *Basic Four* to highlight a fifth food group, fats, sweets, and alcoholic beverages, targeted for moderation. Also in 1979, the Department of Health, Education, and Welfare (now the Department of Health and Human Services [DHHS]) released a study by the American Society for Clinical Nutrition (ASCN) on the relationship between dietary practices and health outcomes (DHHS Task Force 1979).

Responding to the need for authoritative, consistent guidance on diet and health, the USDA and DHHS together issued seven principles for a healthful diet intended for healthy Americans aged 2 and older. They were based in part on the 1979 Surgeon General's Report suggesting that people reduce consumption of excess calories, fat and cholesterol, salt, and sugar to lower disease rates. It was published in 1980 as the first edition of *Nutrition and Your Health: Dietary Guidelines for Americans*.

That edition emphasized total diet rather than the earlier basic "foundation diet." It taught food selections to lower intake of constituents connected to risk of chronic diseases and suggested the numbers of servings from each of five major food groups:

- The bread, cereal, rice, and pasta group
- The vegetable group

- The fruit group
- The milk, yogurt, and cheese group
- The meat, poultry, fish, dry beans, eggs, and nuts group

It also recommended sparing use of a sixth food group: fats, oils, and sweets. Its release prompted some concern among consumer, commodity, and food industry groups, as well as nutrition scientists who questioned the causal relationship between certain guidelines and health. A Pattern for Daily Food Choices was then presented to consumers in a *food wheel* as part of a 1984 nutrition course developed by the USDA in cooperation with the then American National Red Cross (Anonymous 1984).

6.7   1984 FOOD WHEEL: A PATTERN FOR DAILY FOOD CHOICES

The "pattern" covered:

- A total diet approach, which included goals for both nutrient adequacy and moderation
- Five food groups and amounts, forming the basis of the Food Guide Pyramid
- Daily amounts of food provided at three calorie levels

The second edition in 1985 warned about unsafe weight-loss diets, using large-dose supplements, and the consumption of alcoholic beverages by pregnant women. This edition was adopted as a guide for healthy diets by scientific, consumer, and industry groups.

In 1988, a graphic presentation of the USDA food guide, A Pattern for Daily Food Choices, was prepared to promote the key concepts of *variety*, *proportionality*, and *moderation*. After testing on high school-educated adults, the food guide was presented as a pyramid in 1992 (see Figure 6.1).

6.7.1   THE 1992 FOOD GUIDE PYRAMID

In the 1992 Food Guide Pyramid, *variety* among food groups is shown by the name of the food groups and by the separate sections of the pyramid. Variety within food groups is illustrated by pictures of typical food items. *Proportionality* is conveyed by the size of the food group sections and the text stating numbers of servings.

Moderation of consumption of foods high in fat and added sugars is represented by the small tip of the pyramid and text specifying that they be used sparingly. Moderation related to food choices within food groups is shown by the density of the fat and sugars symbols in the food groups.

The pyramid:

- Presented a total diet approach with goals for both nutrient adequacy and moderation
- Was developed using consumer research to raise awareness of the new food patterns

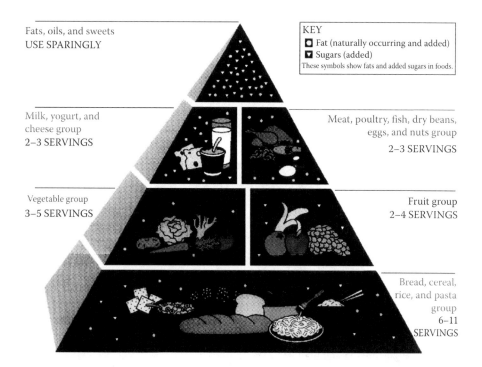

Fats, oils, and sweets
USE SPARINGLY

KEY
☐ Fat (naturally occurring and added)
☑ Sugars (added)
These symbols show fats and added sugars in foods.

Milk, yogurt, and
cheese group
2–3 SERVINGS

Meat, poultry, fish, dry beans,
eggs, and nuts group
2–3 SERVINGS

Vegetable group
3–5 SERVINGS

Fruit group
2–4 SERVINGS

Bread, cereal,
rice, and pasta
group
6–11
SERVINGS

FIGURE 6.1 (See color insert.) The 1992 Food Guide Pyramid. (Courtesy of USDA, Washington, DC.)

- Used illustration to focus on concepts of variety, moderation, and proportion
- Included visualization of added fats and sugars throughout five food groups and in the pyramid tip
- Included the range for daily amounts of food required across three calorie levels

The text of the guide booklet provides additional information on food choices that are low in fat, saturated fat, cholesterol, added sugars, or sodium within each food group. Since its release, the Food Guide Pyramid has been widely used by nutrition and health professionals, educators, the media, and the food industry.

6.7.2 THE NUTRITION FACTS LABEL

The Nutrition Labeling and Education Act of 1990 (NLEA) mandated the use of nutrition information and was implemented in 1994, with the Nutrition Facts label on virtually all packaged and processed foods that one could use to select a healthy diet within the framework of the Food Guide Pyramid.

The Nutrition Facts label gives per serving quantities of food constituents and targets suspects in cardiovascular and heart diseases, hypertension, obesity, metabolic syndrome, and type 2 diabetes. The website http://www.fda.gov/Food/

IngredientsPackagingLabeling/LabelingNutrition/ucm274593.htm, clearly explains the use of the label.

It is a very modestly useful device because few consumers who pick up a package can readily relate *per serving* in grams or liters to how much they will actually consume. We are, after all, on the oz/lb standard. In any case, few could pick out an 8 oz glass from a selection of glasses holding different volumes of liquid.

There are no known scientific clinical outcome studies on the value of the Nutrition Facts label in lowering the incidence of any of the targeted diseases. In fact, rising mortality statistics for these diseases tell a different story.

6.8   SOME BASIC RELEVANT HEALTH HAZARD STATISTICS

According to the National Health Interview Survey, 1999–2000 and 2009–2010:

- Between 1999–2000 and 2009–2010, the percentage of adults aged 45–64 and 65 and over with two or more of nine selected chronic conditions including hypertension, heart disease, diabetes, and cancer, increased in both men and women, in all racial and ethnic groups examined, and for most income groups.
- During the 10-year period, the percentage of adults aged 65 and over with both hypertension and diabetes increased from 9% to 15%, the prevalence of hypertension and heart disease increased from 18% to 21%, and the prevalence of hypertension and cancer increased from 8% to 11% (Freid et al. 2012; Yach et al. 2015).

What is more, projection into the future (2020) is not encouraging, despite the ready availability of the Nutrition Facts label and warnings about the role of diet from health authorities.

6.9   FROM 1995 TO THE PRESENT

The 1995 edition, unlike earlier voluntary guides, was the first mandated by statute: the 1990 National Nutrition Monitoring and Related Research Act (7 U.S.C. 5341). It requires the Secretaries of Agriculture and Health and Human Services jointly to publish a report titled "Dietary guidelines" for Americans at least every 5 years.

Recent research shows that consumers are frustrated when they hear different nutrition messages from different sources. In a USDA survey of main meal planners/preparers, over 40% strongly agreed with the statement, "There are so many recommendations about healthy ways to eat, it's hard to know what to believe" (Cypel et al. 1996).

Almost half of respondents to an American Dietetic Association (ADA) telephone survey of adults said that they found news reports on nutrition to be confusing. Some 81% of respondents reported that they would prefer to hear about new research only after there is acceptance among nutrition and health professionals (versus hearing about all studies individually) (Anonymous 1995).

Last came the USDA MyPlate *Dietary Guidelines for Americans 2015–2020.* MyPlate recommended a diet containing:

- 30% Grains
- 30% Vegetables
- 20% Fruits
- 20% Protein

It does not specify the source of the meat protein (i.e., beef, lamb, fish, etc.) or vegetable proteins (i.e., beans or lentils) except to say to vary them. It also provided tips such as:

- Eat less.
- Enjoy your food.
- Switch to skim or 1% milk.
- Vary your protein food choices.
- Look out for salt (sodium) in foods.
- Make at least half your grains whole.
- Drink water instead of sugary drinks.
- Eat fewer foods that are high in solid fats.
- Make half your plate fruits and vegetables.
- When eating out, choose lower calorie menu options.
- Choose foods and drinks with little or no added sugars.
- Cook more often at home, where you can control what is in your food.

The USDA holds that since the initial release of the *Dietary Guidelines for Americans* in 1980, each edition has gained in acceptance and use by both professionals and consumers:

> As nutrition guidance advances into the 21st century, the underlying themes of variety, proportionality, and moderation—initiated about 100 years ago and reinforced by the dietary guidelines—should likely still apply to choosing healthful diets for many years to come. (Frazão 1999)

The systematic development and publication of dietary guidelines, and the emergence of a Prudent diet, should have resulted in a savvy consumer public inclined to healthful nutrition. In fact, it seems to have had little if any impact on a population largely inclined to violate virtually all of the guidelines in its headlong rush to consume a Western pattern diet. The upshot of this trend is poor health and extravagantly costly health care.

Data from 2009–2010 indicate that over 78 million US adults and about 12.5 million children and adolescents (16.9%) are obese (Ogden et al. 2012). In the early 1970s, this figure was 15% but by 2007 it had doubled to 34% (http://www.fitness.gov/resource-center/facts-and-statistics/0). To underscore this trend, since the 1970s, the number of fast food restaurants in the US has more than doubled. What are the health consequences of this nutrition trend?

6.10   THE CARNIVAL MIRROR

As the nutritionist Chris Woolston put it on the website HealthDay News for Healthy Living:

> The Western diet is the Prudent diet reflected in a carnival mirror. Everything is backwards: red meat and other fatty foods take the forefront, while fruits, vegetables, and whole grains are pushed aside. In addition to fat and calories, the Western diet is loaded with cholesterol, salt, and sugar.

He pointed out, furthermore, that the Western diet is also deficient in dietary fiber and plant-based nutrients that protect us from many health hazards including cancer. (Dan McKillen; https://consumer.healthday.com/encyclopedia/weight-control-39/obesity-health-news-505/what-s-wrong-with-the-american-diet-644659.htm.)

6.11   A NOTE ON OMISSION OF ANTIOXIDANT CAPACITY IN FOOD GUIDELINES

The USDA and other health agencies generally seem to hesitate to provide specific information on the antioxidant capacity of different common foods. As noted in Chapter 3 on antioxidants, a branch of the USDA, the Nutrient Data Laboratory (NDL) of the Agricultural Research Service (ARS), published research on antioxidants in the document *USDA Database for the Oxygen Radical Absorbance Capacity (ORAC) of Selected Foods* in 2007 and listed the ORAC values of 171 foods (Ames et al. 1993).

ORAC is a measure of the quantity of free radicals that the antioxidants in a given food can absorb or neutralize—therefore, the more antioxidant capacity, presumably, the better. But in all fairness, that is not absolutely certain. Then, in 2012, the USDA repudiated the research on ORAC and the NDL removed the USDA ORAC database of selected foods from the NDL website, allegedly because of "mounting evidence that the values indicating antioxidant capacity have no relevance to the effects of specific bioactive compounds, including polyphenols on human health" (http://www.ars.usda.gov/nutrientdata/ORAC).

Removal of the antioxidant database is unfortunate, as many medical sources including the highly respected *Nutrition Journal* (2010) point out:

> This [antioxidant] database is to our best knowledge the most comprehensive Antioxidant Food Database published and it shows that plant-based foods introduce significantly more antioxidants into human diet than non-plant foods. Because of the large variations observed between otherwise comparable food samples the study emphasizes the importance of using a comprehensive database combined with a detailed system for food registration in clinical and epidemiological studies. The present antioxidant database is therefore an essential research tool to further elucidate the potential health effects of phytochemical antioxidants in diet. (Carlsen et al. 2010)

However, to put this skirmish in context, science now tells us that ORAC alone—any antioxidant measure, for that matter—is not an altogether reliable indication of the antioxidant capacity of a given food. There are of course other constituents in the food and biochemical characteristics of the food that also contribute to how antioxidants circulate—or do not circulate—in the body, how long they last there, and how they interact and function. This is their "pharmacokinetics."

6.12 THE PHARMACOKINETICS OF ANTIOXIDANTS

When one consumes some broccoli fleurets at dinner, what happens to the antioxidants they contain? A study published in the journal *Clinical Pharmacokinetics*, in 2003, evaluated a number of micronutrients as antioxidant constituents in the human diet.

This article addressed data from clinical trials, highlighting the clinical pharmacokinetics of vitamin C, vitamin E, beta-carotene, lycopene, lutein, quercetin, rutin, catechins, and selenium. In summary and in part, they found, for instance, that:

- The bioavailability of vitamin C is dose-dependent: saturation of transport occurs with dosages of 200–400 mg/day.
- Vitamin C is not protein-bound and is eliminated with a half-life of 10 hours.
- Alpha-tocopherol is the most abundant tocopherol in human tissue. Elimination of alpha-tocopherol takes several days.
- Elimination of carotenoids takes several days.
- The bioconversion of beta-carotene is dose-dependent, and ranges between 27% and 2% for 6 and 126 mg doses, respectively.
- Several oxidized metabolites of carotenoids are known.
- Flavonols such as quercetin glycosides and rutin are predominantly absorbed bound to plasma proteins.
- The bioavailability of catechins is low and they are eliminated within 2–4 hours (Schwedhelm et al. 2003).

It is beyond the scope of this book to detail antioxidant pharmacokinetics, but here is the tantalizing title of a study published in the journal *Free Radical Biology & Medicine*, in 2007: "Why clinical trials of vitamin E and cardiovascular diseases may be fatally flawed. Commentary on 'The relationship between dose of vitamin e and suppression of oxidative stress in humans'" (Blumberg and Frei 2007).

Here is another one of many examples: the *Journal of Agriculture and Food Chemistry* reported, in 2008, on "Pharmacokinetics of anthocyanins and antioxidant effects after the consumption of anthocyanin-rich acai juice and pulp (*Euterpe oleracea* Mart.) in human healthy volunteers." The antioxidant capacity of acai pulp in applesauce was compared to just applesauce and a non-antioxidant beverage. It was found that plasma antioxidant capacity was significantly increased by the acai pulp and applesauce compared to the plain applesauce and non-antioxidant beverage (Mertens-Talcott et al. 2008). It is likely that anyone might have guessed that, but the study actually provided specific quantities and values.

Clearly, there is no simple explanation of the absorption of antioxidants and their use by the body. To all extents and purposes, it is reasonable to assume, barring unforeseen conditions, that one will get all the exogenous antioxidants needed in the

Proactive Nutrition Program, although it may never be known exactly how many free radicals are being zapped at the lunch counter or the dinner table.

6.13 THE PRUDENT DIET

The term "Heart-Healthy diet" is commonly associated with the American Heart Association (AHA) (http://circ.ahajournals.org/content/94/7/1795.full). Introduced in 1956 as the "Prudent diet," it proposed to reduce the incidence of coronary heart disease (CHD) at a time when that condition had become the leading cause of disability and death in the US. Excessive alcohol intake was added because of its association with hypertension, stroke, and other diseases (Krauss et al. 1996).

It is a fat- and cholesterol-controlled diet, curtailing the intake of eggs, whole milk, and whole milk-based dairy products, liver, shellfish, and commercial pastry products. Lean meats are permitted, but preference is given to fish recommended for use at least four or five times a week (Livingston 1973).

The diet was found to result in a 24% decrease in the risk of cardiovascular and heart disease compared to the 46% increased risk from the Western diet—a net difference of 70% (Adams and Standridge 2006; Fung et al. 2001b; Hu 2003) (see Table 6.1).

The Prudent diet/Heart-Healthy diet is in some respects similar to the Mediterranean diet discussed below and stands in stark contrast to the Western diet, also known as the Standard American Diet (SAD).

What is the contribution of this diet to longevity via preserving telomere length? As noted previously, telomere length is ordinarily observed in *leukocytes*, white immune system blood cells. In a study published in 2015 in the *European Journal of Clinical Nutrition*, investigators compared the "Prudent dietary pattern" to the "Western dietary pattern" characterized by high intake of refined grain, red meat or processed meat, and sweetened carbonated beverages. They found that in Korean adults, the Prudent dietary pattern was associated with longer telomeres. Furthermore, they concluded that a diet over the remote past, that is even 10 years earlier, may affect the degree of biological aging in middle-aged and older adults (Lee et al. 2015).

Although there is some evidence that the Prudent/Heart-Healthy dietary pattern can exert a protective influence on telomere length, a search of the US National Library of Medicine PubMed databases for "Prudent diet AND sirtuin" and "Heart Healthy Diet AND sirtuin" did not turn up support for its activating Sirtuin 1, per se, unlike the Mediterranean diet.

6.14 THE WESTERN DIET, ALSO KNOWN AS THE SAD

The Western dietary pattern originally identified isolated commonly associated foods in the diets of several independent cohorts in the United States (and elsewhere) with a very similar "Western" pattern. It has higher intakes of red and processed meat, butter, high-fat dairy products, eggs, refined grains, white potatoes and French fries, and high-sugar drinks. That is in contrast to a Prudent pattern diet found in the same populations, that has higher levels of fruits, vegetables, whole-grain foods, poultry, and fish (Fung et al. 2001a; Hu 2002).

TABLE 6.1

The Benefits and Sources of Selected Heart-Healthy Foods

Category	Benefits	Sources/Preferred foods
Whole grains	Good source of fiber, minerals, and vitamins E and B	Whole wheat, oats, rye, barley, corn, brown rice and wild rice
	Delay gastric emptying and blunts postprandial insulin response	Whole-grain oatmeal, whole-grain, pumpernickel, rye or dark bread
	Improve insulin sensitivity	Whole-grain, ready-to-eat cereal
	$\Downarrow$ Insulin secretion	Cooked cereal
	$\Downarrow$ Insulin resistance, and diabetes	Pasta
	Improve lipids ($\Uparrow$ HDL)	Popcorn
	$\Downarrow$ Hypertension	Bran
	$\Downarrow$ CVD incidence and CVD mortality	Buckwheat, cracked wheat, wheat germ
Fruits and vegetables	Rich in fiber, flavonoids, and antioxidants	Green leafy vegetables
	$\Downarrow$ Blood pressure	Carotenoid vegetables (carrots,
	$\Downarrow$ LDL	broccoli, spinach, lettuce, tomato, and
	$\Uparrow$ HDL	yellow squash)
	$\Downarrow$ Homocysteine	Citrus (vitamin C-rich) fruits
	$\Downarrow$ CVD and mortality	Temperate fruits (cantaloupe, apple, pear)
	$\Downarrow$ Cancer, especially GI tract	Tropical fruits (mango, papaya,
	$\Downarrow$ All-cause mortality	pineapple, jackfruit, guava, banana)
Viscous fiber	$\Downarrow$ LDL	Cereal grain (oats-beta glucan)
	$\Downarrow$ Postprandial glycemia	Legumes, psyllium (Metamucil)
Soy protein	$\Downarrow$ LDL	Soy bean
Plant sterols and stanols	$\Downarrow$ LDL	Low-fat plant stanols containing margarines
Nuts	$\Downarrow$ LDL	
	$\Uparrow$ HDL	

Source: From Kavita Chhibber. 2007. *The Benefits and Sources of Selected Heart-Healthy Foods.* Available at http://www.kavitachhibber.com/main/main.jsp?id=health-Jul2007. With permission.
Note: CVD, cardiovascular disease; GI, gastrointestinal tract

The Western diet, also known as SAD, features high calories and low antioxidant foods, and low intake of vegetables (and to a lesser extent, low consumption of fruit).

6.14.1 The Western Diet Compromises Health

There is little doubt that the Western pattern diet compromises health and longevity by its emphasis on high sugar, high carbohydrates, high saturated fats, and low concentrations of antioxidants. These factors have been linked to poor health. The diet pattern is nutrient poor and energy dense. In a report appearing in 2005 in the *American Journal of Clinical Nutrition*, investigators propose that the nutritional qualities of the foods in that diet pattern may underlie many of the chronic diseases of Western civilization (Cordain et al. 2005).

In the United States, chronic illnesses and health problems either wholly or partially attributable to diet represent by far the most serious threat to public health: 65% of adults in the United States, aged 20 years or older, are either overweight or obese (Hedley et al. 2004) and the estimated number of deaths attributable to obesity is 280,184 per year (Allison et al. 1999).

The following examples describe clinical research findings pointing to the Western pattern diet as a hazard causally implicated in major chronic medical disorders. It should be noted that each of the reports that follows is only one of the many that are readily available on medical databases including PubMed.gov, the website of the US National Library of Medicine, National Institutes of Health (NIH), all websites accessible to the consumer public as well.

6.14.2   THE WESTERN DIET AND OBESITY

Researchers from the Department of Nutrition, Harvard School of Public Health compared the Western and Prudent diets for indications of obesity and cardiovascular disease (CVD) risk. They isolated dietary patterns in men participants in the Health Professionals Follow-up Study using dietary information from food-frequency questionnaires (FFQs). They report finding significant correlations between the Western pattern and insulin response deficiency, and other markers of obesity and metabolic dysfunction which also increase CVD risk (Fung et al. 2001a).

In another study, one with an unusual twist, individuals having a high Western pattern score were more likely to be obese, while those having a high Prudent pattern score were less so. The findings also indicated that obesity following a Western pattern diet was linked to those participants having at least one obese first-degree relative. This interesting observation suggests that the adverse impact of a Western pattern diet is most likely to impact individuals with an inherited obesity *phenotype*, that is, an observable inherited characteristic that is, however, not due solely to genes (Paradis et al. 2009). It should be noted that the general impact of the Western diet in promoting obesity is not a geographically isolated phenomenon: it was reported in such disparate locations as Brazil (Sichieri 2002) and Iran (Esmaillzadeh and Azadbakht 2008).

6.14.3   THE WESTERN DIET AND METABOLIC SYNDROME

A significant predictive association exists between dietary patterns, metabolic syndrome, and insulin resistance; participants in one nutrition study who ranked in the upper 20% of Prudent dietary pattern scores had a lower odds ratio (OR) for metabolic syndrome and insulin resistance than did those in the lowest 20%. Compared with those in the lowest 20%, women in the highest 20% of Western dietary pattern scores had greater odds for developing metabolic syndrome and insulin resistance (Esmaillzadeh et al. 2007).

Investigators from the Division of Epidemiology and Community Health, University of Minnesota, School of Public Health, Minneapolis, and the Department of Nutrition, University of North Carolina, Chapel Hill, examined the role of diet in the origin of metabolic syndrome using prospective data from participants enrolled in the Atherosclerosis Risk in Communities (ARIC) study. They found that a Western dietary pattern was adversely associated with incident metabolic syndrome.

After further adjustment for intake of meat, dairy, fruit and vegetables, refined grains, and whole grains, analysis of individual food groups revealed that meat, fried foods, and diet soda also were adversely associated with incident metabolic syndrome. No such associations were observed in connection with a Prudent dietary pattern or intakes of whole grains, refined grains, fruit and vegetables, nuts, coffee, or sweetened beverages. The authors concluded that consuming Western dietary pattern foods promotes the incidence of metabolic syndrome (Lutsey et al. 2008).

The prevalence of metabolic syndrome has increased even in Korea, making it a public health issue. In a study, it was found that the Prudent dietary pattern was inversely associated with the risk of metabolic syndrome; the highest 20% adhering to the Prudent dietary pattern were significantly less likely to develop metabolic syndrome than the lowest 20%. This finding was similar for all metabolic syndrome diagnostic criteria: abdominal obesity, elevated blood pressure, elevated triglycerides, elevated fasting glucose, and high-density lipoprotein cholesterol (Choi et al. 2015).

6.14.4 Metabolic Syndrome Shortens Telomeres

Researchers from the University Medical Center in Amsterdam and the University of California, San Francisco found that hallmarks of metabolic syndrome, higher waist circumference, elevated glucose, and lower HDL were consistently associated with shorter leukocyte telomeres during follow-up. A greater 6-year increase in waist circumference was associated with greater telomere attrition (Révész et al. 2015).

6.14.5 The Western Diet and Hypertension

The Western diet pattern combination of foods that promotes hypertension does not respect geographical boundaries. For instance, participants in Australia who had high blood pressure also had a higher intake of Western pattern foods and a lower intake of Prudent dietary pattern foods. Intake of Western and snack and alcohol dietary patterns increases the likelihood of having high blood pressure (Khalesi et al. 2016). Similar findings were reported from Korea (Shin et al. 2013).

The objective of this study is to identify the dietary patterns associated with the risk of hypertensions among Korean adults using data from the Korean National Health and Nutrition Examination Survey (KNHANES 2008–2010). This study analyzes data from 11,883 subjects who participated in the health and nutrition survey, aging from 20 to 64 years. We performed factor analysis based on the weekly mean intake frequencies of 36 food groups to identify major dietary patterns. We identified three major dietary patterns in both sexes, namely "traditional," "western," and "dairy and carbohydrate" patterns. Participants in the highest quartile of Western pattern scores had significantly higher blood pressure, serum total cholesterol, and triglyceride levels than those in the lowest quartile. Although not statistically significant, a trend (P for trend = 0.0732) toward a positive association between the western dietary pattern and hypertension risk was observed after adjustments for age, sex, education, income, body mass index (BMI), smoking, physical activity, and energy intake. The dairy and carbohydrate pattern was inversely related with BMI and blood pressures and positively associated with serum high-density lipoprotein (HDL)-cholesterol. After adjusting the age, sex, education, income, BMI, smoking, physical activity, and energy intake, the dairy and carbohydrate pattern showed inverse associations with hypertension prevalence (OR = 0.64, 95% CI = 0.55-0.75;P for trend < 0.0001). Intakes of fiber, sodium, and antioxidant vitamins were significantly higher in the top quartile for the traditional pattern than in the lowest quartile for the traditional pattern (P for trend < 0.0001). Intakes of fiber (P for trend < 0.0001), calcium (P for trend < 0.0001), retinol (P for trend = 0.0164), vitamin B_1 (P for trend = 0.001), vitamin B_2 (P for trend < 0.0001), niacin (P for trend = 0.0025), and vitamin C (P for trend < 0.0001) were significantly increased across quartiles for the dairy and carbohydrate pattern, whereas sodium (P for trend < 0.0001) intake was decreased for this pattern. In conclusion, the dairy and carbohydrate pattern may be associated with a reduced risk of hypertension, whereas the western pattern may be associated with an increased risk of hypertension among Korean adults.

6.14.6 THE WESTERN DIET AND CARDIOVASCULAR AND HEART DISEASE

In 2014, the *British Medical Journal* published a meta-analysis of data from scientific publications reporting the relationship between the telomere length of white blood immune cells (leukocytes) and cardiovascular and heart disease. The analysis summarizes the findings of many similar studies. The authors concluded that the greater the risk of coronary heart disease, the shorter the telomeres (Haycock et al. 2014).

Diet is acknowledged to be a major modifiable risk factor for cardiovascular disease, but it varies markedly in different regions of the world. One of the objectives of the INTERHEART study was to assess the association between dietary patterns and acute myocardial infarction (AMI) in participants from 52 countries. Three major dietary patterns were identified: the Oriental (high intake of tofu and soy and other sauces), the Western (high in fried foods, salty snacks, eggs, and meat), and the Prudent diets (high in fruit and vegetables). The investigators concluded that there is an inverse relationship between the Prudent pattern and AMI, with higher levels being protective. An unhealthy dietary intake increases the risk of AMI globally and may account for as much as 30% of the population-attributable risk (Iqbal et al. 2008).

In another study, researchers documented more than 1000 cases of nonfatal myocardial infarction and fatal coronary heart disease (CHD) over an 8-year follow-up period. They identified two major dietary patterns using dietary data collected through a food questionnaire: a Prudent pattern and a Western pattern. After adjustment for age and CHD risk factors, the relative risks of those scoring high in the Prudent pattern were lower than for those scoring high in the Western pattern. These associations persisted in subgroup analyses according to cigarette smoking, body mass index, and parental history of myocardial infarction.

These data suggest that major dietary patterns predict risk of CHD, independent of other lifestyle variables (Hu et al. 2000). Similar results were obtained in a study using data from the 1984 Nurses' Health Study cited earlier. The Western diet raises the risk of CHD in women (Hu 2003).

6.14.6.1 Cardiovascular and Heart Disease Shorten Telomeres

The journal of the American Heart Association (AHA), *Circulation*, reported in 2000 that mean telomere length (TL) in white blood cells is shorter in those who are developing coronary heart disease (CHD), data also noted above. The study examined telomere length in young men (mean age 25 years), older men (mean age 65 years), healthy male volunteers, and age-matched patients with CHD (mean age 65 years). It was also found that telomere shortening is not restricted to any particular type of cell as it was found comparably in many types.

Finally, telomere shortening was correlated with the decrease in left ventricular function in CHD patients and showed a very strong correlation with cardiac dysfunction. This suggests a link between CHD and immune cell senescence due to more rapid cycling (Spyridopoulos et al. 2000).

6.14.7 THE WESTERN DIET AND TYPE 2 DIABETES

Major dietary patterns were studied for their ability to predict type 2 diabetes mellitus in a cohort of over 4000 Finnish men and women aged 40–69 years, and free of diabetes at baseline in 1967–1972. Dietary patterns were identified from dietary data collected using a 1-year dietary history interview. A total of 383 incident cases of type 2 diabetes occurred during a 23-year follow-up. Two major dietary patterns were identified, the typical Prudent and the "conservative" pattern similar to the Western pattern.

The Prudent dietary pattern score was associated with a reduced risk of type 2 diabetes, whereas the "conservative" pattern score was associated with an increased risk. The authors conclude that in light of these results, it is conceivable that the risk of developing type 2 diabetes can be reduced by changing dietary patterns (Montonen et al. 2005).

The Western diet is known to be a major risk factor in type 2 diabetes. However, as in other instances of the adverse impact of that diet, a genetic link may predispose some people more than others. In 2009, investigators from the Harvard School of Public Health, Boston, the Department of Epidemiology, Harvard School of Public Health, Boston, and related institutions reported finding that a variant in the form of a *genetic risk score* (GRS) raised the risk created by adherence to a Western pattern diet. The diet–diabetes connection was more evident among men with a high GRS than among those with a low GRS (Qi et al. 2009).

6.14.7.1 Type 2 Diabetes Shortens Telomeres

Investigators conducted a *meta-analysis* (analysis of data published previously and reported in PubMed, Embase, and Web of Science databases) of studies on the association between telomere length and type 2 diabetes. Their results indicated that shortened telomere length was significantly associated with type 2 diabetes risk (Zhao et al. 2013). It is believed that the association is causal.

In another study, it was also found that type 2 diabetes and atherosclerosis shortens telomeres: the average measure of telomere length was significantly lower in those with impaired glucose tolerance, and still lower in type 2 diabetic individuals without plaque, and lowest in type 2 diabetic subjects with atherosclerotic plaque. Measures of telomere length were higher in those with higher HDL cholesterol, and lower in those with high glycated hemoglobin (HbA1c). Among participants with type 2 diabetes, those with atherosclerotic plaque had greater shortening of telomere length compared to those without plaque (Adaikalakoteswar et al. 2006). The bottom line is that the Western diet, also known as SAD, is poor in antioxidants and shortens telomeres (Hallows et al. 2012).

It was shown in Chapter 1 that many basic functions normally decline with age. But the degree of decline that precipitates premature aging, as it relates to the rate of cell cycling, is clearly strongly affected by regular dietary pattern. As can be seen, evidence of the hazards of an imprudent diet such as the Western diet pattern is well documented. Scientific evidence is often controversial but is not invariably controversial; it would be very difficult to find conventional clinical research studies that conclude that the Western diet is the ideal diet for maximum health and longevity.

Furthermore, the Western diet does not activate the life-prolonging protein, Sirtuin 1. Activating Sirtuin 1 requires either calorie restriction—for which that diet is not noted—and/or specific foods in the diet, which has been previously mentioned as the main feature of the Proactive Nutrition Program.

6.15 THE PROACTIVE NUTRITION PROGRAM

The Proactive Nutrition Program is the Mediterranean diet enhanced by sirtfoods in addition to those already in that diet. A food plan and recipes are given in Chapter 7.

6.15.1 The Mediterranean Pattern Diet

The Mediterranean diet, developed by Dr. Ancel Keys (1904–2004) in connection with the Seven Countries Study (SCS) in 1958, examined the relationship between dietary pattern and the prevalence of coronary heart disease in Greece, Italy, Spain, South Africa, Japan, and Finland. This diet is beneficial because of its low energy (calories), low glycemic index, high fiber content, high L-arginine, high nitrates, high polyphenolic, anthocyanidin and other antioxidants, and its activation of sirtuin 1 (Chatzianagnostou et al. 2015).

The Mediterranean diet consists largely of:

- Minimally processed foods
- Olive oil as the principal fat, replacing other fats and oils (including butter and margarine), with total fat ranging from less than 25% to over 35% of energy, and saturated fat providing no more than 7–8% of energy (calories)
- Daily consumption of low to moderate amounts of cheese and yogurt
- Twice weekly consumption of fish and poultry (up to seven eggs per week)
- Fresh fruit as the typical daily dessert
- Red meat limited to a maximum of 12–16 oz (340–450 g) per month, and moderate consumption of wine

6.15.1.1   The Mediterranean Pattern Diet Protects Telomeres

The white immune system cell (leukocyte) telomere length (LTL) and the rate of telomere shortening are known biological markers of aging. Using these markers as indicators, numerous studies have demonstrated that the Mediterranean diet may boost longevity. The following study was conducted to test the correspondence between LTL and adherence to a Mediterranean diet and its effects on health status.

In a study reported in the journal *PLoS One*, in 2013, LTL was measured in a large number of elderly people with low, medium, and high Mediterranean diet adherence scores. Those in the high adherence-score group showed longer LTL compared with the others (Boccardi et al. 2013).

The Nurses' Health Study, an ongoing prospective cohort study of over 120,000 women that began in 1976, also aimed to determine whether adherence to the Mediterranean diet was associated with longer telomere length. Each participant provided blood samples used to measure telomere length, and a completed food frequency questionnaire. It was found that greater adherence to the Mediterranean diet was associated with longer telomeres (Crous-Bou et al. 2014).

6.15.1.2   The Mediterranean Diet Activates Sirtuin 1

According to a recent medical research report, the Mediterranean diet has anti-aging as well as many other beneficial effects such as a reduced risk of age-related medical conditions including cardiovascular, metabolic and neurodegenerative diseases, and cancer. The effects are not limited to the reduction in oxidative stress by compounds present in the diet.

New studies have shown that activating sirtuins has anti-aging effects. For instance, resveratrol, a polyphenol present in grapes, nuts, and berries, has been shown to activate sirtuins, and such activation is said to explain most of the beneficial effects of the diet because it mimics calorie restriction, a factor in longevity (López-Miranda et al. 2012; Pallauf et al. 2013; Russo et al. 2014).

6.15.1.3   The Mediterranean Diet and Obesity

Another study (Schroder et al. 2004) examined the relationship between body mass index (BMI) and obesity based on the level of adherence to the traditional Mediterranean diet. About 1500 Spanish men and 1600 Spanish women ranging in age group from 25 to 74 years participated in the study. A Mediterranean pattern diet score, including foods considered to be characteristic components of the traditional Mediterranean diet (vegetables, fruits, pulses, nuts, fish, meat, cereals, olive oil, and wine), was developed.

The obesity risk decreased in men and women with increasing adherence to the traditional Mediterranean dietary pattern. Both men and women with the top third scores were less likely to be obese. These data suggest that BMI and obesity decrease as the traditional Mediterranean dietary pattern score increases (Schroder et al. 2004).

During the period 2005—2007, elderly men and elderly women (mean age 74 years) from eight Mediterranean islands in Greece and Cyprus participated in a study on demographic, clinical, and dietary characteristics. The conventional MedDietScore was used to assess adherence to the Mediterranean dietary pattern.

The prevalence of diabetes, hypercholesterolemia, and hypertension was higher in the obese elderly than in the simply overweight or in those with normal weight. It was found that a one unit increase in the MedDietScore resulted in an 88% decrease in the likelihood of being obese. The authors concluded that greater adherence to the Mediterranean diet may reduce the burden of obesity among elderly individuals (Tyrovolas et al. 2009).

In a study conducted in Naples, Italy, and published in the *Journal of the American Medical Association* (*JAMA*) in 2003, investigators found that after 2 years, women randomly assigned to an intervention group who received detailed advice on weight reduction through a low-energy Mediterranean-style diet, consumed more foods rich in complex carbohydrates, monounsaturated fat, and fiber, had a lower ratio of omega-6 to omega-3 fatty acids, and had lower energy (calories), saturated fat, and cholesterol intake than a control group. Their BMI decreased and so did serum insulin sensitivity. The authors also noted that there was a significant reduction in markers of blood vessel inflammation and in insulin resistance (Esposito et al. 2003).

6.15.1.4 The Mediterranean Diet and Metabolic Syndrome

Mounting evidence suggests that the Mediterranean diet could help fight diseases that are related to chronic inflammation, including visceral obesity, type 2 diabetes, and metabolic syndrome (Giugliano and Esposito 2008). Because the Mediterranean diet has long been associated with low cardiovascular disease risk in the adult population, investigators conducted a large-scale meta-analysis of epidemiological and clinical studies from databases such as PubMed, Embase, Web of Science, and the Cochrane Central Register of Controlled Trials until April 30, 2010. The database covered about 534,900 participants.

Analysis showed that adherence to the Mediterranean diet was associated with reduced risk of metabolic syndrome and, in addition, results from clinical studies revealed the protective role of the Mediterranean diet on waist circumference, HDL cholesterol, triglycerides, systolic and diastolic blood pressure, and insulin/glucose. Results from epidemiological studies confirmed those of clinical trials (Kastorini et al. 2011).

This study appearing in the journal *Diabetes Care* was a prospective longitudinal cohort study, a study that follows, over time, a group of similar individuals (cohorts) who differ with respect to certain factors under study, to determine how these factors affect rates of outcome. It reported an inverse relationship between adherence to a Mediterranean diet pattern and cumulative incidence of metabolic syndrome. The results are consistent with previous findings of an inverse association between adherence to a Mediterranean diet and obesity, diabetes, insulin resistance, or hypertension. The "prospective" aspect of the study means that information about risk factors for metabolic syndrome, food habits, and lifestyles was collected before the diagnosis of the disease (Tortosa et al. 2007).

6.16 PROMOTING SIRTUINS

The beneficial effects of the Mediterranean diet in reducing insulin resistance, a component of metabolic syndrome, play a significant role in promoting expression of the longevity-promoting sirtuin 1 (de Kreutzenberg et al. 2010). Sirtfoods in a Mediterranean-style diet combat metabolic syndrome, thus reducing the risk factors leading to premature aging, even premature death (Guarente 2006).

6.17 HYPERTENSION AND CARDIOVASCULAR AND HEART FUNCTION: COMPARING THE MEDITERRANEAN DIET TO ANOTHER LOW-FAT DIET

This study published in 2006 in the journal *Annals of Internal Medicine* was designed to compare the short-term effects on cardiovascular risk of two Mediterranean diets versus those of another low-fat diet. Ten teaching hospitals were involved in the study.

Participants were to follow a low-fat diet or one of two Mediterranean diets. Those allocated to Mediterranean diets received nutritional education and either free virgin olive oil (1 liter per week) or free nuts (30 g/day). Outcome was evaluated after 3 months.

Compared with the low-fat diet, the two Mediterranean diets produced beneficial changes in most outcomes.

Compared with the low-fat diet, the mean changes in the Mediterranean diet with olive oil group and the Mediterranean diet with nuts group were significant reductions in plasma glucose levels, blood pressure, and the cholesterol to HDL cholesterol ratio. The Mediterranean diet with olive oil significantly reduced C-reactive protein (CRP), a marker of inflammation, compared with the low-fat diet (see Chapter 8 on functional foods) (Estruch et al. 2006).

In another study appearing in *The New England Journal of Medicine*, a Mediterranean diet supplemented with extra-virgin olive oil or nuts reduced the incidence of major cardiovascular events in persons at high cardiovascular risk. It was therefore recommended as a primary prevention of cardiovascular disease (Estruch et al. 2013).

6.18 THE MEDITERRANEAN DIET AND ELEVATED SERUM CHOLESTEROL

Investigators reported in 2007 that men and women participants at high cardiovascular risk (age range: 55–80 years) were recruited into a large, multicenter, clinical trial directed at testing the efficacy of the traditional Mediterranean diet (TMD) for the primary prevention of coronary heart disease. The participants were assigned to a low-fat diet or one of two TMDs (TMD+virgin olive oil or TMD+nuts). The TMD participants received nutritional education and either free virgin olive oil for all the family (1 L/week) or free nuts (30 g/day). Changes were evaluated after 3 months.

After the 3-month interventions, mean oxidized low-density lipoprotein (LDL) levels decreased significantly in the TMD+virgin olive oil and TMD+nuts groups, with no such changes in the low-fat diet group. The decrease in oxidized LDL levels in the TMD+virgin olive oil group was greater than that of the low-fat group.

The investigators concluded that individuals at high cardiovascular risk who improved their diet toward a TMD pattern showed significant reductions in cellular lipid levels and LDL oxidation: "Results provide further evidence to recommend the Traditional Mediterranean Diet as a useful tool against risk factors for CHD" (Fitó et al. 2007).

6.19 THE MEDITERRANEAN DIET AND HYPERTENSION

The *Journal of Hypertension*, in 2003, reported the prevalence, awareness, treatment, and control of hypertension in Greece, in a random sample of adults free of cardiovascular disease, and evaluated the association between hypertension and adoption of the Mediterranean diet.

The prevalence of hypertension was 38.2% in men and 23.9% in women. The majority of men and women were untreated, and of those who were treated, only 109 of 319 (34%) had their blood pressure adequately controlled. Thus, only 15% of the hypertensive population had their blood pressure well controlled.

Consumption of a Mediterranean diet was associated with a 26% lower risk of being hypertensive, and with a 36% greater probability of having the blood pressure controlled. It was concluded that consumption of a Mediterranean type diet seems to reduce rates of hypertension in the population (Panagiotakos et al. 2003).

As previously noted, the endothelium is the cell inner-lining of blood vessels that regulates their function by producing the gas nitric oxide (NO). Hypertension and cardiovascular and heart disease have been linked to dysfunction of the endothelium/NO mechanism. In fact, one of the newer anti-hypertensive beta-blocker prescription medications, Bystolic (nebivolol), is a nitric oxide (NO)-potentiating medication (Weiss 2006).

6.20 THE MEDITERRANEAN DIET AND ENDOTHELIUM FUNCTION

Patients with metabolic syndrome were assigned to follow either a Mediterranean diet or a Prudent low-fat diet for 2½ years. At the end of the study, 44% of patients in the Mediterranean diet group still had metabolic syndrome, compared with 86% in the control group. The Mediterranean diet group also had improvements in several risk factors:

- Body weight decreased by 8.8 lbs in the Mediterranean diet group compared with 2.6 lbs in the low-fat control group.
- Endothelial function score improved in the Mediterranean diet group, but remained stable in the low-fat control group.
- Inflammatory markers (hs-CRP) and insulin resistance decreased significantly in the Mediterranean diet group (Esposito et al. 2004).

6.20.1 AVERTING PREMATURE AGING OF THE ENDOTHELIUM

Just like the other functions mentioned in Chapter 1, the lining of blood vessels, the endothelium, is subject to progressive age-related decline in its ability to synthesize the nitric oxide (NO) needed to control blood flow and blood pressure. As NO production declines with age (see Chapter 5), the risk of hypertension rises.

By age 40 years, blood vessels can produce only about half the NO that they could produce when younger. And so, systolic blood pressure naturally just keeps rising and there is good reason to believe that it is because, simultaneously, NO formation by the endothelium is declining (Izzo et al. 2000).

It is advisable therefore to prevent premature aging of the endothelium and preserve control of blood pressure. This can be accomplished with the sirtuin activators-enhanced Mediterranean diet, that is, the Proactive Nutrition Program.

NO performs many functions in the body including retarding the formation of atherosclerotic plaque in blood vessels. As the journal *Circulation Research* reported in 2000, age-related impairment in NO formation leads to cell senescence (Vasa et al. 2000). However, the Mediterranean diet, rich in leafy vegetables high in nitrates, and other foods rich in the amino acid, L-arginine, can actually reverse impairment in the formation of NO, thus protecting blood vessels and preventing premature cell senescence (Chauhan et al. 1996; Fried and Edlen-Nezin 2006; Lidder and Webb 2013).

6.21   SIRTUINS AND BLOOD VESSEL AND HEART HEALTH

There are many reports of the protective effect of activating sirtuins on cardiovascular and heart health. For instance, the *European Heart Journal*, in 2015, reported that sirtuins decrease inflammation, reduce serum cholesterol, and beneficially impact numerous aspects of cardiovascular disease (Winnik et al. 2015). Other investigators propose that there may be a decline in cardiac mitochondrial function due to oxidative stress damage and that this decline might be responsible, at least in part, for the decline in cardiac performance with age. They speculate that in cardiac function, sirtuins reduce the accumulation of oxidative damage due to free radicals as we age (Shinmura 2013).

6.21.1   SIRTUIN 1 AND CORONARY HEART DISEASE

A recent article in the *European Heart Journal* describes the *proactive* effects of activating SIRT1 on coronary arteries (Winnik et al. 2015; see also Matsushima and Sadoshima 2015).

6.22   THE MEDITERRANEAN DIET AND TYPE 2 DIABETES

The journal *Diabetic Medicine* reported a study of the relationship between glycated hemoglobin (HbA1c) and adherence to a Mediterranean-type diet assessed by a 9-point scale that incorporated the salient characteristics of this diet (range of scores 0–9, with higher scores indicating greater adherence).

Diabetic patients with the highest scores (6–9) had lower body mass index and waist circumferences, a lower prevalence of metabolic syndrome, and lower HbA1c and post-meal glucose levels than diabetic patients with the lowest scores (0–3). Mean HbA1c and 2-hour post-meal glucose concentrations were significantly lower in diabetic patients with high adherence to a Mediterranean-type diet than those with low adherence.

In type 2 diabetes, greater adherence to a Mediterranean-type diet is associated with lower HbA1c and post-meal glucose levels (Esposito et al. 2009). In a subsequent report published in *Diabetes Research and Clinical Practice*, the authors concluded that not only does adopting a Mediterranean diet help prevent type 2 diabetes, but it also improves glycemic control and reduces cardiovascular risk in patients with established diabetes (Esposito et al. 2010).

6.23   ACTIVATING SIRTUINS IMPROVES TYPE 2 DIABETES

A report published in the journal *Nature*, in 2007, concludes that activating sirtuin 1 has beneficial effects on glucose balance and insulin sensitivity: sirtuin activators improve whole-body glucose balance and insulin sensitivity in adipose (fat) tissue, skeletal muscle, and liver. The authors of the study conclude that "SIRT1 activation is a promising new therapeutic approach for treating diseases of aging such as type 2 diabetes" (Milne et al. 2007).

6.24   A NOTE ON CALORIC RESTRICTION

Caloric restriction is known under certain circumstances to retard aging and delay functional decline as well as the onset of disease in most organisms. Studies have implicated the sirtuins (SIRT1–SIRT7) as mediators of key effects of caloric restriction during aging (see discussion on xenohormesis in Chapter 7). Two unrelated molecules have been shown to increase SIRT1 activity in some settings. First, resveratrol, found in red wine, was shown to be an excellent protector against metabolic stress in mammals: scientists reported in the *Journal of Cell Biology*, in 2010, that sirtuin 1 protects us from DNA damage (Mattson 2008).

Second, an additional reason why the Mediterranean diet offers health benefits is that it supplies a high concentration of green vegetables and colorful fruits with some fish and relatively little red meat. This diet is a rich source of antioxidants and nitrate.

The 1998 Nobel Prize in Medicine was awarded to three American scientists who discovered the secret of healthy cardiovascular and heart function to be formation of a gas, nitric oxide (NO), in our body. NO keeps blood flowing unimpaired in our blood vessels, thus controlling blood pressure and heart function. NO is formed from two major sources, dietary nitrates and the amino acid L-arginine (Fried and Merrell 1999). The science of NO and its value to our health is described in Chapter 5.

The Mediterranean diet is rich in vegetables high in nitrate, and is therefore a rich source of NO. The fish, meat (mostly lamb), and nuts in that diet are high in the amino acid L-arginine, another rich source of NO. In addition, the polyphenols and anthocyanidins in fruits and many vegetables in the diet are natural antioxidants that reduce oxidative stress, thus protecting the heart and blood vessels.

6.25   THE SECRET REVEALED

The Mediterranean diet is a healthy approach to eating because it also supplies NO to protect telomeres by promoting activation of sirtuin 1. In a report published in the journal *Circulation Research* in 2000, it is revealed that formation of nitric oxide

(NO)—which we can promote with the Proactive Nutrition Program—can prevent premature aging of blood vessels: "NO prevents... EC senescence." ("EC" stands for *endothelial cells*, the cells that line and regulate arterial blood vessels and blood flow throughout the body and in the heart.) Furthermore, the diet activates sirtuin 1 that, in turn, promotes NO in blood vessels (Cantó and Auwerx 2011; Potente 2010; Vasa et al. 2000).

6.26 THE CASE FOR THE PROACTIVE NUTRITION PROGRAM

It was shown that natural age-related decline in major body functions, such as control of blood pressure and blood sugar, does not in itself constitute disease. However, that is not the case with accelerated decline of functions. That is a hallmark of disease and is strongly associated with adherence to the Western pattern diet. Accelerated decline in function can be prevented by the Proactive Nutrition Program.

Experts made the case in the journal *PLoS One*, in 2013, that there is strong evidence for an association between adherence to the Mediterranean diet and a slower rate of telomere shortening. They aver that those who adhere to that diet may experience a lower rate of telomere shortening and a healthier life span (Boccardi et al. 2013). Diet makes all the difference.

The next chapter details the Proactive Nutrition Program and provides advice and sample recipes to implement it.

REFERENCES

Adaikalakoteswar, A., M. Balasubramanyam, R. Ravikumar, et al. 2006. Association of telomere shortening with impaired glucose tolerance and diabetic macroangiopathy. *Atherosclerosis*, 195(1):83–89. doi: http://dx.doi.org/10.1016/j.atherosclerosis.2006.12.003.

Adams, S. M., and J. B. Standridge. 2006. What should we eat? Evidence from observational studies. *Southern Medical Journal*, 99(7):744–748.

Allison, D. B., K. R. Fontaine, J. E. Manson, et al. 1999. Annual deaths attributable to obesity in the United States. *Journal of the American Medical Association*, 282:1530–538.

Ames, B. N., M. K. Shigenaga, and T. M. Hagen. 1993. Oxidants, antioxidants, and the degenerative diseases of aging. *Proceedings of the National Academy of Sciences, USA*, 90:7915–7922.

Anonymous. 1941. National nutrition conference for defense. *Proceedings of the National Nutrition Conference for Defense*. Washington, DC: Federal Security Agency.

Anonymous. 1946. *U.S. National Food Guide*. Department of Agriculture. AIS-53.

Anonymous. 1984. *Better Eating for Better Health: Instructor's Guide and Participants Packet*. Washington, DC: American National Red Cross.

Anonymous. 1995. *1995 Nutrition Trends Survey. Executive Summary*. Conducted by the Wirthlin Group for the American Dietetic Association. The American Dietetic Association.

Atwater, W. O. 1894. *Foods: Nutritive Value and Cost*. U.S. Department of Agriculture, Farmers Bulletin No. 23, Washington, DC: Government Printing Office. p. 357.

Blumberg, J. B., and B, Frei B. 2007. Why clinical trials of vitamin E and cardiovascular diseases may be fatally flawed. Commentary on "The Relationship Between Dose of Vitamin E and Suppression of Oxidative Stress in Humans." *Free Radical Biology & Medicine*, 43:1374–1376.

Boccardi, V., A. Esposito, M. R. Rizzo, et al. 2013. Mediterranean diet, telomere maintenance and health status among elderly. *PLoS One*, 8(4):e62781.

Cantó, C., and J. Auwerx. 2011. Targeting sirtuin 1 to improve metabolism: All you need is NAD+? *Pharmacological Reviews*, 64(1):166–187. doi: http://dx.doi.org/10.1124/pr.110.003905.

Carlsen, M. H., B. L. Halvorsen, K. Holte, et al. 2010. The total antioxidant content of more than 3100 foods, beverages, spices, herbs and supplements used worldwide. *Nutrition Journal*, 9:3.

Chatzianagnostou, K., S. Del Turco, A. Pingitore, et al. 2015. The Mediterranean lifestyle as a non-pharmacological and natural antioxidant for healthy aging. *Antioxidants*, 4:719–736.

Chauhan, A., R. S. More, P. A. Mullins, et al. 1996. Aging-associated endothelial dysfunction in humans is reversed by L-arginine. *Journal of the American College of Cardiology*, 28:1796–1804.

Choi, J.-W., H. D. Woo, J.-H. Lee, et al. 2015. Dietary patterns and risk for metabolic syndrome in Korean women. A cross-sectional study. *Medicine (Baltimore)*, 94(34):e1424.

Cleveland, L. E., B. B. Peterkin, A. J. Blum. 1983. Recommended dietary allowances as standards for family food plans. *Journal of Nutrition Education*, 15:8–14.

Cordain, L., S. B. Eaton, A. Sebastian, et al. 2005. Origins and evolution of the Western diet: Health implications for the 21st century. *American Journal of Clinical Nutrition*, 81(2):341–354.

Crous-Bou, M., T. T. Fung, J. Prescott, et al. 2014. Mediterranean diet and telomere length in Nurses' Health Study: Population based cohort study. *British Medical Journal*, 349:g6674.

Cypel, Y. S., J. A. Tamaki, C. W. Enns, et al. 1996. *Nutrition Attitudes and Dietary Status of Main Meal Planners/Preparers, 1989–1991: Results from 1989–1991 Diet and Health. Knowledge Survey and the 1989–1991 Continuing Survey of Food Intakes by Individuals*. U.S. Dept. Agr., Agr. Res. Serv., NFS Report No. 91-1, January.

de Kreutzenberg, S. V., G. Ceolotto, I. Papparella, et al. 2010. Downregulation of the longevity-associated protein sirtuin 1 in insulin resistance and metabolic syndrome: Potential biochemical mechanisms. *Diabetes*, 59(4):1006–1015.

DHHS Task Force sponsored by the American Society for Clinical Nutrition. 1979. The evidence relating six dietary factors to the nation's health. *American Journal of Clinical Nutrition*, 32:2621–2748.

Esmaillzadeh, A., and L. Azadbakht. 2008. Major dietary patterns in relation to general obesity and central adiposity among Iranian women. *The Journal of Nutrition*, 138:358–363.

Esmaillzadeh, A, M. Kimiagar, Y. Mehrabi, et al. 2007. Dietary patterns, insulin resistance, and prevalence of the metabolic syndrome in women. *American Journal of Clinical Nutrition*, 85(3):910–918.

Esposito, K., M. I. Maiorino, A. Ceriello, et al. 2010. Prevention and control of type 2 diabetes by Mediterranean diet: A systematic review. *Diabetes Research & Clinical Practice*, 89(2):97–102.

Esposito, K., M. I. Maiorino, C. Di Palo, et al. 2009. Adherence to a Mediterranean diet and glycaemic control in Type 2 diabetes mellitus. *Diabetic Medicine*, 26(9):900–907.

Esposito, K., R. Marfella, M. Ciotola, et al. 2004. Effect of a mediterranean-style diet on endothelial dysfunction and markers of vascular inflammation in the metabolic syndrome: A randomized trial. *The Journal of the American Medical Association*, 292(12):1440–1446.

Esposito, K., A. Pontillo, C. Di Palo, et al. 2003. Effect of weight loss and lifestyle changes on vascular inflammatory markers in obese women: A randomized trial. *Journal of the American Medical Association*, 289(14):1799–1804.

Estruch, R., M. A. Martinez-Gonzalez, D. Corella, et al. 2006. Effects of a mediterranean-style diet on cardiovascular risk factors. A randomized trial. *Annals of Internal Medicine*, 145:1–11.

Estruch, R., E. Ros, J. Salas-Salvadó, et al. 2013. Primary prevention of cardiovascular disease with a Mediterranean diet. *New England Journal of Medicine*, 368:1279–1290.

Fitó, M. L, M. Guxens, D. Corella, et al. 2007. Effect of a traditional Mediterranean diet on lipoprotein oxidation: A randomized controlled trial. *Archives of Internal Medicine*, 167(11):1195–1203.

Frazão. 1999. America's eating habits: Changes and consequences. In Davis, C., and E. Saltos, eds. *Dietary Recommendations and How They Have Changed Over Time*. Agriculture Information Bulletin 750. Washington, DC: Economic Research Service, US Department of Agriculture. pp. 33–50.

Freid, V. M., A. B. Bernstein, and A. Bush. 2012. *Multiple Chronic Conditions among Adults Aged 45 and over: Trends over the Past 10 Years*. NCHS Data Brief No. 100, CDC National Center for Health Statistics. http://www.cdc.gov/nchs/products/databriefs/ db100.htm.

Fried R., and L. Edlen-Nezin. 2006. *Great Food/Great Sex*. New York: Ballantine Books.

Fried, R., and W. C. Merrell. 1999. *The Arginine Solution*. New York: Time/Warner Books.

Fung, T. T., E. B. Rimm, D. Spiegelman et al. 2001a. Association between dietary patterns and plasma biomarkers of obesity and cardiovascular disease risk. *The American Journal of Clinical Nutrition*, 73(1):61–67.

Fung, T. T., W. C. Willett, M. J. Stampfer, et al. 2001b. Dietary patterns and the risk of coronary heart disease in women. *Archives of Internal Medicine*, 161(15):1857–1862.

Giugliano, D., and K. Esposito. 2008. Mediterranean diet and metabolic diseases. *Current Opinion in Lipidology*, 19(1):63–68.

Guarente, L. 2006. Sirtuins as potential targets for metabolic syndrome. *Nature*, 444:868–874.

Hallows, S. E., T. R. H. Regnault, and D. H. Betts. 2012. The long and short of it: The role of telomeres in fetal origins of adult disease. *Journal of Pregnancy*, 2012:638476. doi: http://dx.doi.org/10.1155/2012/638476.

Haycock, P. C., E. E. Heydon, S. Kaptoge, et al. 2014. Leucocyte telomere length and risk of cardiovascular disease: Systematic review and meta-analysis. *British Medical Journal*, 349:g4227.

Hedley, A. A., C. L. Ogden, C. L. Johnson, et al. 2004. Prevalence of overweight and obesity among US children, adolescents, and adults, 1999–2002. *Journal of the American Medical Association*, 291:2847–2850.

Hu, F. B. 2002. Dietary pattern analysis: A new direction in nutritional epidemiology. *Current Opinion in Lipidology*, 13(1):3–9.

Hu, F. B. 2003. Plant-based foods and prevention of cardiovascular disease: An overview. *American Journal of Clinical Nutrition*, 78(3 Suppl):544S–551S.

Hu, F. B., E. B. Rimm, M. J. Stampfer, et al. 2000. Prospective study of major dietary patterns and risk of coronary heart disease in men. *American Journal of Clinical Nutrition*, 72:912–921. Washington, DC: U.S. Department of Agriculture.

Hunt, C. L. 1916. *Food for Young Children*. Farmers' Bulletin No. 717, Washington, DC: U.S. Department of Agriculture. p. 21.

Hunt, C. L. 1921. *A Week's Food for an Average Family*. Farmers Bulletin No. 1228, Washington, DC: U.S. Department of Agriculture. p. 25.

Hunt, C. L., and H. W. Atwater. 1917. *How to Select Foods*. Farmers Bulletin No. 808, Washington, DC: U.S. Department of Agriculture. p. 14.

Iqbal, R., S. S. Anand, Ounpuu, et al. 2008. Dietary patterns and the risk of acute myocardial infarction in 52 countries: Results of the INTERHEART study. *Circulation*, 118:1929–1937.

Izzo, J. L., D. Levy, and H. R. Black. 2000. Importance of systolic blood pressure in older Americans. *Hypertension*, 35:1021–1024.

Kastorini, C-M., H. J. Milionis, K. Esposito, et al. 2011. The effect of Mediterranean diet on metabolic syndrome and its components: A meta-analysis of 50 studies and 534,906 individuals. *Journal of the American College of Cardiology*, 57(11):1299–1313.

Khalesi, S., S. Sharma, C. Irwin, et al. 2016. Dietary patterns, nutrition knowledge and lifestyle: Associations with blood pressure in a sample of Australian adults (the Food BP study). *Journal of Human Hypertension*, 30(10):581–590. doi: http://dx.doi.org/10.1038/jhh.2016.22.

Knopp, R. H. and B. M. Retzlaff. 2004. Saturated fat prevents coronary artery disease? An American paradox. *American Journal of Clinical Nutrition*, 80(5):1102–1103.

Krauss, R. M., R. J. Deckelbaum, N. Ernst, et al. 1996. Dietary guidelines for healthy American adults. A statement for health professionals from the Nutrition Committee, American Heart Association. *Circulation*, 94:1795–1800.

Lee, J. Y., N. R. Jun, D. Yoon, et al. 2015. Association between dietary patterns in the remote past and telomere length. *European Journal of Clinical Nutrition*, 69(9):1048–1052.

Lidder, S., and A. J. Webb. 2013. Vascular effects of dietary nitrate (as found in green leafy vegetables and beetroot) via the nitrate-nitrite-nitric oxide pathway. *British Journal of Clinical Pharmacology*, 75(3):677–696.

Livingston, G. E. 1973. The prudent diet: What? Why? How? *Preventive Medicine*, 2(3):321–328.

López-Miranda, V., M. L. Soto-Montenegro, G. Vera, et al. 2012. Resveratrol: A neuroprotective polyphenol in the Mediterranean diet. *Revista de Neurologia*, 54(6):349–356.

Lutsey, P. L., L. M. Steffen, and J. Stevens. 2008. Dietary intake and the development of the metabolic syndrome. The Atherosclerosis Risk in Communities study. *Circulation*, (117):754–761.

Matsushima, S., and J. Sadoshima. 2015. The role of sirtuins in cardiac disease. *American Journal of Physiology. Heart & Circulation Physiology*, 309(9):H1375–H1389.

Mattson, M. P. 2008. Dietary factors, hormesis and health. *Ageing Research Reviews*, 7(1):43–48.

Mertens-Talcott, S. U., J. Rios, P. Jilma-Stohlawetz, et al. 2008. Pharmacokinetics of anthocyanins and antioxidant effects after the consumption of anthocyanin-rich acai juice and pulp (*Euterpe oleracea Mart.*) in human healthy volunteers. *Journal of Agriculture & Food Chemistry*, 56(17):7796–7802.

Miettinen, M., O. Turpeinen, M. J. Karvonen, et al. 1972. Effect of cholesterol-lowering diet on mortality from coronary heart-disease and other causes. A twelve-year clinical trial in men and women. *Lancet*, 2:835–838.

Milne, J. C., P. D. Lambert, S. Schenk, et al. 2007. Small molecule activators of SIRT1 as therapeutics for the treatment of type 2 diabetes. *Nature*, 450(7170):712–716.

Montonen, J., P. Knekt, J. Härkänen, et al. 2005. Dietary patterns and the incidence of Type 2 diabetes. *American Journal of Epidemiology*, 161(3):219–227.

Ogden, C. L., M. D. Carroll, B. K. Kit, et al. 2012. Prevalence of obesity and trends in body mass index among US children and adolescents, 1999–2010. *Journal of the American Medical Association*, 307(5):483–490.

Page. L., and E. F. Phipard. 1956. *Essentials of an Adequate Diet. Facts for Nutrition Programs*. Washington, DC: U.S. Department of Agriculture, ARS-62-4.

Pallauf, K., K. Giller, P. Huebbe, et al. 2013. Nutrition and healthy ageing: Calorie restriction or polyphenol-rich "MediterrAsian" diet? *Oxidative Medicine & Cellular Longevity*, 2013:707421.

Panagiotakos, D. B., C. H. Pitsavos, C. Chrysohoou, et al. 2003. Status and management of hypertension in Greece: Role of the adoption of a Mediterranean diet: The ATTICA study. *Journal of Hypertension*, 21:1483–1489.

Paradis, A. M., G. Godin, L. Pérusse, et al. 2009. Associations between dietary patterns and obesity phenotypes. *International Journal of Obesity*, 33:1419–1426.

Potente, M. 2010. An energy-sensor network takes center stage during endothelial aging. *Circulation Research*, 106:1316–1318.

Qi, L., M. C. Cornelis, C. Zhang et al. 2009. Genetic predisposition, Western dietary pattern, and the risk of type 2 diabetes in men. *American Journal of Clinical Nutrition*, 89(5):1453–1458.

Révész, D., Y. Milaneschi, J. E. Verhoeven, et al. 2015. Longitudinal associations between metabolic syndrome components and telomere shortening. *Journal of Clinical Endocrinology & Metabolism*, 100(8):3050–3059.

Russo, M. A., L. Sansone, L. Polletta, et al. 2014. Sirtuins and resveratrol-derived compounds: A model for understanding the beneficial effects of the Mediterranean diet. *Endocrine, Metabolic & Immune Disorders Drug Targets*, 14(4):300–308.

Schroder, H., J. Marrugat, J. Vila, et al. 2004. Adherence to the traditional Mediterranean diet is inversely associated with body mass index and obesity in a Spanish population. *Journal of Nutrition*, 134:3355–3361.

Schwedhelm, E., R. Maas, R. Troost, et al. 2003. Clinical pharmacokinetics of antioxidants and their impact on systemic oxidative stress. *Clinical Pharmacokinetics*, 42(5):437–459.

Shin, J.-Y, J-M. Kim, and Y. Kim. 2013. Associations between dietary patterns and hypertension among Korean adults: The Korean National Health and Nutrition Examination Survey (2008–2010). *Nutrition Research & Practice*, 7(3):224–232.

Shinmura, K. 2013. Effects of caloric restriction on cardiac oxidative stress and mitochondrial bioenergetics: Potential role of cardiac sirtuins. *Oxidative Stress & Cellular Longevity*, 2013: 528935.

Sichieri, R. 2002. Dietary patterns and their associations with obesity in the Brazilian city of Rio de Janeiro. *Obesity Research*, 10(1):42–48. doi: http://dx.doi.org/10.1038/oby.2002.6.

Spyridopoulos, I., J. Hoffmann, A. Aicher, et al. 2000. Accelerated telomere shortening in leukocyte subpopulations of patients with coronary heart disease. Role of cytomegalovirus seropositivity. *Circulation*, 120:1364–1372.

Stiebeling, H. K., and M. Ward. 1933. *Diets at Four Levels of Nutrition Content and Cost*. U.S. Department of Agriculture, Circulation No. 296, p. 59.

Tortosa, A., M. Bes-Rastrollo, A. Sanchez-Villegas, et al. 2007. Mediterranean diet inversely associated with the incidence of metabolic syndrome: The SUN prospective cohort. *Diabetes Care*, 30(11):2957–2959.

Tyrovolas, S., V. Bountziouka, N. Papairakleous, et al. 2009. Adherence to the Mediterranean diet is associated with lower prevalence of obesity among elderly people living in Mediterranean islands: The MEDIS study. *International Journal of Food Science & Nutrition*, 60(Suppl 6):137–150.

Vasa, M., K. Breitschopf, A. M. Zeiher, et al. 2000. Nitric oxide activates telomerase and delays endothelial cell senescence. *Circulation Research*, 87:540–542.

Weiss, R. 2006. Nebivolol: A novel beta-blocker with nitric oxide-induced vasodilatation. *Health Risk Management*, 2(3):303–308.

Winnik, S., J. Auwerx, D. A. Sinclair, et al. 2015. Protective effects of sirtuins in cardiovascular diseases: Bench to bedside. *European Heart Journal*, 36(48):3404–3412.

Yach, D, C. Hawkes, and C. L. Gould. 2015. *The Global Burden of chronic Diseases. Overcoming Impediments to Prevention and Control*. Special communication, UNCLASSIFIED. Washington, DC: U.S. Department of State Case No. F-2014-20439 Doc No. C05772611.

Zhao, J., K. Miao, H. Wang, et al. 2013. Association between telomere length and type 2 diabetes mellitus: A meta-analysis. *PLoS One*, 8(11):e79993.

7 Proactive Nutrition
Enhancing the Mediterranean Diet

7.1 "THE CANARY IN THE COAL MINE"

In 2006, the authors of this book published *Great Food/Great Sex — The Three Food Factors for Sexual Fitness* (Fried and Edlen-Nezin 2006). This book promotes cardiovascular and heart health because medical science has described those as the basis of healthy and vigorous sexual "performance."

In fact, it became well known then that the Mediterranean diet boosts sexual vitality because it is rich in nitric oxide-donor (NO-donor) foods while, at the same time, it helps avoid atherosclerosis, now acknowledged to be the principal cause of erectile dysfunction—the nemesis of sexual vitality (see Chapter 5). Clinical investigators writing in the *American Journal of Cardiology*, in 2011, titled their publication "The link between erectile and cardiovascular health: the canary in the coal mine" (Meldrum et al. 2011).

More recently, a study reported in the *International Journal of Impotence Research*, in 2006, compared men with erectile dysfunction (ED) to a comparable group of men without ED on a scale indicating the degree of adherence to the Mediterranean diet. The authors concluded that dietary factors may be important in the development of ED. They suggested that adoption of a healthy diet would help prevent ED (Esposito et al. 2006). This study and many like it indicate that adherence to a Mediterranean diet confers a healthy cardiovascular system and heart essential to vitality.

Then, in 2010, the authors of that study followed with a report that in clinical trials, the Mediterranean diet was more effective than a comparison diet in ameliorating ED or restoring absent ED in men with obesity or metabolic syndrome. They concluded that the adoption of a Mediterranean diet may be associated with an improvement in erectile function (Boccardi et al. 2013).

Although these studies focus on sexual function as an "index" of cardiovascular and heart health in men, they really apply to other health-related functions as well. And, what is learned from them is first, that cardiovascular and heart health will be better in those who adhere to a Mediterranean diet than in those who do not. Second, those who do not adhere to a Mediterranean diet and have poor cardiovascular and heart health will see improvement by switching to and then adhering to a Mediterranean diet.

7.2   THE LINK TO AVERTING PREMATURE AGING

The link between cardiovascular and heart health and telomere length was not known then. But, it is known now that the same diet, the Mediterranean diet that prolongs life by conferring cardiovascular and heart health, and sexual vitality, also contributes to prevention of premature aging by preventing early and rapid cell cycling and shortening of telomeres. In fact, that is exactly what a recent publication reveals. A report in *PLoS One* in 2013 is aptly titled "Mediterranean diet, telomere maintenance and health status among elderly." It concludes that there is a link between high adherence to the Mediterranean diet and a slower rate of cellular aging. The authors aver that a lower rate of telomere shortening might be involved in lifespan and, most importantly, healthspan among populations adhering to a traditional Mediterranean diet (Boccardi et al. 2013).

7.3   THREE FOOD FACTORS IN THE MEDITERRANEAN DIET ENHANCE HEALTH, VITALITY, AND LONGEVITY

The three food factors in the Mediterranean diet that enhance cardiovascular health are:

- **Greens and beans**: Nitrogen-rich foods including artichokes, arugula, beets, broccoli, Brussels sprouts, cabbage, carrots, celery, chicory, collard greens, cucumbers, dandelion greens, eggplant, fennel, kale, leeks, lemons, lettuce, mushrooms, mustard greens, nettles, okra, onions (red, sweet, white), peas, peppers, potatoes, pumpkin, radishes, rutabaga, scallions, shallots, spinach, sweet potatoes, turnips, zucchini, cannellini beans, chickpeas, fava beans, green beans, kidney beans, and lentils.
- **Staminators**: High L-arginine foods including nuts and seeds such as almonds, hazelnuts, pine nuts, pistachios, sesame seeds, and walnuts

  Fish and shellfish such as abalone, clams, cockles, crab, eel, flounder, lobster, mackerel, mussels, octopus, oysters, salmon, sardines, sea bass, shrimp, squid, tilapia, tuna, and yellowtail.

  Poultry and red meat such as beef, chicken, duck, goat, guinea fowl, lamb, mutton, and pork.
- **The Brights**: Super-antioxidant foods including apples, avocados, cherries, clementines, dates, figs, grapefruits, grapes, melons, nectarines, olives, oranges, peaches, pears, pomegranates, strawberries, tangerines, and tomatoes (yes, tomatoes are fruits).

  The main components of the Mediterranean diet also include:
  - Eggs, dairy including yogurt and cheese such as brie, chevre, Corvo, feta, haloumi, manchego, Parmigiano-Reggiano, pecorino, ricotta, yogurt (including Greek yogurt), and olive oil (extra-virgin olive oil is the principal source of dietary fat used for cooking, baking, and for dressing salads and vegetables).
  - Herbs and spices common to the traditional Mediterranean diet include: anise, basil, bay leaf, chilies, cloves, cumin, fennel, garlic, lavender, marjoram, mint, oregano, parsley, pepper, rosemary, sage, savory, tarragon, and thyme. Most are also rich in antioxidants.

The consumption of alcohol, especially wines, is not bound by region and is popular in the wider Mediterranean cultures. It is acknowledged that many health authorities ascribe health benefits to wine consumption. One study published in the *European Journal of Clinical Nutrition*, in 2002, reports that consuming red wine reduces plasma homocysteine, a major contributor to atherosclerosis (Dixon et al. 2002). Some sources go so far as to recommend daily consumption of two glasses per day.

For instance, a study published in the *International Journal of Angiology*, in 2009, is titled "Polyphenols are medicine: is it time to prescribe red wine for our patients?" (Cordova and Sumpio 2009). Many studies that recommend the "two glasses per day" as "moderate drinking" cite its effects only in terms other than its potential hazards. Case in point: a study in the *Journal of the American College of Nutrition*, in 1997, concluded that:

> In free-living subjects over a 6-week period, the addition of two glasses of red wine to the evening meal does not appear to influence any measured variable which may adversely affect body weight or promote the development of obesity during this time period. (Cordain et al. 1997)

No consideration is given to the possibility that continuous consumption of that quantity of alcohol may lead to addiction.

Therefore, and while wine has demonstrated health benefits, for reasons given earlier, not the least that alcohol is a neurotoxin, we'll pass on that one.

In any case, it cannot be said with certainty what constitutes "healthy" moderate drinking, but clinical evidence suggests that alcohol is not telomere friendly. In a study published in the *International Journal of Cancer*, in 2011, investigators categorized "alcohol abusers" as those who consume more than four alcoholic drinks per day. They compared the telomere length (TL) of their immune system cells (leukocytes) with that in a comparison group of individuals whose alcohol consumption was less than four drinks per day. TL was nearly half that in alcohol *abusers* compared to controls and it decreased in proportion to increasing drink-units/day. Individuals drinking more than four drink-units per day had substantially shorter TL than those drinking less than four drink-units/day or less (Pavanello et al. 2011).

It might help to keep in mind that Nature *invented* the polyphenol antioxidant resveratrol in wine to protect plants from leaf, vine, and root fungi, and other pests, not to protect human telomeres. The useful aspects of resveratrol might well serve better in another medium. And, while there is no doubt that fruits are antioxidant and healthful, one may wish to consider "serving size" because fructose is pro-inflammatory: it induces inflammatory changes in vascular cells and it is, therefore, not telomere friendly either (Glushakova et al. 2008).

7.4   THE ENHANCED MEDITERRANEAN DIET IS THE PROACTIVE NUTRITION PROGRAM

The proposed Proactive Nutrition Program is then, first and foremost, a basic Mediterranean diet assuring the comprehensive "three food factors," foods rich in nitrates and in the amino acid L-arginine, both of which supply nitric oxide (NO), the "anti-aging miracle molecule" that protects our blood vessels and strengthens immune defense. In addition, it is rich in polyphenolic antioxidants and, not least, in oleic acid found in olive oil. More on that later.

Third, the Proactive Nutrition Program also integrates sirtfoods, which are said to regulate energy management and storage in the body and impact longevity. The *Handbook of Experimental Pharmacology* states that sirtuins regulate metabolism and response to stress, two key factors in aging. The activation of SIRT1 reduces the risk of such age-related disorders as type 2 diabetes. The authors further report that "SIRT1 activation has clear potential to not only prevent age-associated diseases but also to extend healthspan and perhaps lifespan" (Satoh et al. 2011).

7.5   A NOTE ON "SIRTFOODS"

"Sirtfoods" is now a popular *buzzword*. The terms "sirtfood" and "sirtuin-rich food" are common and misleading: to be clear, there is no sirtuin of any kind in any food per se. Sirtuins are protein molecules derived from the activation of genes that influence cellular processes such as food storage in the body and aging. They are activated by certain foods, foods that contain constituents that signal those genes that affected controlled metabolism and energy storage (as fat) in ancient times of dire food shortage. Seven types are known. Therefore, what is really meant by "sirtfoods" is that they are foods that activate the formation of sirtuin; likewise, "sirtuin-rich foods" mean foods rich in constituents that *activate* sirtuin.

Another report in the journal *Advances in Experimental Medicine and Biology*, in 2012, notes that sirtuin plays a crucial role during the aging process as a key regulator of metabolic stress and cell cycle control (Mahlknecht and Zschoernig 2012). The good news is that sirtfoods, which are a core component of the Proactive Nutrition Program, are not only nutritious but also tasty.

7.6   THE PROACTIVE NUTRITION PROGRAM IS NOT SIMPLY A DIET

Most people think of a diet as a way of eating that is undertaken for a specific period of time, to try to achieve a specific goal. And also, when most hear the word "diet," they think of restrictions, limits on the foods they like to eat, and behaviors that only need to be adhered to until goals are achieved.

The Proactive Nutrition Program is a way of eating for a better and longer life and it is an easy-to-implement guide to food selection, rather than a rigid regimen. The Proactive Nutrition Program can help one to select healthy sirtfoods and learn to incorporate them into their meals on a daily basis.

7.6.1   THE SMART SHOPPING CART

The Mediterranean diet emphasizes healthy, unprocessed foods (see Figure 7.1). These include:

- Vegetables: Tomatoes, broccoli, kale, spinach, onions, cauliflower, carrots, Brussels sprouts, cucumbers, etc.

- Fruits: Apples, bananas, oranges, pears, strawberries, grapes, dates, figs, melons, peaches, etc.
- Nuts and seeds: Almonds, walnuts, macadamia nuts, hazelnuts, cashews, sunflower seeds, pumpkin seeds, and more
- Legumes: Beans, peas, lentils, pulses, peanuts, chickpeas, etc.
- Tubers: Potatoes, sweet potatoes, turnips, yams, etc.
- Whole grains: Whole oats, brown rice, rye, barley, corn, buckwheat, whole wheat, whole grain bread, and pasta
- Fish and seafood: Salmon, sardines, trout, tuna, mackerel, shrimp, oysters, clams, crab, mussels, etc.
- Poultry: Chicken, duck, turkey, etc.
- Eggs: Chicken, quail, and duck eggs
- Dairy: Cheese, yogurt, Greek yogurt, etc.
- Herbs and spices: Garlic, basil, mint, rosemary, sage, nutmeg, cinnamon, pepper, etc.
- Healthy fats: Extra-virgin olive oil, olives, avocados, and avocado oil
And:
- Eating primarily plant-based foods, such as fruits and vegetables, whole grains, legumes, and nuts
- Replacing butter with healthy unsaturated fats such as olive oil and canola oil*
- Using herbs and spices instead of salt to flavor foods
- Limiting red meat to no more than a few times a month

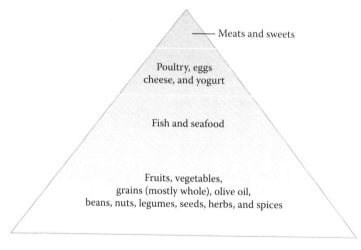

FIGURE 7.1 Mediterranean Diet Pyramid. (© 2009 Oldways Preservation & Exchange Trust, www.oldwayspt.org. With permission.)

---

* All vegetable oils contain a mix of polyunsaturated, monounsaturated, and saturated fatty acids. Canola oil consists mostly of monounsaturated fats (61%, almost as much as olive oil) and polyunsaturated fats (32%). Of all vegetable oils, it is lowest in saturated fats (7%) and is second highest in alpha-linolenic acid (ALA), an omega-3 polyunsaturated fat related to the omega-3s in fish (11% ALA, compared to 57% in flaxseed oil).

Water should be the main beverage in a Mediterranean diet. Coffee and tea are also acceptable, but it is best to avoid sugar-sweetened beverages and fruit juices that are very high in sugar.

Wherever possible, sirtfoods should be included in every meal. This is simpler than one may think, because these are common, delicious foods that can easily become part of the daily intake. A list of sirtfoods is given below.

The goal is to try to consume at least five sirtfoods per day. It will be a pleasant surprise to find many delicious sirtfoods incorporated in the recipes that follow, especially as *smoothies*.

7.6.2   A Basic Shopping List for the Diet

Here is a recommended shopping list to help implement a Proactive Nutrition Program centering on basic Mediterranean diet plan foods:

- Vegetables: Carrots, onions, broccoli, spinach, kale, garlic, etc.
- Fruits: Apples, bananas, oranges, grapes, etc.
- Berries: Strawberries, blueberries, etc.
- Frozen vegetables: Mixes with healthy vegetables
- Grains: Whole grain bread, whole grain pasta, etc.
- Legumes: Lentils, pulses, beans, etc.
- Nuts: Almonds, walnuts, cashews, etc.
- Seeds: Sunflower seeds, pumpkin seeds, etc.
- Condiments: Sea salt, pepper, turmeric, cinnamon, etc.
- Fish: Salmon, sardines, mackerel, trout
- Shrimp and shellfish
- Potatoes and sweet potatoes
- Cheese
- Greek yogurt
- Red meat common to the traditional Mediterranean diet includes beef, chicken, duck, goat, guinea fowl, lamb, mutton, and pork
- Pastured or omega-3-enriched eggs
- Olives
- Extra-virgin olive oil

It is best to remove "unhealthy" foods from your home, thus eliminating the temptation of sodas, ice cream, candy, pastries, white bread, crackers, and processed foods.

A "smart shopping list" can be made before going to the grocery store so as to be sure to include sirtfoods in the cart. The cart should be full of colorful, healthy foods every time one shops. An easy way to start incorporating sirtfoods into the diet is to start cooking with extra-virgin olive oil or canola oil. Onions can be sautéed to add to most main dishes, and parsley can be added as a garnish. Chopped kale can be added to a salad, or if preferred cooked, it can be steamed and then tossed with a tablespoon of olive oil. And using turmeric, the spice that gives curry dishes the beautiful yellow color, is a great way to ramp up the sirtuin-activating levels of the dishes.

Berries, citrus fruit, and apples are great sirtfood desserts. These delicious fruits will not only boost sirtuin activation but also help to avoid the high-fat, high-calorie desserts that many have become accustomed to at the end of a meal. Blackcurrants and passion fruit are also sirtfoods but not as readily available in many markets. A small piece of dark chocolate can be added, thereby not only satisfying a "sweet tooth" but bumping up the sirtuin-activation value of the meal.

Whenever possible, green tea can be substituted for black tea or coffee. Iced green tea is an excellent substitute for sugary sodas. It can be sweetened with a little honey when hot, and then kept in the refrigerator for a refreshing drink.

7.7 THE ABCs OF EATING

There are three core principles to the Proactive Nutrition Program that constitute the ABCs of eating: Attention, Beauty, and Choice. These rules are the key to better digestion, better weight management, and true enjoyment of the foods one eats.

Attention means being aware of the meal whenever one is eating, whether it is a formal meal or a snack grabbed on the run. Attention means trying only to taste, chew, and swallow when putting food into your mouth. This means not watching television, not answering email, not browsing Facebook, etc. The exception to this is having a conversation with anyone with whom one is sharing the meal.

When eating on *auto-pilot*, as so many do in our time-challenged lives, not only does one risk overeating, but it also puts a strain on the digestive system. There are enzymes in the mouth that are specifically designed to help break down the food being eaten. This is also dependent on properly chewing the food. Air is meant to be inhaled, and food is meant to be chewed as thoroughly as possible before swallowing.

Thoroughly chewed food not only releases flavors and increases enjoyment but also protects against swallowing a piece of food large enough to cause choking, and helps ensure proper digestion. For those who suffer from gas after eating, it is quite likely because they are eating too quickly and swallowing air along with partially chewed food.

Beauty refers to the appearance of the meal being served. It is common to pay a lot of attention to "presentation" when eating in restaurants, because beautifully presented food adds to the enjoyment of the meal. But many pay little or no attention to the appearance of the foods on the plate served at home. A slab of meat and a mound of potatoes seem more like putting food down for the dog than an attractive meal for a family.

A plate can be like an artist's palette, and imagination can add color and variety. The easiest way to do this is by adding an array of brightly colored vegetables that creates not only a plate that is appealing to the eye but also a meal that is rich in antioxidants.

Choice is a reminder that most have a fair degree of freedom in selecting foods. Even with dietary restrictions, there are numerous options at almost every meal. This process of selection will help to establish the habit of creating meals that are not only healthy but also attractive.

"Choice" can be thought of as a swap-out challenge—for example, if potatoes are a core component of the dinner, a baked sweet potato can be substituted for mashed white potatoes. This will not only save calories but also bump up the nutritional value of the carbohydrate in the meal. A colorful swap contributes to the beauty of the plate, while adding valuable antioxidants to the meal.

A high omega-3-content fish can be served instead of meat at least three times per week, and if eating grains such as rice or bread, "brown" is better than "white." Also, one can increase the proportion of vegetables versus starch in as many meals as possible so that vegetables represent at least one-third of the space on the dinner plate as often as possible.

7.8 "THE EYES ARE BIGGER THAN THE STOMACH"

Our Paleolithic ancestors are thought to have often been faced with limited and unpredictable food supplies. They must have learned to feast on as much food as possible whenever it was available, so that they could endure the fast that followed when the food supply failed. This is not a useful modern approach to eating in times when food tends to be readily accessible for most 24/7.

Most of us are now still conditioned to be delighted by larger and larger portions. Over time, average portion size in Western societies has dramatically increased. It is no surprise that average weight gain has risen as well. There has also been a dramatic increase in cardiovascular disease, diabetes, and weight-bearing arthritis as portion sizes have increased, and higher percentages of the calories in the common diet are contributed by fat and simple sugars like high-fructose corn syrup.

Many authorities now point to portion size as one culprit in overeating. There is an excellent teaching tool on the site created by the National Heart, Lung, and Blood Institute (NHLBI) of the National Institutes of Health (NIH): www.choosemyplate. gov/ tools-portion-distortion. It is astonishing to see how "super-sized" so many food portions have become.

For instance, the authors of a study titled "Portion size of food affects energy intake in normal-weight and overweight men and women," published in *The American Journal of Clinical Nutrition*, in 2002, concluded that the amount of food that is presented during a single meal directly affects energy intake (the amount of food one will eat) (Rolls et al. 2002).

ESHA Research offers an online Food Processor Nutrition Analysis Software program (http://www.esha.com/products/food-processor-nutrition-analysis-software/) that facilitates analysis of foods and ingredient in a meal plan. It has a database with an uncluttered, easy-to-use interface for accurate and comprehensive nutrition analysis. The site reports that "For more than 30 years, Nutritionists, Dietitians, Restaurants, and Educational Facilities have used the Food Processor Analysis tool to analyze menus, diets, foods, recipes, and even fitness needs of their clients."

7.8.1 THE "COMPLETION COMPULSION"

One of the easy ways to combat portion-creep is to serve meals on smaller plates and bowls. We are conditioned to want to eat everything in front of us. This tendency has been termed the "completion compulsion" (Siegel 1957). Smaller portions look bigger on smaller plates. Over time, one can learn to be satisfied with portions that will help one either lose or maintain weight, without feeling deprived.

If it is difficult to control how much one is eating at home, food can be served restaurant-style. A plate with a reasonable portion can be prepared in the kitchen, rather than the meal served from a large dish at the table. This can be easily done, regardless of how many people are eating at the table, and will help guard against overeating.

When eating out, unless it is at a restaurant that serves reasonably sized portions (as in many Japanese restaurants), the following tips may be helpful: First, if bread is served before the meal, it can be sent back. Most people will overeat bread and butter in restaurants before their meal arrives. One can opt to drink water before the meal arrives. Oftentimes, thirst is mistaken for hunger and unless one routinely drinks water throughout the day, that is likely to lead to dehydration. Being dehydrated can also lead to overeating.

When eating in a restaurant that serves large portions, the waiter can be asked to bring an extra plate. Half of the meal can be put on that extra plate and then the waiter can be asked to have it wrapped up so that it can be taken home for a later meal.

7.8.2 COUNTING CALORIES

The Proactive Nutrition Program does not include counting calories. The program is not about weight control. For the overweight, weight loss is certainly desirable, but this program is about overall health leading to normal aging through cellular health. That means "counting" antioxidants and not calories. As noted previously, weight affects health only in the extremes—at both ends of the weight continuum.

We do not suggest counting calories, per se, because that can become an onerous task, which can take the enjoyment out of eating, but that does not mean that the number of calories consumed is inconsequential. The goal of our approach to meal planning is to try to ensure that key food groups are well represented and foods of low nutritional value are under-represented.

In general, the key to weight loss is portion control, and trying to finish a meal feeling satisfied but not stuffed. The vast array of vegetables and fruits that comprise a core part of this plan is satiating as well as nutritionally sound. We suggest trying to limit refined carbohydrates which are often found in processed foods, as well as baking and grilling proteins rather than frying, which not only reduces fat intake but also more importantly, fat that has been subjected to high heat.

Maintaining a healthy weight has many benefits of course, including a positive body image. Therefore, including sirtfoods whenever possible in the daily eating plan is one of the easiest and most satisfying ways to both lose and control weight. The key is swapping high-calorie, high-fat foods for sirtfoods, and following the suggestions for portion control discussed earlier.

7.8.3 PUTTING THE "E" BACK INTO EATING

Putting the "e" back into eating encourages *enjoying* meals. Making a beautiful plate, taking time to taste all the flavors, and relaxing rather than rushing through meals are all as important as what is eaten. One can be adventurous and challenged to try a new recipe or dish at least once a month. One can be inventive and think of all the ways that sirtfoods can be incorporated in everyday meals. One can be consistent and stop eating before becoming uncomfortably full. It is helpful to let meals last longer by taking the time to relax and not rush through them.

7.9   THE SECRET OF THE MEDITERRANEAN DIET: GREENS AND BEANS, AND NO DONORS

It was indicated in a previous chapter that medical science did not know why the Mediterranean diet is beneficial until it became clear that its cornucopia of foods were a rich source of nitric oxide (NO) from two of the three food factors cited above that are rich in antioxidants, support healthy blood vessel and heart function, and combat inflammation. In addition, the oleic acid found in olive oil, plentiful in the diet, can help reduce the damage to blood vessels caused by type 2 diabetes (see below)

The two NO-donor food factors are the L-arginine-rich "staminators" and the nitrate-rich "greens and beans":

- The staminators are one of the two food sources of nitric oxide (NO). They are rich in L-arginine from which cells in the lining of blood vessels, the endothelium, form nitric oxide (Palmer et al. 1988). The process of NO formation from L-arginine is detailed in Chapter 5 on nitric oxide.
- The greens and beans (and beets) are also rich in L-arginine, but most importantly, they are rich in nitrate (Lidder and Webb 2013), another source of NO.

Dietary source nitrate is metabolized to nitrite in the body to form nitric oxide (NO). An article titled "Nitrate and nitrite in biology, nutrition and therapeutics," published in *Nature Chemical Biology*, in 2009, says the following about dietary nitrate:

> Certain vegetables in daily diet are our principal source of nitrate. Much of the nitrate in foods is actively taken up by the salivary glands as we consume the foods and concentrated in saliva. Bacteria in the mouth then reduce salivary nitrate to nitrite. Continuously swallowing nitrite in saliva forms different nitrogen compounds in the stomach and in particular, nitric oxide (NO). This is the second "pathway" for forming NO and it is called the "entero-salivary circulation of nitrate." (Lundberg and Govoni 2004; Lundberg et al. 2009)

Figure 7.2 shows the entero-salivary circulation cycle: inorganic nitrate in foods is rapidly absorbed in the small intestine. Much of the circulating nitrate is eventually excreted in the urine, but up to 25% is actively extracted by the salivary glands and concentrated in saliva. Bacteria in the mouth effectively reduce nitrate to nitrite by the action of enzymes, leading to a thousand-fold higher concentrations of nitrite in saliva than in plasma. In the acidic stomach, nitrite is spontaneously decomposed

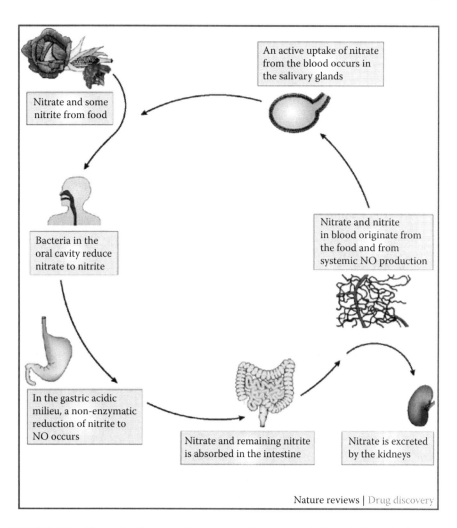

FIGURE 7.2 (**See color insert.**) The entero-salivary circulation of nitrate in humans. (From Lundberg, J.O., *Nat. Rev. Drug Discov.*, 7, 156–167, 2009. With permission.)

to form nitric oxide (NO) and other nitrogen compounds that regulate important physiological functions. Nitrate and the remaining nitrite are absorbed from the intestine into the circulation and can convert to NO in blood and tissues (Lundberg et al. 2009).

It is possible to determine one's NO availability level indirectly as a function of the concentration of nitrite in saliva because it has been shown (1) that consuming nitrate actually raises NO availability in the body (McKnight et al. 1997), and (2) that salivary nitrate and nitrite levels reflect the amount ingested.

In a study published in the journal *Food and Cosmetics Toxicology* in 1997, volunteers consumed vegetables and vegetable juices with high concentrations of nitrate.

Nitrate and nitrite concentrations in saliva were determined for up to 7 hours at intervals of 30 or 60 minutes.

- First, the amount of nitrate secreted by the salivary glands increased directly with the amount of nitrate ingested.
- Second, nitrite concentration in saliva correlated directly with salivary nitrate content, indicating a direct relationship between the salivary nitrite concentrations and the amounts of nitrate ingested in the diet (Spiegelhalder et al. 1976).

The results of this, and similar studies, support the use of a salivary nitrite assay to estimate nitric oxide availability.

7.10   A SALIVARY MARKER OF NO AVAILABILITY: THE HumanN™ N-O INDICATOR STRIPS

There are usually many different ways to determine whether a nutrition plan or a diet is effective. For instance, if one wishes to lose weight, a scale can be used to monitor weight loss efforts, or *keto sticks* that detect the presence of ketones in urine (ketones are formed in the liver when burning fat). To determine whether one is getting the full NO benefit of the Proactive Nutrition Program, there is a simple saliva test that can assess the effects of adequate nitrate consumption because, as noted above, saliva nitrite is a biomarker of nitric oxide status. This test was briefly mentioned in Chapter 5.

HumanN™ (formerly Neogenis Labs®) (https://www.humann.com/products/) is a leader in nitric oxide research and invented the world's first standard non-invasive salivary nitric oxide test strip that can be used to measure nitric oxide levels at home. Using one's own saliva, it is quick and easy to conduct the test; saliva is applied to a strip and its coloration is then compared with a color code on the side of the strip container. This yields a measure of NOx concentration. The use of such a test strip provides *"feedback"*—knowledge of results—insofar as it may help to determine sooner the positive outcome of attention to nutrition (Figure 7.3).

Directions are given on the website https://www.humann.com/products/nitric-oxide-indicator-strips/. It is suggested that the user place a drop of saliva on the indicator strip first thing in the morning, before eating and drinking anything. Then compare the indicator strip with the accompanying color chart on the N-O indicator strip packaging. Results are practically instantaneous, and one can tell at a glance if one is getting sufficient nitric oxide–activating nutrients from the diet.

Results are easy to read by comparing the test strip coloration with the four color-coded reading indicators on the package. The more nitric oxide in the body, the deeper red the indicator pad will appear.

Note: When using the indicator strips, a high (N-O Optimal) reading may, or may not, indicate the concentration of endothelium-derived NO. It could also be

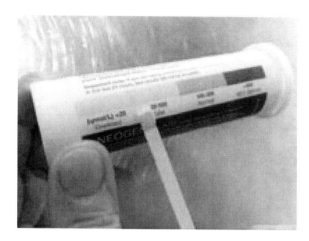

FIGURE 7.3 **(See color insert.)** N-O indicator strips. HumanN® N-O indicator strips are used to assess nitrite levels in saliva as an index of NOx availability. (With permission.)

confounded by a number of factors including recently consuming high L-arginine foods including meats, fish, nuts, or beans, and/or high nitrate foods including green leafy vegetables, or beans, beets, carrots; or if one has a lung, bowel, or other form of inflammatory disease. Immune system cells go into overdrive production of NO in serious infections and inflammation—potentially fatally in the case of septicemia. On the other hand, a low reading may be a clear indication that endothelial NO formation is simply inadequate. To ensure the proper use of the test, it is therefore very important to follow the instructions that accompany the test strips.

Regular use of such "feedback" about the status of NO availability will help support motivation to adhere to the Proactive Nutrition Program. It will confirm that one is on the right nutrition track to:

- Combat chronic systemic inflammation
- Lower blood pressure
- Lower, or even avert, atherosclerosis
- Enhance insulin function/sensitivity to reduce or avert type 2 diabetes
- Reduce, or even avert, metabolic syndrome
- Enhance heart action
- Enhance kidney function
- Enhance sexual performance vitality
- Avert premature, accelerated cell cycling, thus protecting telomeres and averting premature aging, which is the bottom line

Disclaimer: The authors have no commercial interest in the HumanN™ nitric oxide saliva test strips, nor are they in any way commercially involved with any other products of that company.

7.11　IMPLEMENTING THE BASIC MEDITERRANEAN FOOD PLAN AND SAMPLE RECIPES

Keeping in mind that the authors are scientists and not *haute cuisine* chefs, and that this book is about longevity and not culinary arts, nevertheless carefully selected recipes from reliable sources are offered to illustrate the Proactive Nutrition Program. There are two sets of recipes: the Mediterranean diet pattern recipes, followed by sirtfood recipes that enhance the Proactive Nutrition Program.

First, the US Department of Agriculture provides nutrition guidelines for the implementation of a Mediterranean diet pattern. To follow this pattern, see Table 7.1: identify the appropriate calorie level, choose a variety of foods in each group and subgroup over time in recommended amounts, and limit choices that are not in nutrient-dense forms so that the overall calorie limit is not exceeded.

TABLE 7.1
Healthy Mediterranean-style Eating Pattern: Recommended Amounts of Food from Each Food Group at 12 Calorie Levels

Calorie Level of Pattern	1000	1200	1400	1600	1800
Food Group	Daily Amount of Food from Each Group (vegetable and protein foods subgroup amounts are per week)				
Vegetables	1 c-eq	1½ c-eq	1½ c-eq	2 c-eq	2½ c-eq
Dark-green vegetables (c-eq/wk)	½	1	1	1½	1½
Red and orange vegetables (c-eq/wk)	2½	3	3	4	5½
Legumes (beans and peas) (c-eq/wk)	½	½	½	1	1½
Starchy vegetables (c-eq/wk)	2	3½	3½	4	5
Other vegetables (c-eq/wk)	1½	2½	2½	3½	4
Fruits	1 c-eq	1 c-eq	1½ c-eq	2 c-eq	2 c-eq
Grains	3 oz-eq	4 oz-eq	5 oz-eq	5 oz-eq	6 oz-eq
Whole grains (oz-eq/day)	1½	2	2½	3	3
Refined grains (oz-eq/day)	1½	2	2½	2	3
Dairy	2 c-eq	2½ c-eq	2½ c-eq	2 c-eq	2 c-eq
Protein foods	2 oz-eq	3 oz-eq	4 oz-eq	5½ oz-eq	6 oz-eq
Seafood (oz-eq/wk)	3	4	6	11	15
Meats, poultry, eggs (oz-eq/wk)	10	14	19	23	23
Nuts, seeds, soy products (oz-eq/wk)	2	2	3	4	4
Oils	15 g	17 g	17 g	22 g	24 g
Limit on calories for other uses, calories	150	100	110	140	160
(% of calories)	(15%)	(8%)	(8%)	(9%)	(9%)

Source:　Healthy Mediterranean-Style Eating Pattern: Recommended Amounts of Food from Each Food Group at 12 Calorie Levels, Table A4-1, https://health.gov/dietary guidelines/2015/guidelines/appendix-4/.

7.12 SAMPLE MEDITERRANEAN DIET MEAL PLAN

A Mediterranean diet plan does not necessarily depend on traditional Greek or other *Mediterranean region* cuisine. The "three food factors" mentioned previously incorporate all aspects of the Mediterranean diet plan, yet they do not necessarily rely on *Mediterranean region* recipes. The aspects of such a cuisine specific to preserving telomere length, and cardiovascular health in general, were described in the Chapter 6.

7.12.1 FIRST, A NOTE ON OLIVE OIL

The benefits of the Mediterranean diet depend not only on many of its food constituents rich in phytonutrients and polyphenol antioxidants, but also on the absence of certain deficient and unhealthy foods common in the Standard American Diet. It is often the case that when the merits of the Mediterranean diet are proclaimed, it is as though each of its constituent foods is thought to have an equal value in promoting health and longevity. That is in fact not so. Olive oil is a case in point.

The olive is one of the three "core food" plants in the Mediterranean cuisine yielding olive oil (*Olea europaea*) by a pressing extraction process. Its composition varies with the cultivar, the altitude where it is grown, the time of the year when it is harvested, and the form of extraction. The fat composition of olive oil is shown in Table 7.2.

Olive oil consists mainly of the beneficial oleic acid (up to 83%), with smaller amounts of other fatty acids including linoleic acid (up to 21%) and the not-so-beneficial palmitic acid (up to 20%).

Here are some basic facts about olive oil. *Extra-virgin olive oil* means that the oil was produced by the use of mechanical means only, with no chemical treatment, unlike the common extraction of other oils and fats with the chemical solvent *hexane*. Extra-virgin olive oil may contain no more than 0.8% free acidity, and it is judged to have a superior taste to virgin olive oil.

TABLE 7.2
Fat Composition of Olive Oil

Fat Composition

Saturated Fats	
Total saturated	Palmitic acid: 13.0%
	Stearic acid: 1.5%

Unsaturated Fats	
Total unsaturated	>85%
Monounsaturated	Oleic acid: 70.0%
	Palmitoleic acid: 0.3–3.5%
Polyunsaturated	Linoleic acid: 15.0%
	Alpha-linolenic acid: 0.5%

Virgin olive oil is of slightly lower quality than extra-virgin olive oil, with free acidity up to 1.5%. It is considered to have a good taste, but may include some imperfections.

Cold pressed, or cold extracted, means that the oil was not heated over 27°C (80°F) in the process, thereby retaining more nutrients and undergoing less degradation. The difference between cold extraction and cold pressing is regulated in Europe where oil extracted using a centrifuge, the modern method of extraction for large quantities, must be labeled as cold extracted, while that extracted only by physical pressing may be labeled as cold pressed.

Olive oil contains unsaturated fatty acids including oleic, alpha-linolenic, gamma-linolenic, and ricinoleic acids. These stay liquid at lower temperatures than saturated fats.

Olives also contain saturated fatty acids (lauric, myristic, palmitic, stearic) which are more common in solid fats.

A number of studies have reported that regular consumption of olive oil in the daily diet prevents accelerated aging. For instance, the journal *Molecule* reported in 2016 that the hallmarks of aging, including mitochondrial dysfunction, cellular senescence, and telomere attrition, are targeted by dietary virgin olive oil by virtue of the beneficial effects of the predominant monounsaturated fatty acid, oleic acid. Additional beneficial effects are derived from other constituents, especially secoiridoids.

How olive oil targets accelerated aging could explain the reduced risk of aging-associated diseases, and increased longevity associated with the consumption of a typical Mediterranean diet containing this oil as the predominant fat source. The high concentration of polyphenols is known to have beneficial anti-inflammatory and antioxidant properties (Fernández del Río et al. 2016).

A report in the journal *Rejuvenation Research* in 2014 attributes the "anti-aging" effects of extra-virgin olive oil in the diet to its "nutraceutical" properties in monounsaturated fatty acids and various phenolic compounds, such as oleocanthal, oleuropein, hydroxytyrosol, and tyrosol, its main nutraceutical substances. It was also noted that hydroxytyrosol and oleocanthal inhibit the cyclooxygenases (COX-1 and COX-2) responsible for prostaglandin production, and oleuropein is a radical scavenger that blocks the oxidation of low-density lipoproteins (Virruso et al. 2014).

Most studies of the effects of an anti-inflammatory diet such as the Mediterranean diet on preventing premature aging seldom identify the specific role of its constituent olive oil. More typically, the composite Mediterranean diet is said to stabilize atherosclerotic plaque, thus benefiting cardiovascular and heart health as well as modifying insulin response in type 2 diabetes. The composite diet is then reported to affect telomere length insofar as that varies with inflammatory index and cardiovascular disease risk.

However, the authors of a study published in *The American Journal of Clinical Nutrition* in 2015 reported an association between the inflammatory potential of the diet and telomere shortening in individuals with a high cardiovascular disease risk. Their findings are consistent with other reports of a beneficial effect of adherence to an anti-inflammatory diet on aging and health by slowing down telomere shortening. These results suggest that diet might play a key role as a determinant of telomere length through pro-inflammatory or anti-inflammatory mechanisms (as noted earlier) (García-Calzón et al. 2015). Since such studies often do not point specifically to the beneficial role of olive oil, that role is teased out of reports in many studies as well, supported by those few that single out olive oil.

In a study published in the journal *Cardiovascular Diabetology* in 2015, investigators focused on determining the protective role of oleate in insulin resistance and in the atherosclerotic process at the cellular level because the molecular mechanisms that support the protective role of oleate in cardiovascular cells are poorly known.

It was found that palmitate induced insulin resistance. Furthermore, oleate did not induce insulin resistance but had a protective effect against insulin resistance induced by palmitate. This suggest the differential role of oleate and palmitate, and supports the concept of the cardioprotective role of oleate as the main lipid component of extra-virgin olive oil: oleate protects against cardiovascular insulin resistance, improves endothelial dysfunction in response to proinflammatory signals, and reduces proliferation and apoptosis in vascular smooth muscle cells, thus contributing to an ameliorated atherosclerotic process and plaque stability (Perdomo et al. 2015).

A report in *The Journal of Biological Chemistry* in 2010 proposes that oleic acid (in olive oil), plentiful in the Mediterranean diet, plays a crucial role in abating the damaging (and aging) effects of chronic elevated blood glucose—as in type 2 diabetes—on vascular endothelium: de novo lipogenesis, a highly regulated metabolic pathway whereby excess carbohydrate is converted into fatty acids that are then stored, is an insulin-dependent process driven by the multifunctional enzyme, fatty-acid synthase (FAS).

The study showed that FAS maintains endothelial function by targeting endothelial nitric-oxide synthase (eNOS, crucial to nitric oxide [NO] formation) to the endothelium cell membrane. The ratio of oleic acid to palmitic acid is apparently critical in modulating eNOS.

FAS-deficient endothelial cells show poor tissue repair function. Thus, disrupting eNOS bioavailability may be one mechanism in nutritional status and tissue repair that may contribute to diabetic vascular disease and aging (Wei et al. 2010). And, as reported in the *International Journal of Molecular Science* in 2013, more specific to the focus of this book, the Mediterranean diet goes a long way to reduce oxidative stress also linked to endothelial aging (Marín et al. 2013).

7.12.2 A Note on Palm Oil

Palm oil is an edible vegetable oil derived from the fruit of the oil palms, primarily the African oil palm (*Elaeis guineensis*), and to a lesser extent the American oil palm (*Elaeis oleifera*) and the maripa palm (*Attalea maripa*). It has an especially high concentration of saturated fat, about as much saturated fat as butter, and has been said to be "especially adept at raising cholesterol levels." However, palm oil also contains oleic acid.

Here is the fatty acids composition of palm oil:

- Palmitic saturated C16: 43.5%
- Oleic monounsaturated C18: 36.6%
- Linoleic polyunsaturated C18: 9.1%
- Stearic saturated C18: 4.3%

The average consumer is generally unaware of the ubiquitous nature of palm oil. It is the most widely consumed vegetable oil in supermarket products and can be found under various names on the Nutrition Facts label of about half of all packaged food products. Alternative names include vegetable oil, vegetable fat, palm kernel, palm kernel oil, palm fruit oil, palmate, palmitate, palmolein, glyceryl, stearate, stearic acid, palmitic acid, palm stearine, and palmitoyl oxostearamide, among a wide variety of other names.

Unlike olive oil, the health benefits and safety of consuming palm oil and its derivatives is disputed, with the preponderance of the evidence favoring caution in its use in the diet. For instance, on the positive side, the journal *Oxidative Medicine and Cellular Longevity* reported a study in 2010 on the effects of palm gamma-tocotrienol (GGT) on oxidative stress–induced cellular aging in normal human skin fibroblast cell lines derived from different age groups: young (21-year-old), middle-aged (40-year-old), and old (68-year-old) fibroblasts. Gamma-tocotrienol is a form of vitamin E.

Changes in cell viability, telomere length, and telomerase activity were assessed after treatment with gamma-tocotrienol for 24 hours. Results showed that treatment with different concentrations of gamma-tocotrienol increased fibroblast viability in both middle-aged and old fibroblasts. Curiously, at higher concentrations, gamma-tocotrienol treatment caused a marked decrease in cell viability.

In young and old fibroblasts, pretreatment with gamma-tocotrienol prevented shortening of telomere length and reduction in telomerase activity. In middle-aged fibroblasts, telomerase activity increased while no changes in telomere length were observed. These data suggest that gamma-tocotrienol protects against oxidative stress-induced cellular aging by modulating the telomere length possibly via telomerase (Makpol et al. 2010).

However, visceral adiposity in obesity causes excessive free fatty acid (FFA) flux into the liver and may cause fatty liver disease and hepatic insulin resistance. It is, however, difficult to determine the contribution of free fatty acids to hepatic insulin resistance. Therefore, many investigators including the authors of this study in *The Journal of Biological Chemistry* in 2009 chose to use a cell line. In this case, it was an animal hepatocellular line (H4IIEC3) treated with a monounsaturated fatty acid (oleate) and with a saturated fatty acid (palmitate) to investigate the direct and initial effects of FFAs on hepatocytes.

Hepatocytes make up the main tissue of the liver. They are involved in protein synthesis and storage; transformation of carbohydrates; synthesis of cholesterol, bile salts, and phospholipids; and detoxification, modification, and excretion of exogenous and endogenous substances.

It was found that palmitate but not oleate inhibits insulin, thus causing increased reactive oxygen species (ROS) formation in mitochondria. Mitochondria-derived ROS induced by palmitate may be major contributors to cellular insulin resistance (Nakamura et al. 2009).

It was also shown in a report published in *Acta Physiologica Scandinavica*, in 2005, that pretreatment of myotubes (developing muscle cells) with palmitate, chronic hyperglycemia, and acute high concentrations of insulin changed fatty acid metabolism in favor of accumulation of intracellular lipids. It was concluded that changes in fatty acid metabolism in human muscle are probably crucial for the molecular mechanism behind skeletal muscle insulin resistance and impaired glucose metabolism (Aas et al. 2005).

In 2012, the journal *Archives of Medical Science* published the results of a study conducted in Iran to examine the potential role of a high dietary intake of palmitic and linoleic acid on the risk of atherosclerosis. Chronic activation of endothelial cells in the presence of palmitic and linoleic oil was thought to account for the pathogenesis of cardiovascular events. These findings suggested further support for the detrimental effects of these fatty acids, especially palmitic acid, in the promotion and induction of the cardiovascular diseases that are prevalent in the Iranian population (Sanadgol et al. 2012).

A study on skeletal muscle cells reported in *The Journal of Biological Chemistry*, in 2008, concerned the contribution to insulin resistance and inflammation of two common dietary fatty acids. Exposure of cells to the saturated fatty acid palmitate led to a number of adverse conditions (enhanced diacylglycerol levels leading to activation of the protein kinase Cθ/nuclear factor κB pathway), resulting in enhanced interleukin 6 secretion and down-regulation of the expression of genes involved in the control of the oxidative capacity of skeletal muscle and triglyceride synthesis.

Interleukin 6 acts as both a pro-inflammatory cytokine and an anti-inflammatory myokine. Cytokines are molecules that aid cell-to-cell communication in immune responses, and stimulate the movement of cells toward sites of inflammation, infection, and trauma. Myokines are small proteins produced and released by muscle cells in response to muscular contractions.

In contrast, exposure to the monounsaturated fatty acid oleate did not lead to these changes. Interestingly, co-incubation of cells with palmitate and oleate reversed both inflammation and impairment of insulin signaling by channeling palmitate into triglycerides and by up-regulating the expression of genes involved in mitochondrial beta-oxidation, thus reducing its incorporation into diacylglycerol (a source of prostaglandins).

The findings support a model of cellular lipid metabolism where oleate protects against palmitate-induced inflammation and insulin resistance in skeletal muscle cells (Coll et al. 2008).

7.12.3 And a Note on Coconut Oil

Coconut oil is extracted from the meat of coconuts harvested from the coconut palm (*Cocos nucifera*). It has a high saturated fat content and therefore oxidizes slowly. It is commonly used in cooking, especially for frying. Despite its high saturated fat content, virgin coconut oil has become popular. However, while it works well in baked goods, pastries, and sautés, it also adds substantial calories.

Conventional coconut oil processors use hexane as a solvent to extract up to 10% more oil than produced with just rotary mills and expellers. They then refine the oil to remove certain free fatty acids to reduce its susceptibility to becoming rancid.

Here is the fatty acid content of coconut oil:

Lauric saturated C12 48%
Myristic saturated C14 16%
Palmitic saturated C16 9.5%
Decanoic saturated C10 8%
Caprylic saturated C8 7%
Oleic monounsaturated C18:1 6.5%
Other 5%

A number of health authorities have voiced concerns about the consumption of coconut oil due to its high levels of saturated fat. These include:

- The United States Food and Drug Administration (FDA). Around the block nutrition facts at a glance: more on nutrients to get less of (available from http://archive.fo/BzcW5).
- The World Health Organization (WHO). Avoiding heart attacks and strokes (available from http://www.who.int/cardiovascular_diseases/publications/avoid_heart_attack_report/en/).
- The International College of Nutrition (ICN). Recommendations for the prevention of coronary artery disease in Asians: a scientific statement of the International College of Nutrition (Singh, R. B., Mori, H., Chen, J., et al. 1996. *Journal of Cardiovascular Risk* Dec; (6):489–494).
  - The United States Department of Health and Human Services (DHHS). Dietary guidelines for Americans 2010 (available from https://health.gov/dietaryguidelines/dga2010/DietaryGuidelines2010.pdf)
  - The American Heart Association (AHA). Healthy cooking oils (available from http://www.heart.org/HEARTORG/HealthyLiving/HealthyEating/SimpleCookingandRecipes/Healthy-Cooking-Oils_UCM_445179_Article.jsp#.WOz7xfnyvIU).

Coconut oil contains a large proportion of lauric acid, a saturated fat that raises total blood cholesterol levels by increasing both high-density lipoprotein (HDL) cholesterol, and low-density lipoprotein (LDL) cholesterol (Mensink et al. 2003). On the bright side, this may create a more favorable total blood cholesterol profile. However, this does not mean that persistent consumption of coconut oil may not increase the risk of cardiovascular disease through other mechanisms, particularly the increase in blood cholesterol induced by lauric acid (Mensink et al. 2003).

Medical health authorities generally condemn the consumption of coconut oil, seemingly because of its fat composition. In fairness, that has been strongly linked to cardiovascular hazards, especially dyslipidemia, and insulin resistance. This is in opposition to the "pop" health sources that make health claims for it. Few of the "pop" health sources cite reliable evidence-based research. Admittedly much of that work is based on animal models, but here follow a few examples.

Virgin coconut oil improves blood glucose levels. Coconut does not contain much sugar (a significant proportion of the sugar it contains is in the form of fructose).

In that context, *The Journal of Food Science and Technology* reported in 2016 that high fructose-containing coconut oil (CO) is an established model for insulin resistance and fatty liver disease, characterized by inflammation of the liver with concurrent fat accumulation (steatohepatitis) in rodents.

In this study, replacement of CO with virgin coconut oil (VCO) in a high-fructose diet markedly improved glucose metabolism and dyslipidemia. The animals fed the VCO diet had only a 17% increase in blood glucose level compared with CO-fed animals (46%).

Increased levels of gluthatione (GSH) and antioxidant enzyme activities in VCO-fed rats indicated improved liver status. Reduced lipid peroxidation and carbonyl adducts in VCO-fed rats corroborated tissue analysis findings that liver damage and steatosis were reduced as compared to the CO-fed comparison animals. These results suggest that VCO could be an efficient nutraceutical in preventing the development of diet-induced insulin resistance and associated complications possibly through its antioxidant efficacy (Narayanankutty et al. 2016).

Lauric acid present in coconut oil (CO) may protect against diabetes-induced dyslipidemia. A study published in the *Indian Journal of Pharmacology*, in 2010, reported the effect of saturated fatty acid (SFA)-rich dietary vegetable oils on the lipid profile, endogenous antioxidant enzymes, and glucose tolerance in type 2 diabetic rats. The lipid profile, endogenous antioxidant enzymes, and oral glucose tolerance were monitored.

Type 2 diabetes was induced by administering streptozotocin (90 mg/kg, i.p.) in neonatal rats. Then 28-day-old normal and diabetic rats were fed for 45 days with a fat-enriched special diet (10%) prepared with coconut oil—lauric acid–rich SFA, palm oil—palmitic acid–rich SFA and groundnut oil—comparison animals.

Diabetic rats fed with coconut oil showed a significant decrease in total cholesterol and non-high-density lipoprotein cholesterol. They also exhibited improvement in antioxidant enzymes and glucose tolerance as compared to the diabetic rats in the groundnut oil group. The palm oil regimen aggravated dyslipidemia and resulted in a significant decrease in superoxide dismutase levels when compared to non-diabetic rats fed the ground nut regimen. Groundnut plus palm oil treatment also impaired glucose tolerance compared to diabetic and non-diabetic animals on the groundnut treatment.

The authors concluded that the type of fatty acid (FA) in dietary oil determines its adverse or beneficial effects. Lauric acid present in coconut oil may protect against diabetes-induced dyslipidemia (Mathai Kochikuzhyil et al. 2010).

Similar effects were observed in connection with "contrasting metabolic effects of medium- versus long-chain fatty acids in skeletal muscle" in a report in the *Journal of Lipid Research* in 2013.

The changes were associated with improved insulin action in medium-chain fatty acid (MCFA)-treated myotubes. MCFA-fed mice exhibited increased energy expenditure, reduced adiposity, and better glucose tolerance compared with long-chain fatty acid (LCFA)-fed mice. Dietary MCFAs increased respiration in isolated mitochondria, with a simultaneous reduction in reactive oxygen species (ROS) generation, and subsequently low oxidative damage.

These findings indicate that as compared to LCFAs, MCFAs increase the intrinsic respiratory capacity of mitochondria without increasing oxidative stress. These effects potentially contribute to the beneficial metabolic actions of dietary MCFAs (Magdalene et al. 2013).

Coconut oil is a rich source of medium chain fatty acids, particularly lauric acid.

7.12.4　EXTRA-VIRGIN OLIVE OIL AND THE XENOHORMESIS HYPOTHESIS: WHEN PLANTS "TALK" TO THE ANIMALS, WHAT DO THEY TELL THEM?

We now expect plant foods to not only supply us with nutrients but also to furnish us with antioxidants to protect us from the adverse impact of our environment and the debilitating by-products of our own metabolism. How and why do plants produce antioxidants?

In fact, plant antioxidants are as much a part of their immune system as T-cells and lymphocytes are a part of ours. And, to continue the comparison, we share with plants the property that immune system elements are activated when we are attacked by microbial predators. The challenge to plants by such adversaries typically in the form of bacteria, viruses, fungi, and insects of one sort or another, results in a response that science terms hormesis.

Hormesis describes a favorable, but seemingly paradoxical biological response to exposure to low levels of toxins and microbial or other pest stressors. In other words, a low-dose stressor, biological or chemical, may trigger a response in an organism opposite to that when given a very high dose of the same. We have learned that stress-inducible plant phytochemicals can be passed on to humans to produce a beneficial low-level stress response as well.

The study of hormesis in connection with the biological activity of components of extra-virgin olive oil has led investigators in a laboratory in Spain to the novel conclusion that, in a sense, plants "talk" to the animals that feed on them and convey a very specific molecular message relating to survival in times of food shortage, that is, calorie restriction (CR). The message is about the basic reality that there may be a period of food shortage to come and the animals that feed on them apparently "get it" and seem to prepare their own body defenses to cope with lean times.

When plants are "stressed" by adverse environmental conditions, they increase the production of defense molecules (polyphenols including resveratrol—antioxidants for us) that are thought to pass the message along to the animals that feed on them so that they can, in turn, develop defenses to protect themselves against calorie restriction. The xenohormesis hypothesis, that organisms have evolved to respond to stress signaling molecules produced by other species in their environment, is the explanation for this surprising observation. In this way, organisms can prepare in advance for a deteriorating environment and/or jeopardized food supply.

Xenohormesis also explains how certain molecules such as plant polyphenols that increase with stress in the plants can have a longevity-conferring effect in the animal that consumes the plant because the state of calorie restriction is the only state that we know to contribute to longevity by also promoting the activation of sirtuins, that is, SIRT1 and SIRT2 (Figure 7.4).

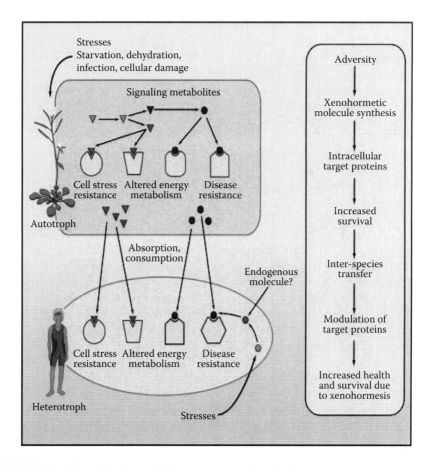

FIGURE 7.4 **(See color insert.)** The xenohormesis hypothesis. (From Howitz and Sinclair, 2008. *Cell*, 133(3), 387–391, 2008. With permission.)

Parenthetically, the term xenohormesis was first reported in the article "Small molecules that regulate lifespan: evidence for xenohormesis," which appeared in the journal *Molecular Biology* in 2004 (Lamming et al. 2004).

If the plants an animal is eating are under stress, their increased polyphenol composition may signal approaching famine conditions. It could be advantageous for the animal to start preparing for the lean times to come. The effects researchers have observed from resveratrol, for instance, may be just such a response (Sajish and Schimmel 2015).

We know that resveratrol in grape leaves and vines increases with attacks on the plant by *Botrytis cinerea*, a grape fungus. In fact, according to a report in the journal *Plant Physiology* in 2003, trans-resveratrol has been successfully applied as a pesticide in *B. cinerea*-infected grapes (Montero et al. 2003).

The hormesis hypothesis of calorie restriction (CR), that low calorie intake is in itself a mild stress that evokes a general stress response, explains why CR animals are more resistant to a broad array of stresses (Lamming et al. 2004). But, where does extra-virgin olive oil fit in this picture?

The authors of a study reported in the journal *Cell Cycle* in 2013 report that the xenohormetic nature of complex polyphenols naturally present in extra-virgin olive oil is a key component of the Mediterranean-style diet that has been repeatedly associated with a reduction in age-related adverse health conditions and longer life expectancy.

They showed for the first time that secoiridoids in extra-virgin olive oil prevent age-related changes in the cell size, structure, and function, leading to senescence. The authors aver that extra-virgin olive oil secoiridoids, which provide an effective defense against plant attack by herbivores and pathogens, are bona fide xenohormetins that are able to activate an enzyme, AMPK, that plays a role in cellular energy homeostasis and trigger numerous resveratrol-like anti-aging (gerosuppressor) factors.

They conclude that extra-virgin olive oil secoiridoids constitute a new family of plant-produced gerosuppressant agents that "repair" the aimless (and harmful) AMPK-driven pathway that leads to aging and aging-related diseases (including cancer) (Menendez et al. 2013).

Polyphenols such as resveratrol and quercetin, which are produced by stressed plants, activate sirtuins, thus extending the lifespan of animals, presumably by mimicking the beneficial effects of caloric restriction (CR). Perhaps, it is because the sirtuins have evolved to respond to plant stress molecules as indicators of an impending deterioration of the environment. This is the xenohormesis hypothesis, the name stemming from the prefix xeno- (for stranger) and hormesis (a protective response induced by mild stress).

Finally, as documented in a report from the Food and Agriculture Organization and the World Health Organization (FAO/WHO), a diet rich in polyunsaturated fats (PUFA) and low in saturated fats (SF) is beneficial to health (no authors listed 2009). It is also well known now that the primary health benefit of olive oil, or for that matter, any oil consumed in the diet, is related to its antioxidant capacity.

However, these oils oxidize readily, that is, they decompose when they are exposed to oxygen to a "rancid" state. And there is some concern by health authorities about possible adverse health consequences from the consumption of oxidized lipids because little is known about how that may constitute a health hazard for humans.

In a study published in the journal *Food and Nutrition Research* in 2011, the authors compared saturated fats in commercially available marine omega-3 supplements and vegetable oils to unsaturated fats with respect to the concentration of reactive oxygen species (ROS).

Assessing the oxidative status of commercially available omega-3 supplements and vegetable oils showed that the degree of oxidation varies. The content of ROS in marine omega-3 supplements is far higher than in fresh vegetable oils. Heating vegetable oils was shown to considerably increase ROS levels. Since there is a larger intake of vegetable oils in the common diet than fish oil supplements, the former is the largest source of primary as well as secondary oxidation products in the diet.

The authors conclude that despite the biological toxicity of lipid oxidation products, an upper limit corresponding to a safe dose of these compounds has not been established and they recommend further study of the potentially harmful effects of oxidized oils (Halvorsen and Blomhoff 2011).

7.13   SEVEN-DAY FOOD PLAN

The majority of the recipes that follow are courtesy of the National Heart, Lung, and Blood Institute (NHLBI) *Stay Young at Heart* program, consistent with the Mediterranean diet plan. Recipes identified with one asterisk (*) are reproduced with permission from the NHLBI of the US National Institutes of Health (NIH). USDA recipes are identified by two asterisks (**).

The reader is encouraged also to try to follow the Mediterranean food pyramid and incorporate dishes that are high in fruits and/or vegetables. When selecting protein, choose nuts and beans, lean meat, poultry and, if possible, fish at least three times per week.

7.13.1   SERVING SIZES, KITCHEN MEASURES, AND METRIC CONVERSION

Serving sizes, kitchen measures, and metric conversion factors are given in Tables 7.3–7.5.

Planning for proactive nutrition can begin with a food plan such as the following 7-day food plan. This is followed by recipes consistent with the nutrition program.

TABLE 7.3
Serving Equivalents

For starches (grains, beans, and starchy vegetables), a serving can equal:
   One slice of bread
   One small potato
   ½ cup cooked cereal or ¾ cup dry cereal
   ⅓ cup of rice
   ½ cup of peas
For fruits, a typical serving might equal:
   One small apple
   ½ cup apple or orange juice
   ½ grapefruit
   ½ banana
   1¼ cup whole strawberries
For vegetables, one serving can equal:
   ½ cup carrots
   ½ cup cooked green beans
   1 cup salad
   ½ cup broccoli
   ½ cup tomato juice
A single serving of milk or yogurt equals one cup of fat-free plain yogurt or one cup of skim milk.
A single serving of protein foods, such as meat or cheese, is generally 2–3 oz after cooking (this is about the size of a deck of cards).
A 2 oz serving of cheese or 4 oz of tofu (about 1/2 cup) also equals a single serving of protein.
A single serving of oil is one teaspoon and a single serving of salad dressing is one tablespoon.

TABLE 7.4

Kitchen Measures

1/16 cup = 1 tablespoon
1/8 cup = 2 tablespoons
1/6 cup = 2 tablespoons + 2 teaspoons
1/4 cup = 4 tablespoons
1/3 cup = 5 tablespoons + 1 teaspoon
3/8 cup = 6 tablespoons
1/2 cup = 8 tablespoons
2/3 cup = 10 tablespoons + 2 teaspoons
3/4 cup = 12 tablespoons
1 cup = 48 teaspoons
1 cup = 16 tablespoons
8 fluid ounces (fl oz) = 1 cup
1 pint (pt) = 2 cups
1 quart (qt) = 2 pints
4 cups = 1 quart
1 gallon (gal) = 4 quarts
16 ounces (oz) = 1 pound (lb)

TABLE 7.5

Metric Conversion Table

Multiply	By	To Get
Fluid Ounces	29.57	grams
Ounces (dry)	28.35	grams
Grams	0.0353	ounces
Grams	0.0022	pounds
Kilograms	2.21	pounds
Pounds	453.6	grams
Pounds	0.4536	kilograms
Quarts	0.946	liters
Quarts (dry)	67.2	cubic inches
Quarts (liquid)	57.7	cubic inches
Liters	1.0567	quarts
Gallons	3,785	cubic centimeters
Gallons	3.785	liters

7.13.2 Monday

- Breakfast: Low-sugar cereal (with at least 5 g of fiber), Greek yogurt, and berries
- Snack: Chai latte made with almond milk
- Lunch: Greek salad (romaine lettuce, cherry tomatoes, olives, and hot pepper) with low-fat feta cheese, and olive oil and balsamic vinegar dressing

- Snack: Raw carrot and celery dippers with hummus
- Dinner: Brown rice with shrimp or tuna, roasted cherry tomatoes, and arugula.

7.13.3 TUESDAY

- Breakfast: Whole grain oatmeal, served with berries
- Snack: A small 4.5 oz pot of plain Greek yogurt with a handful of walnuts
- Lunch: A whole wheat wrap with grilled chicken and mushrooms
- Snack: Blueberries and 1 oz dark chocolate
- Dinner: Baked sea bass with grilled vegetables (eggplant, asparagus, zucchini, and peppers)

7.13.4 WEDNESDAY

- Breakfast: Scrambled eggs with crispbread
- Snack: Fruit smoothie with berries, apple, and banana
- Lunch: Chickpea salad (chickpeas, celery, chopped onion, red pepper, and tomato) on romaine lettuce, with tahini dressing and crispbread
- Snack: Dark chocolate
- Dinner: Chicken, mushroom, and onion kebabs (marinated in garlic and olive oil) with bulgar wheat or couscous salad

7.13.5 THURSDAY

- Breakfast: Two handfuls of chopped fruit with 1–2 tbsp of natural or Greek yogurt and 1 tsp of organic honey (optional 1 tbsp of granola)
- Snack: Handful of nuts
- Lunch: Chicken with hummus and salad in a pita
- Snack: Banana
- Dinner: Salmon salad with lentils, pomegranate, and red onion with a dressing of extra-virgin olive oil, lemon, honey, tarragon, and parsley

7.13.6 FRIDAY

- Breakfast: Low-sugar cereal (with at least 5 g of fiber), milk, and berries
- Snack: Handful of nuts
- Lunch: Spicy veggie or bean burger in a pita with salad and cooling cucumber and mint yogurt
- Snack: Fresh fruit (one piece or one cup)
- Dinner: Tomato fish chowder (white fish, red potatoes, celery, onion, and garlic) with a green salad, and olive oil and balsamic vinegar dressing

7.13.7 SATURDAY

- Breakfast: Baked tomato and spinach eggs with a toasted pita
- Snack: Fruit smoothie (berries, apple, banana, and ice cubes mixed in a blender)

- Lunch: Italian salad (romaine lettuce, hot peppers, olives, and sweet peppers) with mozzarella
- Snack: Handful of nuts
- Dinner: Salmon with brown rice salad (sweetcorn, cherry tomatoes, cucumber, and red onion)

7.13.8 SUNDAY

- Breakfast: Two handfuls of chopped fruit with 1–2 tbsp of natural or Greek yogurt and 1 tsp of organic honey (optional 1 tbsp of granola)
- Snack: Rice cake with apple butter
- Lunch: Whole wheat wrap with chicken salad (steamed chicken breast with celery, raisins, and apple, tossed with 1 tbsp mayonnaise)
- Snack: Chai latte with almond milk
- Dinner: Turkey meatloaf, baked sweet potato, and steamed kale with pine nuts

7.14 SELECTED RECIPES

7.14.1 BREAKFAST DISHES

7.14.1.1 Vegetable Omelet

Ingredients:

- 1 tbsp olive oil
- 2 cups thinly sliced fresh fennel bulb
- 1 Roma tomato, diced
- ¼ cup pitted green brine-cured olives, chopped
- ¼ cup artichoke hearts, marinated in water, rinsed, drained, and chopped
- 6 eggs
- ¼ tsp salt
- ½ tsp pepper
- ½ cup goat cheese, crumbled
- 2 tbsp chopped fresh dill, basil, or parsley

Directions:

- Preheat the oven to 325°F.
- In a large ovenproof skillet, heat the olive oil over medium-high heat.
- Add the fennel and sauté for 5 minutes, until soft.
- Add in the tomato, olives, and artichoke hearts and sauté for 3 minutes, until softened.
- Whisk the eggs in a large bowl and season with the salt and pepper.
- Pour the whisked eggs into the skillet over the vegetables and stir with a heat-proof spoon for 2 minutes.
- Sprinkle the omelet with the cheese and bake for 5 minutes or until the eggs are cooked through and set.

- Top with the dill, basil, or parsley.
- Remove the omelet from the skillet onto a cutting board. Carefully cut the omelet into four wedges, like a pizza, and serve.
- Yield: 4 servings. Per serving: calories 152 (91 from fat), fat 10 g (saturated 4 g), cholesterol 13 mg, sodium 496 mg, carbohydrate 6 g (dietary fiber 2 g), and protein 11 g.

7.14.1.2 Zucchini and Goat Cheese Frittata

Ingredients:

- 2 medium zucchinis
- 8 eggs
- 2 tbsp milk
- ¼ tsp salt
- ⅛ tsp pepper
- 1 tbsp olive oil
- 1 clove garlic, crushed
- 2 oz goat cheese, crumbled

Directions:

- Preheat the oven to 350°F.
- Slice the zucchinis into ¼-inch-thick round slices. In a large bowl, whisk the eggs with the milk, salt, and pepper.
- In a heavy, ovenproof skillet (preferably cast iron), heat the olive oil over a medium heat.
- Add the garlic and cook for 30 seconds. Add the zucchini slices and cook for 5 minutes.
- Pour the whisked eggs over the zucchini and stir for 1 minute.
- Top with the cheese and transfer to the oven. Bake for 10–12 minutes or until the eggs are set. Remove the pan from the oven and let it sit for 3 minutes.
- Transfer the frittata to a cutting board, slice into four pie wedges, and serve hot or at room temperature.
- Yield: 4 servings. Per serving: calories 134 (72 from fat), fat 8 g (saturated 3 g), cholesterol 11 mg, sodium 324 mg, carbohydrate 4 g (dietary fiber 1 g), and protein 12 g.

7.14.1.3 Lemon Scones

Ingredients:

- 2 cups plus ¼ cup flour
- 2 tbsp sugar
- ½ tsp baking soda
- ½ tsp salt
- ¼ cup butter
- Zest of one lemon

- ¾ cup reduced-fat buttermilk
- 1 cup powdered sugar
- 1–2 tsp lemon juice

Directions:

- Heat the oven to 400°F.
- In a medium bowl, combine 2 cups of the flour, the sugar, baking soda, and salt.
- Using a pastry blender or a food processor, cut in the butter until the mixture resembles fine crumbs.
- Add the lemon zest and buttermilk, stirring just until mixed.
- Flour a surface with the remaining flour and turn out the dough and knead gently six times. Shape the dough into a ball and then flatten into a ½-inch-thick circle with a rolling pin.
- Cut the circle into 4 wedges and then cut each wedge into 3 smaller wedges, yielding 12 scones.
- Place the scones on a baking sheet and cook for 12–15 minutes or until golden brown.
- In a small bowl, mix the powder sugar and just enough lemon juice to make a thin frosting. Drizzle the frosting over the hot scones and serve.
- Yield: 12 scones. Per serving: calories 175 (39 from fat), fat 4 g (saturated 3 g), cholesterol 11 mg, sodium 190 mg, carbohydrate 31 g (dietary fiber 1 g), and protein 3 g.

7.14.1.4   Breakfast Mango Smoothies

Ingredients:

- 1 ripe mango, about 1 cup
- ½ cup (125 g) canned sliced peaches
- ½ cup (120 ml) 2% or low-fat milk
- 3 oz (85 g) 0% fat unflavored yogurt
- ½ cup ice

Directions:

- Place all ingredients in a blender and process until smooth.
- Yield: 1 serving: calories 250, total fat 15 g, and saturated fat 2 g.

7.14.1.5   Breakfast Berry Smoothie*

Ingredients:

- 1 cup plain non-fat yogurt
- 6 medium strawberries
- 1 medium banana
- 1 cup crushed pineapple in juice
- 6 ice cubes

Directions:

- Place all ingredients in a blender and purée until smooth.
- Serve in a frosted glass.
- Makes 3 servings. Serving size: 1 cup. Each serving provides: calories 121, fat less than 1 g, saturated fat less than 1 g, cholesterol 1 mg, and sodium 64 mg.

7.14.2 Soups, Salads, and Side Dishes

7.14.2.1 Bean and Macaroni Soup**

Ingredients:

- 2 cans (16 oz) great northern beans
- 1 tbsp extra-virgin olive oil
- ½ lb fresh mushrooms, sliced
- 1 cup onion, coarsely chopped
- 2 cups carrots, sliced
- 1 cup celery, coarsely chopped
- 1 clove garlic, minced
- 3 cups peeled fresh tomatoes, cut up, or 1½ lb canned whole tomatoes, cut up
- 1 tsp dried sage
- 1 tsp dried thyme
- ½ tsp dried oregano
- Black pepper, to taste
- 1 bay leaf, crumbled
- 4 cups elbow macaroni, cooked

Directions:

- Drain the beans and reserve the liquid. Rinse the beans.
- Heat the oil in a 6-quart kettle; add mushrooms, onion, carrots, celery, and garlic and sauté for 5 minutes.
- Add tomatoes, sage, thyme, oregano, pepper, and bay leaf.
- Cover and cook over a medium heat for 20 minutes. Cook the macaroni according to the directions on the package using unsalted water. Drain when cooked. Do not overcook.
- Combine the reserved bean liquid with water to make 4 cups.
- Add liquid, beans, and cooked macaroni to the vegetable mixture.
- Bring to a boil, cover, and simmer until the soup is thoroughly heated. Stir occasionally.
- Yield: 16 servings. Serving size: 1 cup. Each serving provides: calories 158, total fat 1 g, saturated fat 1 g, cholesterol 0 mg, sodium 154 mg,[*] fiber 5 mg, protein 8 mg, carbohydrate 29 g, and potassium 524 mg.

---

[*] If canned tomatoes are used, sodium will be higher.

7.14.2.2 Minestrone Soup

Ingredients:

- ¼ cup extra-virgin olive oil
- 1 clove garlic, minced, or ⅛ tsp garlic powder
- 1⅓ cups onion, coarsely chopped
- 1½ cups celery and leaves, coarsely chopped
- 1 can (6 oz) tomato paste
- 1 tbsp fresh parsley, chopped
- 1 cup sliced carrots, fresh or frozen
- 4¾ cups cabbage, shredded
- 1 can (1 lb) tomatoes, cut up
- 1 cup canned red kidney beans, drained and rinsed
- 1½ cups frozen peas
- 1½ cups fresh green beans
- Dash of hot sauce
- 11 cups water
- 2 cups spaghetti, uncooked and broken

Directions:

- Heat oil in a 4-quart saucepan. Add the garlic, onion, and celery and sauté for about 5 minutes.
- Add all remaining ingredients except the spaghetti, and stir until ingredients are well mixed.
- Bring to a boil. Reduce the heat, cover, and simmer about 45 minutes or until vegetables are tender.
- Add uncooked spaghetti and simmer 2–3 minutes only.
- Yield: 16 servings. Serving size: 1 cup. Each serving provides: calories 112, total fat 4 g, saturated fat 0 g, cholesterol 0 mg, sodium 202 mg, fiber 4 g, protein 4 g, carbohydrate 17 g, and potassium 393 mg.

7.14.2.3 Gazpacho

Ingredients:

- 4 cups tomato juice[*]
- ½ medium onion, peeled and coarsely chopped
- 1 small green pepper, peeled, cored, seeded, and coarsely chopped
- 1 small cucumber, peeled, seeded, and coarsely chopped
- ½ tsp Worcestershire sauce
- 1 clove garlic, minced
- 1 drop hot pepper sauce
- ⅛ tsp cayenne pepper

---

[*] To cut back on sodium, try low-sodium tomato juice.

- ¼ tsp black pepper
- 2 tbsp extra-virgin olive oil
- 1 large tomato, finely diced
- 2 tbsp minced chives or scallion tops
- 1 lemon, cut in 6 wedges

Directions:

- Put 2 cups of tomato juice and all the other ingredients except the diced tomato, chives, and lemon wedges in a blender.
- Purée.
- Slowly add the remaining 2 cups of tomato juice to the puréed mixture. Add the chopped tomato and chill.
- Serve icy cold in individual bowls garnished with chopped chives and lemon wedges.
- Yield: 6 servings. Serving size: 1 cup. Each serving provides: calories 87, total fat 5 g, saturated fat less than 1 g, cholesterol 0 mg, and sodium 593 mg.

7.14.2.4   Rockport Fish Chowder*

Ingredients:

- 2 tbsp extra-virgin olive oil
- ¾ cup coarsely chopped onion
- ½ cup coarsely chopped celery
- 1 cup sliced carrots
- 2 cups potatoes, raw, peeled, and cubed
- ¼ tsp thyme
- ½ tsp paprika
- 2 cups bottled clam juice
- 8 whole peppercorns
- 1 bay leaf
- 1 lb fresh or frozen (thawed) cod or haddock fillets, cut into ¾-inch cubes
- ¼ cup whole wheat flour
- 3 cups low-fat (1%) milk
- 1 tbsp fresh parsley, chopped

Directions:

- Heat the oil in a large saucepan. Add the onion and celery and sauté for about 3 minutes.
- Add the carrots, potatoes, thyme, paprika, and clam broth.
- Wrap the peppercorns and bay leaves in cheese cloth. Add to the pot. Bring to a boil, reduce heat, and simmer for 15 minutes.
- Add the fish and simmer for an additional 15 minutes, or until fish flakes easily and is opaque.

- Remove the fish and vegetables and break the fish into chunks. Bring the broth to a boil and continue boiling until the volume is reduced to 1 cup. Remove the bay leaves and peppercorns.
- Shake the flour and ½ cup low-fat (1%) milk in a container with a tight-fitting lid until smooth. Add to the broth in the saucepan with the remaining milk. Cook over a medium heat, stirring constantly, until the mixture boils.
- Return the vegetables and fish chunks to stock and heat thoroughly. Serve hot, sprinkled with chopped parsley.
- Yield: 8 servings. Serving size: 1 cup. Each serving provides: calories 186, total fat 6 g, and saturated fat 1 g.

7.14.2.5   Cannery Row Soup**

Ingredients:

- 2 lb varied fish fillets (e.g., haddock, perch, flounder, cod, or sole), cut into 1-inch-square cubes
- 2 tbsp olive oil
- 1 clove garlic, minced
- 3 carrots, cut into thin strips
- 2 cups celery, sliced
- ½ cup onion, chopped
- ¼ cup green peppers, chopped
- 1 can (28 oz) whole tomatoes, cut up, with liquid
- 1 cup clam juice
- ¼ tsp dried thyme, crushed
- ¼ tsp dried basil, crushed
- ⅛ tsp black pepper
- ¼ cup fresh parsley, minced

Directions:

- Heat the oil in a large sauce pan. Sauté the garlic, carrots, celery, onion, and green pepper in oil for 3 minutes.
- Add the remaining ingredients except the parsley and fish. Cover and simmer for 10–15 minutes or until the vegetables are fork-tender.
- Add the fish and parsley. Simmer, covered, for 5–10 minutes more or until the fish flakes easily and is opaque. Serve hot.
- Yield: 8 servings. Serving size: 1 cup. Each serving provides: calories 170, total fat 5 g, saturated fat less than 1 g, cholesterol 56 mg, sodium 380 mg, fiber 3 g, protein 22 g, carbohydrate 9 g, and potassium 710 mg.

7.14.2.6   Chicken Salad**

Ingredient

- 3¼ cups chicken, cooked, cubed, and skinned
- ¼ cup celery, chopped

- 1 tbsp lemon juice
- ½ tsp onion powder
- ⅛ tsp salt*
- 3 tbsp mayonnaise, low-fat

Directions:

- Bake the chicken, cut into cubes, and refrigerate.
- In large bowl, combine the rest of ingredients, add the chilled chicken and mix well.
- Yield: 5 servings. Serving size: ¾ cup. Each serving provides: calories 176, total fat 6 g, saturated fat 2 g, cholesterol 77 mg, sodium 179 mg, fiber 0 g, protein 27 g, carbohydrate 2 g, and potassium 236 mg.

7.14.2.7   Spinach Salad**

Ingredients:

- 3 cups baby spinach leaves, well washed and dried
- 1 cup seasonal fresh vegetables or fruits of your choice, such as raw sugar snap peas, strawberry halves, blueberries, or peach slices
- 3 tbsp vinaigrette salad dressing, low-fat
- ½ tsp black pepper

Directions:

- Place the spinach and seasonal fruits or vegetables into a large bowl. The more colors you add to the diet, the more nutrients in it. Toss with the dressing and serve.
- Serves: 2 people. Each serving provides (nutritional information includes strawberries in salad): calories 59, total fat 2 g, saturated fat 0 g, carbohydrate 10 g, sodium 250 mg, and fiber 6 g.

7.14.2.8   Sunshine Salad**

Ingredients:

- 5 cups spinach leaves, packed, washed, and dried well
- ½ red onion, sliced thin
- ½ red pepper, sliced
- 1 whole cucumber, sliced
- 2 oranges, peeled and chopped into bite-size pieces
- ⅓ cup of bottle "lite" vinaigrette dressing (around 15 calories per tablespoon or less)

---

* Reduce sodium by removing the 1/8 tsp of added salt. The new sodium content for each serving is 127 mg.

Directions:

- Toss all ingredients together in a large bowl. Add dressing and toss again. Serve immediately.
- Serves: 5 people. Each serving provides: cholesterol 0 mg, fiber 8 g, sodium 200 mg, calories from protein 18%, calories from carbohydrate 62%, and calories from fat 20%.

7.14.2.9   Fresh Cabbage and Tomato Salad*

Ingredients:

- 1 small head cabbage, sliced thinly
- 2 medium tomatoes, cut in cubes
- 1 cup sliced radishes
- ¼ tsp salt
- 2 tsp extra-virgin olive oil
- 2 tbsp rice vinegar (or lemon juice)
- ½ tsp black pepper
- ½ tsp red pepper
- 2 tbsp fresh cilantro, chopped

Directions:

- In a large bowl, mix together the cabbage, tomatoes, and radishes.
- In another bowl, mix together the rest of the ingredients and pour over the vegetables.
- Yield: 8 servings. Serving size: 1 cup. Each serving provides: calories 41, total fat 1 g, saturated fat less than 1 g, cholesterol 0 mg, sodium 88 mg, calcium 49 mg, and iron 1 mg.

7.14.2.10   Waldorf Salad

Ingredients:

- 2 red-skinned crisp apples, try Jongold or Red Delicious (3 cups)
- 2 tbsp lemon juice
- 2 ribs celery, diced (½ cup)
- 2 tbsp toasted walnuts, chopped
- ¼ cup mayonnaise dressing, low-fat
- 4 cups romaine lettuce, washed and torn into bite-size pieces
- ¼ cup raisins

Directions:

- Wash and cut the apples into quarters, core, then dice into ¾-inch pieces. Toss with the lemon juice.
- Add the celery, walnuts, and mayonnaise dressing. Mix thoroughly.

- Place the lettuce on four plates or into salad bowls.
- Scoop the apple mixture onto each salad and scatter the raisins over the top.
- Yield: 4 servings. Each serving provides: calories 129, total fat 4 g, saturated fat 0 g, carbohydrate 25 g, sodium 163 mg, and fiber 4 g.

7.14.2.11 Stuffed Artichokes

Ingredients:

- 2 cups fresh breadcrumbs, preferably whole wheat (whole meal)
- 1 tbsp olive oil
- 4 large artichokes
- 2 lemons, halved
- ⅓ cup grated Parmesan cheese
- 3 garlic cloves, finely chopped
- 2 tbsp finely chopped fresh flat-leaf (Italian) parsley
- 1 tbsp grated lemon zest
- ¼ tsp freshly ground black pepper
- 1 cup plus 2–4 tbsp vegetable stock, chicken stock, or broth
- 1 cup dry white wine
- 1 tbsp minced shallot
- 1 tsp chopped fresh oregano

Directions

- Preheat the oven to 400°F.
- In a bowl, combine the breadcrumbs and olive oil. Toss to coat. Spread the crumbs in a shallow baking pan and bake, stirring once halfway through, until the crumbs are lightly golden, about 10 minutes. Set aside to cool.
- Working with one artichoke at a time, snap off any tough outer leaves and trim the stem flush with the base. Cut off the top third of the leaves with a serrated knife, and trim off any remaining thorns with scissors. Rub the cut edges with a lemon half to prevent discoloration. Separate the inner leaves and pull out the small leaves from the center. Using a melon baller or spoon, scoop out the fuzzy choke then squeeze some lemon juice into the cavity. Trim the remaining artichokes in the same manner.
- In a large bowl, toss the breadcrumbs with the Parmesan, garlic, parsley, lemon zest, and pepper. Add the 2–4 tbsp stock, 1 tbsp at a time, using just enough for the stuffing to begin to stick together in small clumps.
- Using ⅔ of the stuffing, mound it slightly in the center of the artichokes. Then, starting at the bottom, spread the leaves open and spoon a rounded teaspoon of stuffing near the base of each leaf. (The artichokes can be prepared to this point several hours ahead and kept refrigerated.)
- In a Dutch oven with a tight-fitting lid, combine 1 cup of stock, the wine, shallot, and oregano. Bring to a boil then reduce the heat to low. Arrange the

artichokes, stem end down, in the liquid in a single layer. Cover and simmer for about 45 minutes until the outer leaves are tender (add water if necessary). Transfer the artichokes to a rack and let cool slightly. Cut each artichoke into quarters and serve warm.

- Yield: 8 servings. Each serving provides: 140 calories, total fat 4 g, monounsaturated fat 2 g, sodium 246 mg, and cholesterol 5 mg.

7.14.3 ENTREES

7.14.3.1 Chicken Orientale*

Ingredients:

- 8 boneless, skinless chicken breasts
- 8 fresh mushrooms
- Black pepper to taste
- 8 parboiled whole white onions
- 2 oranges, quartered
- 8 canned pineapple chunks
- 8 cherry tomatoes
- 1 can (6 oz) frozen, concentrated apple juice, thawed
- 1 cup dry white wine
- 2 tbsp soy sauce, low sodium
- Dash ground ginger
- 2 tbsp vinegar
- ¼ cup extra-virgin oil

Directions:

- Sprinkle chicken breasts with pepper.
- Thread 8 skewers as follows: chicken, mushroom, chicken, onion, chicken, orange quarter, chicken, pineapple chunk, and cherry tomato.
- Place the kabobs in a shallow pan.
- Combine remaining the ingredients and spoon over the kabobs. Marinate in a refrigerator for at least 1 hour.
- Drain. Broil 6 inches from heat, 15 minutes on each side, brushing with marinade every 5 minutes. Discard any leftover marinade.
- Yield: 8 servings. Serving size: ½ chicken breast kabob. Each serving provides: calories 359, total fat 11 g, saturated fat 2 g, cholesterol 66 mg, and sodium 226 mg.

7.14.3.2 Chicken Ratatouille*

Ingredients:

- Extra-virgin olive oil
- 4 medium chicken breast halves, skinned, and fat removed, boned, and cut into 1-inch pieces

- 2 zucchini, about 7 inches long, unpeeled and thinly sliced
- 1 small eggplant, peeled and cut into 1-inch cubes
- 1 medium onion, thinly sliced
- 1 medium green pepper, cut into 1-inch pieces
- ½ lb fresh mushrooms, sliced
- 1 can (16 oz) whole tomatoes, cut up
- 1 clove garlic, minced
- 1½ tsp dried basil, crushed
- 1 tbsp fresh parsley, minced
- Black pepper to taste

Directions:

- Heat the oil in a large cast iron skillet. Add the chicken and sauté for about 3 minutes, or until lightly browned.
- Add the zucchini, eggplant, onion, green pepper, and mushrooms. Cook for about 15 minutes, stirring occasionally.
- Add the tomatoes, garlic, basil, parsley, and pepper; stir and continue cooking for about 5 minutes, or until chicken is tender.
- Broil 6 inches from heat, 15 minutes on each side, brushing with marinade every 5 minutes. Discard any leftover marinade.
- Yield: 4 servings. Serving size: 1½ cups. Each serving provides: calories 266, total fat 8 g, saturated fat 2 g, cholesterol 66 mg, and sodium 253 mg.

7.14.3.3   Scallop Kabobs*

Ingredients:

- 3 medium green peppers, cut into 1½-inch squares
- 1½ lb fresh bay scallops
- 1 pint cherry tomatoes
- ¼ cup dry white wine
- ¼ cup vegetable oil
- 3 tbsp lemon juice
- Dash garlic powder
- Black pepper to taste

Directions:

- Parboil the green peppers for 2 minutes. Alternately thread the first three ingredients on skewers. Combine the next five ingredients.
- Brush the kabobs with the wine/oil/lemon mixture, place on a grill (or under a broiler), and grill for 15 minutes, turning and basting frequently.
- Yield: 4 servings Serving size: 6 oz scallop kabob. Each serving provides: calories 224, total fat 6 g, saturated fat less than 1 g, cholesterol 43 mg, and sodium 355 mg.

7.14.3.4 Mediterranean Baked Fish*

Ingredients:

- Extra-virgin olive oil
- 1 large onion, sliced
- 1 can (16 oz) whole tomatoes, drained (reserve the juice), and coarsely chopped
- 1 bay leaf
- 1 clove garlic, minced
- 1 cup dry white wine
- ½ cup reserved tomato juice, from the canned tomatoes
- ¼ cup lemon juice
- ¼ cup orange juice
- 1 tbsp fresh grated orange peel
- 1 tsp fennel seeds, crushed
- ½ tsp dried oregano, crushed
- ½ tsp dried thyme, crushed
- ½ tsp dried basil, crushed
- Black pepper to taste
- 1 lb fish fillets (sole, flounder, or sea perch)

Directions:

- Heat the oil in a large cast iron skillet. Add the onion and sauté over a moderate heat for 5 minutes or until soft.
- Add all remaining ingredients except the fish, stir well and simmer for 30 minutes, uncovered.
- Arrange fish in a 10×6-inch baking dish and cover with sauce.
- Bake, uncovered, at 375°F for about 15 minutes or until the fish flakes easily.
- Yield: 4 servings. Serving size: 4 oz fillet with sauce. Each serving provides: calories 177, total fat 4 g, saturated fat 1 g, cholesterol 56 mg, and sodium 281 mg.

7.14.3.5 Spinach-Stuffed Sole*

Ingredients:

- Extra-virgin olive oil cooking spray as needed
- 1 tsp olive oil
- ½ lb fresh mushrooms, sliced
- ½ lb fresh spinach, chopped
- ¼ tsp oregano leaves, crushed
- 1 clove garlic, minced
- 1½ lb sole fillets or other white fish
- 2 tbsp sherry
- 4 oz part-skim mozzarella cheese, grated

Directions:

- Preheat oven to 400°F.
- Spray a 10×6-inch baking dish with extra-virgin olive oil (the pan can be wiped with oil on a paper towel if a sprayer is not available).
- Heat the oil in a skillet and sauté the mushrooms for about 3 minutes or until tender.
- Add the spinach and continue cooking for about 1 minute or until the spinach is barely wilted. Remove from the heat and drain liquid into the prepared baking dish.
- Add the oregano and garlic to the drained sautéed vegetables and stir to mix the ingredients.
- Divide the vegetable mixture evenly among the fillets, placing the filling in the center of each fillet.
- Roll the fillet around the mixture and place seam-side down in the prepared baking dish.
- Sprinkle with the sherry, then the grated mozzarella cheese. Bake for 15–20 minutes or until the fish flakes easily. Lift out with a slotted spoon.
- Yield: 4 servings. Serving size: 1 fillet roll. Each serving provides: calories 262, total fat 8 g, saturated fat 4 g, cholesterol 95 mg, and sodium 312 mg.

7.14.3.6   Black Beans with Rice*

Ingredients:

- 1 lb dry black beans
- 7 cups water
- 1 medium green pepper, coarsely chopped
- 1½ cups chopped onion
- 1 tbsp extra-virgin olive oil
- 2 bay leaves
- 1½ clove garlic, minced
- ½ tsp salt
- 1 tbsp vinegar (or lemon juice)
- 6 cups rice, cooked in unsalted water
- 1 jar (4 oz) sliced pimento, drained
- 1 lemon cut into wedges

Directions:

- Pick through the beans to remove the bad ones. Soak the beans overnight in cold water. Drain and rinse.
- In large soup pot or Dutch oven, stir together the beans, water, green pepper, onion, oil, bay leaves, garlic, and salt. Cover and boil for 1 hour.
- Reduce the heat and simmer, covered, for 3–4 hours or until the beans are very tender. Stir occasionally and add water if needed.

- Remove about ⅓ of the beans, mash, and return to pot. Stir and heat through.
- Remove the bay leaves and stir in the vinegar or lemon juice when ready to serve.
- Serve over rice. Garnish with sliced pimento and lemon wedges.
- Yield: 6 servings. Serving size: 8 oz. Each serving provides: calories 561, total fat 4 g, saturated fat 1 g, cholesterol 0 mg, and sodium 193 mg.

7.14.3.7 New Orleans Red Beans*

Ingredients:

- 1 lb dry red beans
- 2 quarts water
- 1½ cups chopped onion
- 1 cup chopped celery
- 4 bay leaves
- 1 cup chopped green pepper
- 3 tbsp chopped garlic
- 3 tbsp chopped parsley
- 2 tsp dried thyme, crushed
- 1 tsp salt
- 1 tsp black pepper

Directions:

- Pick through beans to remove the bad ones and rinse thoroughly.
- In a large pot combine the beans, water, onion, celery, and bay leaves. Bring to a boil and reduce heat. Cover and cook over a low heat for about 1½ hours or until the beans are tender. Stir and mash the beans against the side of the pan.
- Add the green pepper, garlic, parsley, thyme, salt, and black pepper. Cook, uncovered, for about 30 minutes over a low heat until creamy. Remove the bay leaves.
- Serve with hot cooked brown rice, if desired.
- Yield: 8 servings. Serving size: 1¼ cup. Each serving provides: calories 171, total fat less than 1 g, saturated fat less than 1 g, cholesterol 0 mg, and sodium 285 mg.

7.14.3.8 Summer Vegetable Spaghetti*

Ingredients:

- 2 cups small yellow onions, cut in eighths
- 2 cups chopped, peeled, fresh, ripe tomatoes (about 1 lb)
- 2 cups thinly sliced yellow and green squash (about 1 lb)
- 1½ cups cut fresh green beans (about ½ lb)
- ⅔ cups water
- 2 tbsp minced fresh parsley

- 1 clove garlic, minced
- ½ tsp chili powder
- ¼ tsp salt
- Black pepper to taste
- 1 can (6 oz) tomato paste
- 1 lb uncooked whole grain spaghetti
- ½ cup grated Parmesan cheese

Directions:

- Combine the first 10 ingredients in a large saucepan; cook for 10 minutes then stir in the tomato paste. Cover and cook gently for 15 minutes, stirring occasionally until the vegetables are tender.
- Cook the spaghetti in unsalted water according to package directions.
- Spoon the sauce over the drained hot spaghetti and sprinkle the parmesan cheese over the top.
- Yield: 9 servings. Serving size: 1 cup spaghetti and ¾ cup sauce with vegetables. Each serving provides: calories 279, total fat 3 g, saturated fat 1 g, cholesterol 4 mg, and sodium 173 mg.

7.14.3.9   Zucchini Lasagna*
Ingredients:

- ½ pound cooked whole grain lasagna noodles (in unsalted water)
- ¾ cup mozzarella cheese, part-skim, grated
- 1½ cup cottage cheese, fat-free
- ¼ cup Parmesan cheese, grated
- 1½ cup zucchini, raw, sliced
- 2½ cup tomato sauce, no salt added
- 2 tsp basil, dried
- 2 tsp oregano, dried
- ¼ cup onion, chopped
- 1 clove garlic
- ⅛ tsp black pepper

Directions:

- Preheat the oven to 350°F.
- Lightly spray a 9×13-inch baking dish with extra-virgin olive oil spray.
- In a small bowl, combine ⅛ cup mozzarella and 1 tbsp Parmesan cheese. Set aside.
- In a medium bowl, combine the remaining mozzarella and Parmesan cheese with all of the cottage cheese. Mix well and set aside.
- Combine the tomato sauce with the remaining ingredients. Spread a thin layer of tomato sauce in the bottom of the baking dish. Add a third of the noodles in a single layer.

- Spread half of the cottage cheese mixture on top. Add a layer of zucchini. Repeat layering.
- Add a thin coating of sauce. Top with noodles, sauce, and reserved cheese mixture.
- Cover with aluminum foil.
- Bake for 30–40 minutes. Cool for 10–15 minutes. Cut into 6 portions.
- Yield: 6 servings. Serving size: 1 piece. Each serving provides: calories 276, total fat 5 g, saturated fat 2 g, cholesterol 11 mg, and sodium 380 mg.

7.14.3.10　Italian Vegetable Bake*

Ingredients:

- 1 can (28 oz) whole tomatoes
- 1 medium onion, sliced
- ½ lb fresh green beans, sliced
- ½ lb fresh okra or 10 oz packet frozen okra, cut into ½-inch pieces
- ¾ cup finely chopped green pepper
- 2 tbsp lemon juice
- 1 tsp chopped fresh basil, or 1 tsp dried basil, crushed
- 1½ tsp chopped fresh oregano leaves, or ½ tsp dried oregano, crushed
- 3 medium (7-inch long) zucchini, cut into 1-inch cubes
- 1 medium eggplant, pared and cut into 1-inch cubes
- 2 tbsp grated parmesan cheese

Directions:

- Drain and coarsely chop the tomatoes. Save the liquid. Mix together the tomatoes and reserved liquid, onion, green beans, okra, green pepper, lemon juice, and herbs. Cover and bake at 325°F for 15 minutes.
- Mix in the zucchini and eggplant and continue baking, covered, for 60–70 more minutes or until vegetables are tender. Stir occasionally.
- Sprinkle top with parmesan cheese just before serving.
- Yield: 18 servings. Serving size: ½ cup. Each serving provides: calories 36, total fat less than 1 g, saturated fat less than 1 g, cholesterol less than 1 mg, and sodium 86 mg.

7.14.3.11　Smothered Greens*

Ingredients:

- 3 cups water
- ¼ lb smoked turkey breast, skinless
- 1 tbsp hot pepper, freshly chopped
- ¼ tsp cayenne pepper
- ¼ tsp cloves, ground

- 2 cloves garlic, crushed
- ½ tsp thyme
- 1 stalk scallion, chopped
- 1 tsp ginger, ground
- ¼ cup onion, chopped
- 2 lb greens (mustard, turnip, collard, kale, or a mixture)

Directions:

- Place all the ingredients except the greens into a large saucepan and bring to the boil.
- Prepare the greens by washing thoroughly and removing stems.
- Tear or slice the leaves into bite-size pieces. Add the greens to the turkey stock.
- Cook for 20–30 minutes until tender.
- Yield: 5 servings. Serving size: 1 cup. Each serving provides: calories 80, fat 2 g, saturated fat less than 1 g, cholesterol 16 mg, and sodium 378 mg.

7.14.3.12   Fusilli Diablo*

Ingredients:

- 2 cloves garlic, minced
- 1 tbsp extra-virgin olive oil
- ¼ cup freshly minced parsley
- 1 tbsp fresh basil, chopped
- ¼ tsp salt
- Ground cayenne pepper to taste
- 4 cups cooked whole grain fusilli
- ½ pound cooked chicken breasts, chopped into 1-inch pieces (optional)

Directions:

- Heat the extra-virgin olive oil in a medium saucepan. Sauté the garlic and parsley until golden.
- Add tomatoes and spices. Cook uncovered over low heat for 15 minutes or until thickened, stirring frequently. If desired, add the chicken and continue cooking for 15 minutes until the chicken is heated through and the sauce is thick.
- Cook the pasta in unsalted water until firm.
- To serve, spoon the sauce over the pasta and sprinkle with coarsely chopped parsley. Serve hot as a main dish or cold for lunch the next day.
- Yield: 4 servings. Serving size: 1 cup. Each serving provides: calories 304, total fat 5 g, saturated fat less than 1 g, cholesterol 0 mg, and sodium 285 mg (with chicken: calories 398, total fat 7 g, saturated fat 1 g, cholesterol 44 mg, and sodium 325 mg).

7.14.3.13   Oriental Rice

Ingredients:

- 1½ cups water
- 1 cup low-fat, low-sodium chicken broth
- 1⅓ cup uncooked long grain brown rice
- 2 tsp extra-virgin olive oil
- 2 tbsp finely chopped onion
- 2 tbsp finely chopped green pepper
- ½ cup chopped pecans
- ¼ tsp sage

Directions:

- Bring the water and stock to a boil in a medium-size saucepan. Add rice and stir. Cover and simmer for 20 minutes.
- Remove the pan from the heat. Let stand, covered, for 5 minutes or until all liquid is absorbed. Reserve.
- Heat the oil in a large cast iron skillet.
- Sauté the onion and celery over moderate heat for 3 minutes. Stir in the remaining ingredients including the reserved cooked rice. Fluff with a fork before serving.
- Yield: 10 servings. Serving size: ½ cup. Each serving provides: calories 139, total fat 5 g, saturated fat less than 1 g, cholesterol 0 mg, and sodium 86 mg.

7.14.4   Sauces and Dressing

7.14.4.1   Fresh Salsa*

Ingredients:

- 6 tomatoes preferably Roma (or 3 large tomatoes)
- ½ medium onion, finely chopped
- 1 clove garlic, finely minced
- 2 serrano or jalapeno peppers, finely chopped
- 3 tbsp cilantro, chopped
- ⅛ tsp oregano, finely crushed
- ⅛ tsp salt
- ⅛ tsp pepper
- ½ avocado diced (black skin)
- Juice of 1 lime

Directions:

- Combine all the ingredients in a glass bowl.
- Serve immediately or refrigerate and serve within 4 or 5 hours.

- Yield: 8 servings. Serving size: ½ cup. Each serving provides: calories 42, total fat 2 g, saturated fat less than 1 g, cholesterol 0 mg, sodium 44 mg, calcium 12 mg, and iron 1 mg.

7.14.4.2   Vinaigrette Salad Dressing*

Ingredients:

- 1 bulb garlic, separated and peeled
- ½ cup water
- 1 tbsp balsamic vinegar
- ¼ tsp honey

Directions:

- Place the garlic cloves into a small saucepan and pour enough water (about ½ cup) to cover them.
- Bring the water to a boil, then reduce the heat and simmer for about 15 minutes until the garlic is tender.
- Reduce the liquid to 2 tablespoons and increase the heat for 3 minutes.
- Pour the contents into a small sieve over a bowl and with a wooden spoon, mash the garlic through the sieve into the bowl.
- Whisk the vinegar into the garlic mixture, and incorporate the oil and seasoning.
- Yield: 4 servings. Serving size: 2 tablespoons. Each serving provides: calories 33, total fat 3 g, saturated fat less than 1 g, cholesterol 0 mg, and sodium 0 mg.

7.14.4.3   Yogurt Salad Dressing*

Ingredients:

- 8 oz plain non-fat Greek yogurt
- ¼ cup non-fat mayonnaise
- 2 tbsp dried chives
- 2 tbsp dried dill

Directions:

- Mix all the ingredients in a bowl and refrigerate.
- Yield: 8 servings. Serving size: 2 tablespoons. Each serving provides: calories 23, total fat 0 g, saturated fat less than 0 g, cholesterol 1 mg, and sodium 84 mg.

7.14.5   Desserts

7.14.5.1   Rainbow Fruit Salad

Ingredients:

Fruit salad:

- 1 large mango, peeled and diced
- 2 cups fresh blueberries

- 2 bananas, sliced
- 2 cups fresh strawberries, halved
- 2 cups seedless grapes
- 2 nectarines, unpeeled and sliced
- 1 kiwi fruit, peeled and sliced

Honey orange sauce:

- ⅓ cup unsweetened orange juice
- 2 tbsp lemon juice
- 1½ tbsp honey
- ¼ tsp ground ginger
- Dash of nutmeg

Directions:

- Prepare the fruit.
- Combine all the ingredients for the sauce and mix.
- Just before serving, pour the honey orange sauce over the fruit.
- Yield: 12 servings. Serving size: 4 oz cup. Each serving provides: calories 96, total fat 1 g, saturated fat less than 1 g, cholesterol 0 mg, and sodium 4 mg.

7.14.5.2 Banana Mousse*

Ingredients:

- 2 tbsp low-fat (1%) milk
- 4 tsp sugar
- 1 tsp vanilla
- 1 medium banana, cut in quarters
- 1 cup plain low-fat yogurt
- Eight ¼- inch banana slices

Directions:

- Place the milk, sugar, vanilla, and banana in a blender. Process for 15 seconds at high speed until smooth.
- Pour the mixture into a small bowl and fold in the yogurt. Chill. Spoon into 4 dessert dishes and garnish each with 2 banana slices just before serving.
- Yield: 4 servings. Serving size: ½ cup. Each serving provides: calories 94, total fat 1 g, saturated fat 1 g, cholesterol 4 mg, and sodium 47 mg.

7.14.5.3 Rice Pudding

Ingredients:

- ½ cup basmati rice
- 4 cups milk

- 3 tbsp sugar
- ¼ cup raisins
- ½ tsp cardamom
- ¼ tsp cinnamon
- ½ tsp rose water (optional)
- ¼ almonds, chopped
- 1 tbsp orange zest

Directions:

- Soak the rice in water for 10 minutes and drain.
- In a heavy saucepan, bring the milk and sugar to a low boil over a medium-high heat.
- Add the rice, raisins, cardamom, and cinnamon and simmer for about 45 minutes over a low heat until thickened, stirring frequently.
- Remove from the heat and add the rose water (if desired).
- Combine the almonds and orange zest. Ladle the pudding into serving bowls and garnish with the almond mixture. Serve hot or cold.
- Yield: 6 servings. Per serving: calories 207 (43 from fat), fat 5 g (saturated 1 g), cholesterol 8 mg, sodium 75 mg, carbohydrate 34 g (dietary fiber 1 g), and protein 8 g.

7.14.5.4 Poached Pears with Raspberries*

Ingredients:

- 4 Bosc pears
- 4 tbsp maple syrup
- 16 oz frozen raspberries or fresh in season
- Cinnamon sugar to taste

Directions:

- Peel the pears and slice the bottoms, so the pears will stand up straight. Place in microwave dish.
- Spoon 1 tsp of maple syrup over each pear, and sprinkle each pear with cinnamon sugar. Cover dish. Put in a microwave oven on high for 10 or 12 minutes or until the pears are tender but not too soft.
- Meanwhile heat the berries and purée in a blender, run through a sieve to remove the seeds, add enough sugar to sweeten and heat on top of the stove. Place the poached pear on a serving plate and cover with the sauce or put the sauce on a plate and set a pear in the center.
- Garnish with a few whole berries.
- Yield: 4 servings. Per serving: calories 249, fat less than 1 g, cholesterol 0 mg, and sodium 5 mg.

7.14.5.5   Baked Apples

Ingredients:

- ⅓ cup dried cherries, coarsely chopped
- 3 tbsp chopped almonds
- 1 tbsp wheat germ
- 1 tbsp firmly packed brown sugar
- ½ tsp ground cinnamon
- ⅛ tsp ground nutmeg
- 6 small Golden Delicious apples, about 1¾ pounds total weight
- ½ cup apple juice
- ¼ cup water
- 2 tbsp dark honey
- 2 tsp walnut oil or canola oil

Directions:

- Preheat the oven to 350°F.
- In a small bowl, toss together the cherries, almonds, wheat germ, brown sugar, cinnamon, and nutmeg until all the ingredients are evenly distributed. Set aside.
- The apples can be left unpeeled, if you like. To peel the apples in a decorative fashion, with a vegetable peeler or a sharp knife, remove the peel from each apple in a circular motion, skipping every other row so that rows of peel alternate with rows of apple flesh. Working from the stem end, core each apple, stopping ¾ inch from the bottom.
- Divide the cherry mixture evenly among the apples, pressing the mixture gently into each cavity. Arrange the apples upright in a heavy ovenproof frying pan or small baking dish just large enough to hold them. Pour the apple juice and water into the pan.
- Drizzle the honey and oil evenly over the apples, and cover the pan snugly with aluminum foil.
- Bake for 50–60 minutes until the apples are tender when pierced with a knife.
- Transfer the apples to individual plates and drizzle with the pan juices. Serve warm or at room temperature.
- Serving size 1 apple: Per serving: calories 200, total fat 4 g, monounsaturated fat 2 g, cholesterol 10 mg, and sodium 7 mg.
- These recipes are provided for convenience and typify reasonably simple means to implement a Proactive Nutrition Program in keeping with the principal food and nutrients elements of a Mediterranean diet plan. There are many recipes available on the internet that may suit readers interested in implementing a more nearly Mediterranean "ethnic"—for lack of a better term—diet plan. Such cuisine may include more comprehensive traditional food plans and recipes including Greek, Italian, Moroccan, Turkish, and Lebanese cuisine, for instance:
  - http://us.hellomagazine.com/cuisine/2013031811663/italian-mediterranean-healthy-recipes/

- http://www.themediterraneandish.com/
- http://www.eatingwell.com/nutrition_health/weight_loss_diet_plans/your_1_day_mediterranean_diet_plan
- http://casaveneracion.com/topic/italian-greek-mediterranean-recipes/
- http://www.theperfectpantry.com/italianmediterranean-dish.html
- http://www.foodnetwork.com/healthy/photos/mediterranean-diet-recipes.page-2.html
- http://allrecipes.com/recipes/731/world-cuisine/european/greek/
- http://ozlemsturkishtable.com/recipes/
- http://moroccan.food.com/
- https://www.pinterest.com/explore/lebanese-recipes/
- http://www.diabetes.org/mfa-recipes/meal-plans/mediterranean-meal-plan.html
- http://www.mayoclinic.org/healthy-lifestyle/nutrition-and-healthy-eating/in-depth/ mediterranean-diet-recipes/art-20046682

- Ingredients may be substituted in the recipes if they contain foods one dislikes—substitute foods with a similar calorie count (see the USDA National Nutrient Database for Standard Reference). For example, if one does not like fish, chicken with the same calories may be substituted; if one dislikes tomatoes, green beans may be substituted. One may prefer peaches to strawberries on cereal.
- Beverages: Calorie-free drinks are allowed anytime including water, flavored seltzer, diet iced tea (lemon wedge is fine), or diet soda.
- Finally, an interesting discussion of whether calories matter can be found on the website http://eatingacademy.com/nutrition/do-calories-matter.

7.15 THE PROACTIVE NUTRITION PROGRAM SAMPLE SIRTFOOD AND SMOOTHIE RECIPES

The following are examples of "sirtfood" recipes. The reader is guided to the following links for a sample of additional recipes:

- http://lifestyle.one/closer/diet-body/diet-recipes/sirtfood-diet-works-recipe-ideas/
- http://www.marieclaire.co.uk/life/health-fitness/the-sirtfood-diet-sounds-a-little-too-good-to-be-true-doesn-t-it-here-s-everything-you-need-to-know-22576
- https://www.amazon.com/Sirtfood-Diet-Recipe-Book-Calorie-Counted/dp/0993320449
- https://www.amazon.com/Essential-Sirt-Food-Diet-Recipe/dp/0993320457/ref=pd_ sbs_14_t_1?ie=UTF8&psc=1&refRID=WXCQJ1326TDC8KM0H8HR
- https://www.amazon.com/Sirtfood-Diet-Beginners-Sirtfoods-enefits/dp/1532724950/ ref=pd_sbs_14_t_2?ie=UTF8&psc=1&refRID=7TTWE1MP4E8F7MSX9YTE

Note: These sources for "sirtfoods," websites and books, primarily target weight loss. They are listed here because, as noted in previous chapters, it has been shown that the same sirtfoods are telomere protective and therefore help to avert premature aging.

7.15.1 SAMPLE SIRTFOODS

Sample sirtfoods are listed in the table.

Apples	Kale
Blueberries	Lovage
Buckwheat	Matcha green tea
Capers	Medjool dates
Celery	Parsley
Chili	Red onion
Cocoa	Red wine
Coffee	Dark chocolate
Extra-virgin olive oil	Tofu and other soy products
Turmeric	Strawberries
Walnuts	Green tea
Olives and extra-virgin olive oil	Blackcurrants
Passion fruit	Citrus fruit
Onions	

7.15.2 SAMPLE RECIPES

7.15.2.1 Turmeric Cauliflower

Ingredients:

- 420 g cauliflower
- 1 jalapeno pepper
- 2 tsp yellow mustard seeds
- 3½ tbsp cold pressed extra-virgin olive oil
- 1½ tbsp ground turmeric

Directions:

- Preheat the oven to 425°F.
- Cut cauliflower into florets. Dice jalapeno pepper, including seeds. Mix the pepper and spices with olive oil until well blended. Toss the cauliflower in the spice mixture until evenly coated.
- Place the cauliflower in a baking tray and bake for 25–30 minutes, or until cauliflower has started to brown and is soft.
- Calorie count: 198 per serving, 3 servings.

7.15.2.2 French Onion Soup

Ingredients:

- 10 medium onions, sliced
- 2 tbsp olive oil
- 1 tbsp dried thyme
- 2 tsp kosher salt
- ¼ tsp ground pepper
- 2 tbsp sugar
- 43½ oz chicken broth
- ¾ cup dry red wine

Directions:

- Preheat the oven to 450°F.
- Put the onions, olive oil, thyme, salt, pepper, and sugar in a roasting pan and mix well. Cover the pan with aluminum foil, and roast for 30 minutes.
- Remove the foil, stir, and roast uncovered for 30 more minutes. Stir again, and roast until onions caramelize.
- Remove from the oven, and add to a stock pot, along with the chicken broth.
- In the empty roasting pan, deglaze any left-over bits with the red wine, reduce by half, and add this to the stock pot. Simmer for about 15 minutes.
- Serve with toasted croutons made with multi-grain baguette, with melted low-fat Swiss cheese. Place the soup in bowls and top with croutons.
- Calorie count: 168 per serving, 6 servings.

7.15.3 SAMPLE SMOOTHIES

7.15.3.1 Cacao Passion Sirt-Smoothie

Ingredients:

- 1 frozen banana
- 2 handfuls spinach
- 1 passion fruit (insides)
- 1 tsp cacao powder
- 2 cups almond milk

Directions:

- Place the ingredients in a blender.
- Calorie count: 761 per serving.

7.15.3.2 Kale-Apple Super Sirt-Smoothie

Ingredients:

- ½ squeezed lemon
- 2 handfuls kale

- 1 apple
- 1 frozen banana
- 1 avocado
- 1 tbsp chia seeds
- 1–2 cups water
- 1 cup ice

Directions:

- Place all the ingredients in a blender
- Calorie count: 485 per serving.

7.15.3.3 Parsley Go Bananas Sirt-Smoothie

Ingredients:

- 1 handful spinach
- ½ handful parsley
- 1 frozen banana
- 1 papaya (without seeds)
- 2–3 ice cubes
- 1–2 cups water

Preparation:

- Place all the ingredients in a blender
- Calorie count: 256 per serving.

Additional recipes can found in a number of books and on websites dedicated specifically to sirtfoods nutrition plans including:

- http://www.redonline.co.uk/health-self/nutrition/why-were-eating-sirt-foods-this-summer
- http://sirtfooddiet.net/best-sirtfood-recipes/

REFERENCES

Aas, V., M. Rokling-Andersen, A. J. Wensaas, et al. 2005. Lipid metabolism in human skeletal muscle cells: Effects of palmitate and chronic hyperglycaemia. *Acta Physiologica Scandinavica*, 183(1):31–41.

Boccardi, V., A. Esposito, M. R. Rizzo, et al. 2013. Mediterranean diet, telomere maintenance and health status among elderly. *PLoS One*, 8(4):e62781.

Coll, T., E. Eyre, R. Rodríguez-Calvo, et al. 2008. Oleate reverses palmitate-induced insulin resistance and inflammation in skeletal muscle cells. *The Journal of Biological Chemistry*, 283(17):11107–11116.

Cordain, L., E. D. Bryan, C. L. Melby, et al. 1997. Influence of moderate daily wine consumption on body weight regulation and metabolism in healthy free-living males. *Journal of the American College of Nutrition*, 16(2):134–139.

Cordova, A. C., and B. E. Sumpio. 2009. Polyphenols are medicine: Is it time to prescribe red wine for our patients? *International Journal of Angiology*, 18(3):111–117.

Dixon, J. B., M. E. Dixon, and P. E. O'Brien. 2002. Reduced plasma homocysteine in obese red wine consumers: A potential contributor to reduced cardiovascular risk status. *European Journal of Clinical Nutrition*, 56(7):608–614.

Esposito, K., F. Giugliano, M. I. Maiorino, et al. 2010. Dietary factors, Mediterranean diet and erectile dysfunction. *Journal of Sexual Medicine*, 7(7):2338–2345.

Fernández del Río, L., E. Gutiérrez-Casado, A. Varela-López, et al. 2016. Olive oil and the hallmarks of aging. *Molecules*, 21(2):163.

Fried, R., and L. Edlen-Nezin. 2006. *Great Food/Great Sex*. New York: Ballantine Books.

García-Calzón, S., G. Zalba, M. Ruiz-Canela, et al. 2015. Dietary inflammatory index and telomere length in subjects with a high cardiovascular disease risk from the PREDIMED-NAVARRA study: Cross-sectional and longitudinal analyses over 5 y. *American Journal of Clinical Nutrition*, 102(4):897–904.

Glushakova, O., T. Kosugi, C. Roncal, et al. 2008. Fructose induces the inflammatory molecule ICAM-1 in endothelial cells. *Journal of the American Society of Nephrology*, 19(9):1712–1720.

Halvorsen, B. L., and R. Blomhoff. 2011. Determination of lipid oxidation products in vegetable oils and marine omega-3 supplements. *Food and Nutrition Research*, 55. doi: 10.3402/fnr.v55i0.5792.

Lamming, D. W., J. G. Wood, and D. A., Sinclair. 2004. MicroReview: Small molecules that regulate lifespan: Evidence for xenohormesis. *Biology*, 53(4):1003–1009.

Lidder, S., and A. J. Webb. 2013. Vascular effects of dietary nitrate (as found in green leafy vegetables and beetroot) via the nitrate-nitrite-nitric oxide pathway. *British Journal of Clinical Pharmacology*, 75(3):677–696.

Lundberg, J. O., M. T. Gladwin, A. Ahluwalia, et al. 2009. Nitrate and nitrite in biology, nutrition and therapeutics. *Nature Chemical Biology*, 5(12):865–869.

Lundberg, J. O., and M. Govoni. 2004. Inorganic nitrate is a possible source for systemic generation of nitric oxide. *Free Radical Biology & Medicine*, 37(3):395–400.

Magdalene, K., M. K. Montgomery, B. Osborne, et al. 2013. Contrasting metabolic effects of medium- versus long-chain fatty acids in skeletal muscle. *Journal of Lipid Research*, 54(12):3322–3333.

Mahlknecht, U., and B. Zschoernig. 2012. Involvement of sirtuins in life-span and aging related diseases. *Advances in Experimental Medicine and Biology*, 739:252–261.

Makpol, S., A. Zainal Abidin, K. Sairin, et al. 2010. γ-Tocotrienol prevents oxidative stress-induced telomere shortening in human fibroblasts derived from different aged individuals. *Oxidative Medicine & Cellullar Longevity*, 3(1):35–43.

Marín, C., E. M. Yubero-Serrano, J. López-Miranda, et al. 2013. Endothelial aging associated with oxidative stress can be modulated by a healthy Mediterranean diet. *International Journal of Molecular Science*, 14(5):8869–8889.

Mathai Kochikuzhyil, B., K. Devi, and S. Raghunandan Fattepur. 2010. Effect of saturated fatty acid-rich dietary vegetable oils on lipid profile, antioxidant enzymes and glucose tolerance in diabetic rats. *Indian Journal of Pharmacology*, 42(3):142–145.

McKnight, G. M., L. M. Smith, R. S. Drummond, et al. 1997. Chemical synthesis of nitric oxide in the stomach from dietary nitrate in humans. *Gut*, 40:211–214.

Meldrum, D. R., J. C. Gambone, M. A. Morris, et al. 2011. The link between erectile and cardiovascular health: The canary in the coal mine. *American Journal of Cardiology*, 108(4):599–606.

Menendez, J. A., J. Joven, G. Aragonès, et al. 2013. Xenohormetic and anti-aging activity of secoiridoid polyphenols present in extra virgin olive oil: A new family of gerosuppressant agents. *Cell Cycle*, 12(4):555–578.

Mensink, R. P., P. L. Zock, A. D. Kester, et al. 2003. Effects of dietary fatty acids and carbohydrates on the ratio of serum total to HDL cholesterol and on serum lipids and apolipoproteins: Meta-analysis of 60 controlled trials (PDF). *American Journal of Clinical Nutrition*, 77(5):1146–1155.

Montero, C., S. M. Cristescu, J. B. Jiménez, et al. 2003. trans-Resveratrol and grape disease resistance. A dynamical study by high-resolution laser-based techniques. *Physiology*, 131(1):129–138.

Nakamura,S., T. Takamura, N. Matsuzawa-Nagata, et al. 2009. Palmitate induces insulin resistance in H4IIEC3 hepatocytes through reactive oxygen species produced by mitochondria. *The Journal of Biological Chemistry*, 284(22):14809–14818.

Narayanankutty, A., R. K. Mukesh, S. K. Ayoob, et al. 2016. Virgin coconut oil maintains redox status and improves glycemic conditions in high fructose fed rats. *Journal of Food Science & Technology*, 53(1):895–901.

No authors listed. 2009. Fats and fatty acids in human nutrition. Proceedings of the Joint FAO/WHO Expert Consultation. November 10–14, 2008. Geneva, Switzerland. *Annals of Nutrition and Metabolism*, 55(1–3):5–300.

Palmer, R. M., D. S. Ashton, and S. Moncada. 1988. Vascular endothelial cells synthesize nitric oxide from L-arginine. *Nature*, 333(6174):664–666.

Pavanello, S., M. Hoxha, L. Dioni, et al. 2011. Shortened telomeres in individuals with abuse in alcohol consumption. *International Journal of Cancer*, 129(4):983–992.

Perdomo, L., N. Beneit, Y. F. Otero, et al. 2015. Protective role of oleic acid against cardiovascular insulin resistance and in the early and late cellular atherosclerotic process. *Cardiovascular Diabetology*, 14:75.

Rolls, B. J., E. L. Morris, and L.S. Roe. 2002. Portion size of food affects energy intake in normal-weight and overweight men and women. *American Journal of Clinical Nutrition*, 76(6):1207–1213.

Sajish, M., and P. Schimmel. 2015. A human tRNA synthetase is a potent PARP1-activating effector target for resveratrol. *Nature*, 519(7543):370–373.

Sanadgol, N., A. Mostafaie, K. Mansouri, et al. 2012. Effect of palmitic acid and linoleic acid on expression of ICAM-1 and VCAM-1 in human bone marrow endothelial cells (HBMECs). *Archives of Medical Science*, 8(2):192–198.

Satoh, A., L. Stein, and S, Imai. 2011. The role of mammalian sirtuins in the regulation of metabolism, aging, and longevity. *Handbook of Experimental Pharmacology*, 206:125–162.

Siegel, P. S. 1957. The completion compulsion in human eating. *Psychological Reports*, 3:15–16.

Spiegelhalder, B., G. Eisenbrand, & R. Preussmann. 1976. Influence of dietary nitrate on nitrite content of human saliva: Possible relevance to in vivo formation of N-nitroso compounds. *Food and Cosmetics Toxicology*, 14(6):545–548.

Virruso, C., G. Accardi, G. Colonna-Romano, et al. 2014. Nutraceutical properties of extra-virgin olive oil: A natural remedy for age-related disease? *Rejuvenation Research*, 17(2):217–220.

Wei, X., J. G. Schneider, S. M. Shenouda, et al. 2010. De Novo lipogenesis maintains vascular homeostasis through endothelial nitric-oxide synthase (eNOS) palmitoylation. *The Journal of Biological Chemistry*, 286:2933–2945.

8 Selected Functional Foods That Combat Inflammation

The Lord hath created medicines out of the earth; and he that is wise will not abhor them. (Ecclesiasticus 38:4KJV)

8.1 INTRODUCTION

The consistent theme in this book is that aging is normal, whereas premature aging is not normal and is, indeed, preventable. Published evidence supports the theory that premature aging may result from accumulating free radical damage to our cells causing them to cycle or die—often way before their time. This can be seen in the comparative telltale abbreviation of telomeres in cells subjected to oxidative stress in both controlled laboratory studies and clinical studies.

It has been shown that premature cell cycling, and therefore premature telomere shortening, can be avoided with a consistently antioxidant-rich diet. To that end, this book proposes a Proactive Nutrition Program that also supplies ample nitrates and L-arginine to help the body antioxidant defenses; plus, the program is enhanced with foods that promote Sirtuin1. In addition, a simple and inexpensive do-it-yourself at home saliva/nitrate test to ensure that one is on the right nutritional track is described.

This may be the best plan there is to meet the requirements of a telomere protection program. What's more, it was left to the experts to speak about their relevant findings through their scientific journal publications to support the diet program.

Health authorities urge the public to be sure to have a "healthy diet" because a "healthy diet" is the best source of all the nutrients needed. However, most consumers are not sufficiently well informed about food science to evaluate the validity of this assertion. And, besides, many health authorities also tend to ridicule dietary supplements and dismiss their use as faddist, which, making matters worse, in many cases may actually be true.

Having reviewed as much as possible of what has been published by conventional scientists about the oxidant/antioxidant balance and its impact on oxidative stress, and therefore aging, it is not clear how strongly one can come down in favor of exogenous antioxidant supplementation without resorting to some caveats, as noted in Chapter 3 on antioxidants. It is one thing to read about that balance in controlled laboratory or clinical studies, but it is another thing to guess about it in individuals going about their daily routine.

It seems likely, however, that in most cases where the body may need it, supplementation with antioxidants in various forms and at moderate concentrations may be helpful rather than harmful. However, it is possible that antioxidant supplements that tout a sky-high ORAC or FRAP value may tip the scale. After all it is not known to what extent the body needs exogenous antioxidant supplementation and how much and what kind should be supplemented. Nor is it possible to know the consequences of overindulgence.

Bearing this in mind, here follow some common types of foods, condiments, berries, and beverages that are rich in antioxidants and that are generally considered safe to consume and healthful, which meet specific needs. These are selected primarily on the basis that they help combat *chronic systemic inflammation*, a well-known, reliable generator of a consistent and dense stream of free radicals.

8.2 FUNCTIONAL FOODS

The term "functional foods" was chosen rather than *supplements*, or *nutraceuticals*, to distance this category from the common definition of those terms. First, "supplements" imply solitary substances that take up the slack for inadequate supply in the diet. Second, "nutraceutical" implies stepping through a loophole in federal medicine claims limitations statutes. Foods proposed here, especially those in this section, are not intended to replace pharmaceutical prescription medications. In fact, no known prescription medications are considered to prevent accelerated cell cycling, and, what is most telling is that none target chronic inflammation.

Non-steroidal anti-inflammatory drugs (NSAIDs) are intended for relatively short-term use, becoming hazardous over time with continued use. Furthermore, chronic inflammation, albeit described in detail by medical professionals, is not currently recognized as a routinely treatable clinical disorder. One can rest assured that were the medical world to decide to diagnose and treat chronic inflammation, there would soon be a spate of prescription drugs to do it.

In that vein, two types of functional foods were selected: foods that have a potentially positive effect on health beyond basic nutrition, and foods that help the body in its struggle with the effects of chronic inflammation. In the first case, there is no known deficiency of the active constituents of the functional food. For instance, although there is no known deficiency of gingerols in the body, ginger helps to reduce chronic inflammation and in some cases it does that also by its bactericidal activity.

Our body also hosts bacteria and other microorganisms that the immune system keeps in check but does not eradicate. There are many potentially deadly microorganisms that do us no harm unless they reach a "quorum sensing" critical concentration in the body (Waters and Bassler 2005). Perhaps, they are symbiotic in controlled numbers, but many are often the source of chronic inflammation that adds to free radical load.

In the second case, the functional food supplies a constituent that makes up a known deficiency. Iodine should be a regular constituent of diet but is often inadequate if not entirely absent. Perhaps because less salt is consumed now, iodine deficiency is reaching epidemic proportions, resulting in thyroid malfunction. Iodine deficiency is also strongly implicated in the chronic inflammation that leads to early formation of atherosclerosis which leads to cardiovascular and heart disease.

Here follows a small selection of common foods likely to be readily available in most homes or nearby health food stores that have been scientifically shown to be helpful in reducing chronic systemic inflammation. The list is not comprehensive because that is not the aim of this book. However, even this brief list may raise awareness that there are helpful foods at home and nearby and the reader may be encouraged to look further: One helpful source is the US Department of Health and Human Services, National Center for Complementary and Integrative Health, Dietary and Herbal Supplements website: https://nccih.nih.gov/health/supplements. There are also others.

8.3 THE TWO-PRONGED APPROACH TO ANTIOXIDATION

This chapter will describe some foods and their function in reducing free radicals by a second pathway, whereas in previous chapters, the focus was on "neutralizing" free radicals by the action of endogenous and exogenous antioxidants, as in all other books on antioxidation. As an analogy, it is common practice to protect ourselves from the damage caused by the heat of a fire, or alternatively, we can put out the fire.

Benjamin Franklin put it wisely: "An ounce of prevention is worth a pound of cure." So, in this chapter, the focus is on the alternative, eliminating the formation of free radicals at their source. This is done by *quenching* inflammation—chronic or acute. Here also, the experts express their clinical opinion through their scientific publications.

But first, a disclaimer: The information in this book is neither intended to diagnose nor treat any disease, nor is it a substitute for medical guidance. The authors do not propose that anyone who is undergoing treatment for any medical condition under the care of a physician, or any other qualified healthcare provider, should terminate such treatment in favor of any treatment or substance described here. Rather, where it may seem helpful to adopt a nutrition strategy based on foods described here, the authors urge the reader to do so only with the advice and the supervision of his/her physician or other qualified healthcare provider. The information provided here is intended only to educate the reader to what may be available and not to suggest self-treatment. The authors shall not be held liable or responsible for any misunderstanding or misuse of the information contained in this book or for any loss, damage, or injury caused or alleged to be caused directly or indirectly by any treatment, action, or application of any food or food source discussed in this book.

8.4 INFLAMMATION CAUSES OXIDATIVE STRESS

Inflammation is the natural reaction of the body to infection by bacteria, viruses, fungi, etc., to toxins, or to physical, chemical, or traumatic injury. Inflammation is a complex process that aims to protect against injury while the body is figuring out how to heal itself. It usually, but not invariably, causes pain. Inflammation is the way that the body responds to infection and is not to be confused with the infection, rather it is the response of the body to the cause of the infection. Inflammatory conditions can range from minor nuisances to those leading to fatality, as in *sepsis*. Some sources even hold that chronic inflammation can set the stage for cancer (Salzano et al. 2014).

In many instances, chronic systemic (i.e., "whole body") inflammation is not confined to a particular tissue, but may involve the lining of blood vessels, the lining of joints, the digestive tract, and many other internal organs and systems including the brain. This inflammatory process is the source of oxidative stress and may not cause pain, as some internal organs do not relay pain. When there is no pain, one may simply remain unaware of the serious damage that the systemic inflammation may be causing. In many cases, it leads to debilitating and even life-threatening diseases.

Clinical investigators made that point clear in the title of their publication, "Inflammation as a cardiovascular risk factor," published in *Circulation*, the journal of the American Heart Association (AHA), in 2004. Their report emphasizes that inflammation occurs in our blood vessels in response to injury, including that caused by lipid peroxidation and infection. Various risk factors, including hypertension, diabetes, and smoking, are aggravated by the harmful effects of oxidized low-density-lipoprotein cholesterol, initiating a chronic inflammatory reaction that may result in unstable plaque prone to rupture and thrombosis. Epidemiological and clinical studies have shown strong and consistent relationships between arkers of inflammation and the risk of future cardiovascular events (Willerson and Ridker 2004).

A report published in *Diabetes*, the journal of the American Diabetes Association, in 2003, is titled, "Inflammatory cytokines and the risk to develop Type 2 diabetes." Cytokines are protein molecules that affect the function of other cells, in this case, immune system cells in inflammation. The report tells us that a subclinical inflammatory reaction has been shown to precede the onset of type 2 diabetes. In other words, type 2 diabetes may result from activation of the immune system consonant with chronic inflammation (Spranger et al. 2003). However, note the term "subclinical," which means that it goes largely undetected. Many conditions that are clinical disorders seem to also harbor chronic inflammation.

Here is a title from the journal *Circulation* (2000): "Chronic subclinical inflammation as part of the insulin resistance syndrome. The Insulin Resistance Atherosclerosis Study (IRAS)" (Festa et al. 2000). It certainly speaks for itself.

A report titled "Metabolic syndrome, inflammation and atherosclerosis," published in the journal *Vascular Health and Risk Management*, in 2006, states that we are beginning to become aware that chronic inflammation may underlie all phases of atherosclerosis. In addition, central obesity and insulin resistance, common underlying factors of metabolic syndrome, are accompanied by a chronic low-grade inflammation. The authors propose that treatment should aim to reduce the levels of inflammation biomarkers and address traditional risk factors.

To the extent that there is chronic inflammation, it is to be expected that there will be significant formation of free radicals and reactive oxygen species (ROS). If endogenous antioxidants are swamped, then cell cycling may accelerate and with that comes telomere shortening and premature aging. This line of reasoning is supported by studies that find a connection between systemic inflammation and accelerated telomere shortening.

In states of inflammation, subsequent increases in oxidative stress and cellular division may lead to the accelerated abbreviation of telomeres that protect chromosomes from decay. However, findings on the association between plasma inflammatory marker concentrations and telomere length have been inconsistent. For that reason, a study published in the journal *PLoS One*, in 2014, summarized the longitudinal association between telomere length and plasma inflammatory biomarker concentrations over a 2-year period. The study assessed a number of chronic inflammation markers including C-reactive protein (CRP, see below) and various interleukins, proteins produced by white blood cells (leukocytes) for regulating immune responses.

At all follow-up times, each increase in plasma CRP concentration was associated with a measurable decrease in telomere length. The authors concluded that increased systemic inflammation, consistent with blood vessel injury, is associated with decreased leukocyte telomere length (Wong et al. 2014).

For instance also in the following study published in the journal *Tanaffos* (Respiration), in 2015, the authors reported that chronic obstructive pulmonary disease (COPD) is characterized by airflow limitation that is not completely reversible by administration of inhaled bronchodilators. COPD is also considered a chronic inflammation disease. In this study, it was found that telomere length in COPD patients was shorter even than that in smokers irrespective of age, gender, and history of cigarette smoking (Sadr et al. 2015).

Likewise, chronic inflammation induces telomere dysfunction and accelerates aging, albeit in mice: systemic chronic inflammation can accelerate aging via ROS-mediated telomere dysfunction and cell senescence in the absence of any other genetic or environmental factor (Jurk et al. 2014).

Leukocyte telomere length (LTL) is an emerging marker of biological age. Chronic inflammatory activity is commonly proposed as a promoter of biological aging in general, and of leukocyte telomere shortening in particular. In addition, senescent cells with critically short telomeres produce pro-inflammatory factors (O'Donovan et al. 2011).

8.5 C-REACTIVE PROTEIN: A STANDARD MARKER OF INFLAMMATION

One way to assess the severity of inflammation is by observing CRP, principal among the biomarkers of inflammation. It is a protein made by the liver and released into the blood within a few hours after tissue injury, after the start of an infection, or following other causes of inflammation. CRP is most commonly thought of in connection with the detection of heart "events" (Ridker 2003). However, many conventional routine blood panel tests include CRP, and it is a good idea to keep track of that value and, if it is elevated without an obvious cause, it might be well to ask for further testing to detect possible chronic inflammation.

8.5.1 CRP AND COPD

A study published in the journal *Thorax*, in 2004, aimed at evaluating CRP in chronic obstructive pulmonary disease (COPD) because it predicts increased risk of cardiovascular disease, osteoporosis, and muscle wasting suggesting systemic inflammation.

It was found that CRP was a stronger predictor of cardiovascular events than serum level of LDL cholesterol (Gan et al. 2004).

8.5.2   CRP AND PERIODONTAL DISEASE

Periodontal disease is a chronic inflammation of the gums characterized by a loss of attachment between the tooth and bone, and bone loss. CRP elevation is a part of the acute phase response to acute and chronic inflammation. Many epidemiological studies have shown that serum CRP levels are elevated also in patients with chronic periodontitis. In fact, CRP levels increase rapidly within hours following infection (Bansal et al. 2014).

8.5.3   CRP AND *HELICOBACTER PYLORI* INFECTION

Helicobacter pylori found in about two-thirds of the world's population is a type of bacterium that can cause infection in the stomach. It is best known as the most common cause of gastritis, peptic ulcers, and even cancer.

In a recent report in the *Journal of Investigational Biochemistry*, it was shown that the mean serum level of hs-CRP in patients with *H. pylori* infection was significantly higher than in matched healthy comparison participants not so infected (Al-Fawaeir and Abu Zaid 2013). And, by the way, anyone with gastritis who thinks that *H. pylori* infection is at best a great nuisance should consider the title of a report in the journal *Oncology*, in 2003, "*Helicobactor* [sic] *pylori* infection is closely associated with telomere reduction in gastric mucosa" (Kuniyasu et al. 2003).

A variety of over-the-counter medications are taken by gastritis sufferers, many of whom are infected with *H. pylori*. They often do not come to the attention of medical professionals as they ascribe their indigestion and heartburn to their eating habits. The point is that there are also many other types of chronic inflammation and that CRP does not distinguish between sources if there is more than one. It does however point to existing inflammation and that deserves a heads-up.

Here are two more reports that go to the heart of the matter (pun intended). A study published in the journal *Aging and Disease*, in 2016, stated that the consequence of chronic inflammation is endothelial dysfunction. This is very bad news for nitric oxide formation (see Chapter 5 on nitric oxide). Furthermore, the authors aver that chronic inflammatory diseases are associated with increases in cardiovascular diseases and subclinical atherosclerosis as well as early-stage endothelial dysfunction (Castellon and Bogdanova 2016).

A report in the *International Journal of Molecular Science*, in 2014, tells us that as the cause of atherosclerosis is increasingly being recognized to be chronic inflammation, similarities arise between atherosclerosis and systemic inflammatory diseases such as rheumatoid arthritis, inflammatory bowel diseases, lupus, psoriasis, and others. But, the bottom line is that chronic inflammation diseases are associated with accelerating atherosclerosis and increased risk of cardiovascular diseases (CVD), likely due to endothelial dysfunction (Steyers and Miller 2014).

8.6 "INFLAMM-AGING"

The theory by Dr. Harman that aging is a function of the aggregate result of free radical damage, especially to mitochondria, was mentioned earlier (Harman 1992). In the year 2000, a report appeared in the *Annals of the New York Academy of Sciences*, titled "Inflamm-aging. An evolutionary perspective on immunosenescence." It would appear that the authors may have described the "accelerant."

In their report, they tell us that a reduction in the capacity to cope with a variety of stressors and the resulting progressive increase in systemic inflammation, are major characteristics of the aging process. They called this "inflamm-aging." Their argument is based in part on the idea that immune and stress responses are equivalent and that antigens are nothing other than particular types of stressors (antigens are any substances that cause the immune system to produce antibodies against it). In other words, provoking our immune system to defend us may be life-saving, but at a cost: the concomitant inflammation is stressful, and that stress is cumulative and damaging to the cells in the body. They then implicate macrophages as "actors" in the stress response (Franceschi et al. 2000).

Can inflamm-aging be "cured"? Franceschi writing in *Nutrition Reviews*, in 2007, said that "The key to successful aging and longevity is to decrease chronic inflammation without compromising an acute response when exposed to pathogens" (Franceschi 2007). It sounds plausible, but how does one do that? Given the strong possibility—the likelihood, actually—that inflammation is a major contributor to "aging," as well as to cardiovascular and heart and related diseases, what do functional foods offer us for relief?

8.6.1 Chronic Inflammation Shortens Telomeres

Many clinical and research reports attest to the fact that chronic systemic inflammation damages telomeres. Information about that damaging process can be found by searching online libraries such as PubMed (US National Library of Medicine) or NCBI (National Center for Biotechnology Information) for "chronic inflammation shortens/damages telomeres" or "oxidative stress shortens/damages telomeres" because the bottom line is, regardless of the cause of the damage, that telomere shortening is shown to result from unopposed free radicals. The following sample of studies and reports underscore that assertion.

A recent clinical study reported in *PLoS One*, in 2015, concluded that telomere length (TL) was shortened in Cushing syndrome patients who also had abnormal blood lipid profiles. Where hypertension and/or obesity were also present, there was a notable increase in inflammation markers. The authors concluded that increased lipids and chronic low grade inflammation may contribute to telomere shortening, and consequently to premature aging and increased risk of death (Aulinas et al. 2015) .

Cushing syndrome, sometimes called hypercortisolism, may occur when the body makes too much cortisol on its own or by the use of oral corticosteroid medication. Hallmark signs of Cushing syndrome are a fatty hump between the shoulders, a rounded face, and pink or purple stretch marks on the skin.

The author of a report published in the journal *Trends in Biochemical Sciences*, in 2002, put it bluntly in the title of the report: "Oxidative stress shortens telomeres." He asserts that oxidative stress damage accelerates telomere shortening, whereas antioxidants reduce the rate of shortening. He proposes that oxidative stress is an important modulator of telomere loss and that telomere-driven replication cell senescence is primarily a stress response. He further proposes that this might have evolved to block the growth of cells that have been exposed to a high risk of mutation (von Zglinicki 2002).

8.7 FUNCTIONAL FOODS THAT FIGHT INFLAMMATION

The following is a partial list and description of functional foods that science reveals may help to reduce chronic systemic inflammation. While some of these "foods" have different applicable properties, most are primarily antioxidant. The focus here is primarily on their anti-inflammatory action.

8.7.1 GINGER (*ZINGIBER OFFICINALE* ROSCOE)

Ginger (*Zingiber officinale* Roscoe) is a flowering perennial plant whose rhizome, ginger root or simply ginger, is widely used as a spice or as folk medicine. It contains pungent phenolic substances known as gingerols. 6-Gingerol is the major pharmacologically active component of ginger known to be anti-inflammatory and antioxidant. Due to its efficacy and regulation of multiple targets, as well as its safety for human use, 6-gingerol has received considerable interest as a potential therapeutic agent for the prevention and/or treatment of various medical conditions (von Zglinicki. 2002).

Gingerols are reportedly counter inflammatory including the analgesic and anti-inflammatory effects of [6]-gingerol (the pungent constituent of ginger) (Semwal et al. 2015; Young et al. 2005). In fact, investigators reported in the journal *Planta Medica*, in 2007, that ginger dry extract, used as a solution and in plasters for topical application, likewise showed anti-inflammatory action (Minghetti et al. 2007).

The original discovery in the early 1970s that ginger can inhibit the formation of prostaglandins that mediate inflammation has been repeatedly confirmed. This discovery identified ginger as an herbal medicinal product that shares pharmacological properties with NSAID drugs. The pharmacological property of ginger distinguishes it from NSAIDs though it may have a better therapeutic profile and fewer side effects than NSAIDs (Grzanna et al. 2005).

In fact, a report in *Food & Function*, in 2013, affirms the gastro-protective effects of ginger: it has been shown to be effective in preventing gastric ulcers induced by NSAIDs, such as indomethacin and aspirin, and by *H. pylori* (in laboratory animals) (see Section 8.11 on Mastic). Various studies have also shown ginger possesses anti-emetic effects, although there are conflicting reports in connection with the prevention of chemotherapy-induced nausea and vomiting, and motion sickness.

Ginger has been shown to possess free radical scavenging antioxidants and promotes inhibition of lipid peroxidation. These properties might have contributed to the observed gastro-protective effects (Haniadka et al. 2013). Gingerol easily undergoes dehydration reactions to form the corresponding shogaols, which impart the characteristic taste to dried ginger. Both gingerols and shogaols are anti-inflammatory, antioxidant, antimicrobial, and anti-allergic. Shogaols appear to be more potent than the gingerols.

The numerous reports that ginger counters inflammation led to the following study appearing in the journal *Advanced Pharmaceutical Bulletin* in 2013. It aimed to evaluate the effects of ginger on pro-inflammatory cytokines (substances, such as interferon and interleukin, that are secreted by immune system cells) and the acute phase protein hs-CRP in type 2 diabetes (the notation "hs" stands for "high sensitivity").

Patients were assigned to ginger or placebo comparison groups and received two tablets per day for 2 months. The concentrations of cytokines and hs-CRP were analyzed in blood samples before and after the intervention. It was found that supplementation with ginger significantly reduced the levels of both cytokines and hs-CRP in the ginger group in comparison with the comparison group (Mahluji et al. 2013). Also concerning inflammation biomarkers, a study published in the *Journal of Traditional and Complementary Medicine*, in 2015, aimed to test the effects of ginger powder supplementation on nitric oxide (NO) and CRP in elderly knee osteoarthritis patients. The study was designed to determine the effect of ginger powder supplementation on some inflammatory markers (NO and hs-CRP) in these patients. This was a clinical trial with a follow-up period of 3 months conducted on outpatients with moderately painful knee osteoarthritis given 500 mg of ginger powder compared to a comparison group given placebo for 3 months.

There was no significant difference in inflammatory markers (i.e., NO and hs-CRP) between the two groups prior to the intervention. However, after 3 months of supplementation, serum concentrations of NO and hs-CRP had decreased in the ginger group, and after 12 weeks, the concentration of these markers had declined even more in the ginger group. Ginger powder supplementation at a dose of 1 g/day can reduce inflammatory markers in patients with knee osteoarthritis, and it was recommended as a suitable supplement for these patients (Naderi et al. 2015).

8.7.1.1 Ginger and Type 2 Diabetes

A study reported in the *Iranian Journal of Pharmaceutical Research*, in 2015, aimed to investigate the effects of ginger on fasting blood sugar, hemoglobin A1c, and malondialdehyde (a marker of ROS concentration) in type 2 diabetic patients. Diabetic patients assigned to a ginger group received 2 g/day of ginger powder supplement, while a comparison group received lactose as placebo for 12 weeks. The serum concentrations of fasting blood sugar, hemoglobin A1c, and malondialdehyde were analyzed before and after the intervention.

Ginger supplementation significantly reduced the levels of fasting blood sugar, hemoglobin A1c, and malondialdehyde in the ginger treatment group in comparison to baseline, as well as the control comparison group. It seems that oral administration of ginger powder supplement can improve fasting blood sugar and hemoglobin A1c and lower malondialdehyde level in type 2 diabetic patients (Khandouzi et al. 2015).

Insulin resistance is also a prime feature of metabolic syndrome. A study published in the journal *Complementary Therapies in Medicine*, in 2015, aimed to identify the effect of ginger on insulin resistance. Participants with diabetes were assigned to a ginger (GG) or a comparison (CG) groups. The GG group received three 1-gram capsules containing ginger powder, while the CG group received three 1 g comparison placebo capsules daily for 8 weeks.

Mean fasting blood sugar (FBS) declined by 10.5% in the ginger group, whereas the placebo comparison group showed a mean increase of 21%. The change in mean HbA1c level showed the same trend as the FBS. The authors concluded that daily consumption of 3 g of ginger powder for 8 weeks helps patients with type 2 diabetes by reducing fasting blood sugar and HbA1c, as well as improving insulin resistance indices (via QUICKI index) (Mozaffari-Khosravi et al. 2014).

8.7.1.2 Ginger and Periodontal Disease

As previously noted, periodontal disease results in chronic inflammation. The gingerol-related components of ginger have been reported to possess antimicrobial and antifungal properties. A study appearing in the journal *Phytotherapy Research*, in 2008, reported that extracts of ginger exhibited antibacterial activities against three anaerobic Gram-negative bacteria causing periodontal disease. One ginger compound destroyed oral pathogens at a minimum bactericidal concentration (Park et al. 2008).

8.7.1.3 Periodontal Disease Is Associated with Shorter Telomeres

The title, "Oxidative stress, chronic inflammation, and telomere length in patients with periodontitis" speaks for itself. It comes from a study published in the journal *Free Radical Biology & Medicine*, in 2011. The authors concluded that "shorter telomere lengths are associated with a diagnosis of periodontitis and their measures correlate with the oxidative stress and severity of disease" (Masi et al. 2011).

There are many online sources that provide free recipes for cooking with ginger. However, crystalized ginger is often sold smothered in sugar. It is recommended that the sugar be shaken off—perhaps even washed off—before consuming it.

8.7.1.4 How Safe Is Consumption of Ginger?

Ginger is said by the US Food and Drug Administration (FDA) to be a food additive that is "generally recognized as safe." Observational human studies have provided no evidence that it causes fetal malformation when used as a treatment for early pregnancy nausea. According to a report in the *American Journal of Obstetrics & Gynecology*, in 2003, administration of ginger beginning at the first trimester of pregnancy showed no increase in the rates of major malformations above the baseline rate of 1–3%.

The Motherisk Program aimed also to establish the safety of ginger in the treatment of nausea and vomiting of pregnancy (NVP). The primary objective of the study was to examine the safety, while the secondary objective was to examine the effectiveness of ginger for NVP. The women taking ginger were compared with a group of women who were exposed to non-teratogenic drugs that were not antiemetic medications (teratogenic means causing fetal deformity). The women were followed up to ascertain the outcome of the pregnancy and the health of their infants. They were also asked on a scale of 0 to 10 how effective the ginger was for their symptoms of NVP.

There was no significant difference between the ginger group and the comparison group other than that there were more infants weighing less than 2500 g in the comparison group. These results suggested that ginger does not appear to increase the rates of major malformations above the baseline rate of 1–3% and that it has a mild effect in the treatment of nausea and vomiting in pregnancy (Portnoi et al. 2003a).

Overall, clinical studies indicate that ginger consumption appears to be quite safe with very limited side effects (Bode and Dong 2011). However, it should be noted that a study appearing in the *Archives of Pharmacal Research*, in 2008, reported some cytotoxic components were extracted from the dried rhizomes of *Zingiber officinale* Roscoe (Portnoi et al. 2003b).

8.7.2 Mostly Green Tea

Drinking a daily cup of tea will surely starve the apothecary. (Chinese proverb)

Green tea is made from *Camellia sinensis* leaves that have not undergone the same withering and oxidation applied when processing it into oolong tea and black tea. It is loaded with polyphenols like flavonoids and catechins, which are antioxidants. Black tea is the tea most commonly consumed in the Western world. It is fully fermented before drying and more oxidized than oolong, green, and white teas. It is generally stronger in flavor than the less oxidized teas.

Researchers from the College of Medicine, National Taiwan University, Taipei, reported in the *Journal of Agricultural and Food Chemistry*, in 2003, on "Factors affecting the levels of tea polyphenols and caffeine in tea leaves." They tell us that a laboratory procedure was developed for the simultaneous determination of caffeine and six catechins in tea samples.

When 31 commercial teas extracted by boiling water, or 75% ethanol, were analyzed by this technique, the levels of (–)-epigallocatechin 3-gallate (EGCG) and total catechins were higher in green tea (old leaves) than in green tea (young leaves), and higher in oolong tea than in black tea or pu-erh tea.

Note: (–)-Epigallocatechin 3-gallate is a type of catechin and the main catechin in tea. Catechin is a natural phenol and antioxidant. It is a plant secondary metabolite that belongs to the group of flavan-3-ols, part of the chemical family of flavonoids.

The contents of caffeine and catechins also have been measured in fresh tea leaves from the tea experiment stations in Wen-Shan and Taitung. Old tea leaves were found to contain less caffeine but more EGCG and total catechins than young leaves.

To compare caffeine and catechins in the same tea but manufactured by different fermentation processes, the level of caffeine in different manufactured teas was in the following order of concentration: black tea > oolong tea > green tea > fresh tea leaf.

The levels of EGCG and total catechins were in the order of concentration: green tea > oolong tea > fresh tea leaf > black tea. In addition, six commercial tea extracts were used to assess their biological functions including hydroxyl radical scavenging, nitric oxide suppressing, and apoptotic effects. The pu-erh tea extracts protected plasmid DNA from damage as well as the comparison control at a concentration of 100 µg/ml (Lin et al. 2003).

8.7.2.1   Tea Lowers Inflammation

Green tea has been shown to combat inflammation. An unusual property of green tea is described in an article in the journal *Food & Function*, in 2013. Flavanols from tea were shown to have an unusual affinity for cell nuclei and have been reported to accumulate in the cell nucleus in considerable concentrations.

The nature of this phenomenon, which could provide novel approaches for understanding the well-known beneficial health effects of tea phenols, is investigated in this study which found that selected polyphenols displayed affinity for all of the selected cell nuclear structures. Theaflavin-digallate was shown to display the highest affinity for DNA of any naturally occurring molecule reported so far. This finding may have implications for understanding the role of tea phenolics as "life span essentials" (Mikutis et al. 2013a).

Writing in the journal *Current Medicinal Chemistry*, investigators concluded that catechins, the major polyphenolic compounds in green tea, exert vascular protective antioxidative, anti-hypertensive, anti-inflammatory, anti-proliferative, anti-thrombosis, and lipid lowering effects. They aver that tea catechins are free radical scavengers; reduce intestinal lipid absorption, thereby improving blood lipid profile; activate endothelial nitric oxide; prevent the vascular inflammation that plays a critical role in the progression of atherosclerotic lesions; and suppress platelet adhesion, thereby inhibiting the formation of blood clots (Mikutis et al. 2013).

In 2007, the journal *Cardiovascular & Hematological Disorders - Drug Targets* confirmed that epigallocatechin gallate (EGCG) in green tea polyphenols is a free radical scavenger and the major and most active component in green tea. It protects against cellular damage by inhibiting DNA damage and oxidation of LDL. EGCG can also reduce the inflammatory response associated with local tissue by lowering lipid peroxidation and oxidative stress, and by inhibiting the overproduction of pro-inflammatory cytokines and mediators, and reducing the formation of ROS.

EGCG effectively prevents cellular damage by lowering the inflammatory reaction, reducing lipid peroxidation and NO generated radicals leading to oxidative stress (Tipoe et al. 2007).

8.7.2.2   Tea Normalizes Insulin Sensitivity and Sugar Metabolism

Glucose control and insulin sensitivity play a significant role in metabolic syndrome, a source of chronic systemic inflammation. In fact, low-grade inflammation is characteristic of metabolic syndrome (Devaraj et al. 2009). That point is driven home by the title of a study, "Low-grade systemic inflammation connects aging, metabolic syndrome and cardiovascular disease," appearing in the journal *Interdisciplinary Topics in Gerontology*, in 2015.

The authors reported that aging is accompanied by a chronic inflammatory state that contributes to metabolic syndrome, diabetes, and their cardiovascular consequences. Risk factors for cardiovascular diseases (CVDs) and diabetes overlap, leading to the conclusion that they share an inflammatory basis (Guarner and Rubio-Ruiz 2015). The *Journal of the American College of Nutrition*, in 2009, concluded that "green tea may be beneficial for people with decreased insulin sensitivity and increased oxidative stress, such as those with the metabolic syndrome or type 2 diabetes" (Hininger-Favier et al. 2009).

A more recent (2013) study in the same journal reported the outcome of a meta-analysis of the effect of green tea on human insulin sensitivity. The authors concluded that green tea significantly decreased fasting glucose and HbA1c concentrations (Liu et al. 2013). Insulin sensitivity is a component of metabolic syndrome, in turn a major contributor to oxidative stress and chronic inflammation. That makes tea a valuable functional food in combating oxidative stress-related chronic inflammation.

A study published in the *Journal of Agricultural and Food Chemistry*, reported in 2002 that teas differ in their capacity to enhance insulin activity, although they all do it to a greater or lesser extent. Tea, as normally consumed, was shown to increase insulin activity more than 15-fold in vitro in an experimental fat cell assay. Black, green, and oolong teas were all shown to increase insulin activity (Anderson and Polansky 2002).

8.7.2.3 Tea Reduces Inflammation and Protects Blood Vessels by Promoting Endothelium NO Formation

Epidemiological studies indicate that tea has beneficial cardiovascular effects, but are different types of tea superior in their cardiovascular benefits? In a study published in *Basic Research in Cardiology*, in 2009, investigators compared green and black tea nitric oxide (NO) production, and vasodilation. They chose a highly fermented black tea and determined concentrations of individual tea compounds in both green and black tea of the same type (Assam). The fermented black tea was almost devoid of catechins.

Both types of tea triggered the endothelium NO enzyme, eNOS, and blood vessel relaxation to the same extent in animal models: bovine aortic endothelial cells (BAEC) and rat aortic rings. But, in green tea, only epigallocatechin-3-gallate (EGCG) resulted in pronounced NO production and NO-dependent vasorelaxation in aortic rings. It is thought that during tea processing to produce black tea, the catechins are converted to theaflavins and thearubigins. Individual black tea theaflavins showed a higher potency than EGCG in NO production and vasorelaxation. The thearubigins in black tea are highly efficient stimulators of vasodilation and NO production.

These results show that highly fermented black tea is equally as potent as green tea in promoting beneficial endothelial effects. Theaflavins and thearubigins predominantly counterbalance the lack of catechins in black tea. The findings may underline the contribution of black tea consumption to the prevention of cardiovascular diseases (Lorenz et al. 2009).

8.7.2.4 A Green Tea Constituent Protects Telomeres

A study (in an animal model) published in the *International Journal of Cardiology*, in 2013, investigated the effects of epigallocatechin gallate (EGCG), the major component of polyphenols in green tea, on cardiomyocytes, the cells that make up the heart muscles. Ordinarily, what happens to telomeres in heart dysfunction may lead to cell self-destruction (apoptosis).

In this study, rats were subjected to a surgical procedure that results in the same stress changes to the heart as would prolonged, sustained, hypertension. EGCG 50 or 100 mg/kg, quercetin 100 mg/kg, captopril 50 mg/kg, losartan 30 mg/kg, and carvedilol 30 mg/kg were administered for 6 weeks.

At 3, 5, and 7 weeks after aortic constriction, the heart weight indices had increased progressively. Malondialdehyde (MDA) content progressively increased, while superoxide dismutase (SOD) activities decreased. Progressive cardiomyocyte apoptosis and telomere attrition were also found.

The investigators concluded that blood pressure overload induces cardiac hypertrophy (heart enlargement), initiates oxidative stress, and accelerates telomere shortening in hypertrophic heart muscle. EGCG, quercetin, and carvedilol with a potent antioxidant effect may inhibit cardiac myocyte apoptosis by preventing telomere shortening (Sheng et al. 2013).

8.7.2.5 It Is Best to Leave Out the Milk

One of the more powerful compounds in green tea is the polyphenolic bioflavonoid antioxidant epigallocatechin gallate (EGCG). The aim of a study published in the *European Journal of Clinical Nutrition*, in 1996, was to assess the antioxidant capacity of green and black tea as well as the effect of adding milk to the beverage. Conventional antioxidant capacity assessment methods were used on two groups, each of which consumed 300 ml of either black or green tea, after an overnight fast. The human plasma antioxidant capacity (Total Peroxyl Radical Trapping Capacity) was measured before and 30, 50, and 80 minutes after consuming tea.

Note: In measurement for cooking, a cup is 250 ml (236 ml, or 8 ounces in US).

When the experiment was repeated on a separate day, 100 ml whole milk was added to the tea (ratio 1:4). Both teas inhibited dose-dependent antioxidant capacity but the green tea was sixfold more potent than the black tea until milk was added. The addition of milk totally inhibited antioxidant capacity (Serafini et al. 1996).

Besides leaving out milk if you want the full antioxidant effect, brewing loose tea is probably the best way to consume it in the long run—matcha green tea can also be mixed into cold water without losing its properties. Also, according to a study published in the *International Journal of Food Science & Nutrition*, in 2000, tea bag materials may prevent some extraction of flavonoids into the tea beverage, thus acting as a sort of filter (Langley-Evans 2000).

8.7.2.6 Green Tea versus Black Tea and Brewing "Loose" Tea versus Tea Bags: The Case for Lower Oxalate Levels

For individuals who may have kidney stones, green tea brewed from loose tea leaves may be preferable to tea in other conventional forms including black tea and oolong tea made from both loose leaf tea and from tea bags.

A total of 32 commercially available teas consisting of green, oolong, and black teas purchased in local markets in New Zealand in 2001 were examined for the soluble oxalate content of the infusate made from each of the teas. The mean soluble oxalate content of black tea in tea bags and loose tea leaves was 4.68 and 5.11 mg/g tea, respectively, while green teas and oolong tea had lower oxalate content, ranging from 0.23 to 1.15 mg/g tea.

A regular tea drinker consuming six cups of tea per day would have an intake of 26.46–98.58 mg soluble oxalate/day from loose black tea and 17.88–93.66 mg soluble oxalate/day from black tea in tea bags. The oxalate intake from the regular daily consumption of black teas is modest when compared to the amounts of soluble oxalate that can be found in common foods. However, oxalate in black teas has the potential to bind to a significant proportion of calcium in the milk, which is commonly consumed with black tea (Charrier et al. 2002).

Some tea bags are treated with epichlorohydrin to prevent them from disintegrating or tearing. Epichlorohydrin is mainly used in the production of epoxy resins and when it comes in contact with water, it breaks down to 3-MCPD, a known carcinogen that has also been linked to infertility and suppressed immune function. According to the Institute of Food Science and Technology (UK) Issues Statement on 3-MCPD, on 25 March 2003, its presence in food stuffs should be reduced to an undetectable level (http://www.foodnavigator.com/Science/IFST-issues-statement-on-3-MCPD).

8.7.2.7 Is It Safe to Drink a Lot of Tea?

The authors cautioned about excess consumption of polyphenols in Chapter 3. Some people will say that they drink a lot of tea every day, just as they will say that they drink a lot of coffee. Just how much is "a lot"?

A study in the journal *Clinical Cancer Research*, in 2003, addressed the question, "What is a lot?" in connection with tea as part of a cancer treatment project because green tea and green tea polyphenols were shown to possess cancer preventive activities in preclinical model systems. In preparation for future green tea intervention trials, the investigators conducted a clinical study to determine the safety and the way that green tea polyphenols move through the body (pharmacokinetics) after 4 weeks of daily oral consumption of epigallocatechin gallate (EGCG) or polyphenon E (a defined, decaffeinated green tea polyphenol mixture).

Adverse events reported during the 4-week treatment period included excess gas, upset stomach, nausea, heartburn, stomach ache, abdominal pain, dizziness, headache, and muscle pain. All of the reported events were rated as mild. For most events, the incidence reported in the polyphenol-treated groups was no higher than that reported in a comparison placebo group. No significant changes were observed in blood counts or blood chemistry profiles after repeated administration of green tea polyphenol products.

The investigators concluded that it is safe for healthy individuals to take green tea polyphenol products in amounts equivalent to the EGCG content in 8–16 cups of green tea once a day, or in divided doses twice a day for 4 weeks (Chow et al. 2003).

The journal *Drug Safety* reported, in 2008, that regulatory agencies in France and Spain had suspended market authorization of a weight-loss product containing green tea extract because of concerns about possible liver damage. Adverse event case reports involving green tea products were cited. In response, the US Pharmacopeia (USP) Dietary Supplement Information Expert Committee (DSI EC) systematically reviewed the safety information for green tea products in order to re-evaluate the current safety class to which these products are assigned.

Clinical pharmacokinetics and animal toxicological information indicated that consumption of green tea concentrated extracts on an empty stomach is more likely to lead to adverse effects than consumption in the fed state. However, based on this safety review, the DSI EC determined that when dietary supplement products containing green tea extracts are used and formulated appropriately, they were unaware of significant safety issues that would prohibit monograph development, provided a caution statement is included in the labeling section (Sarma et al. 2008).

8.8 HOT CHILI PEPPERS

Sometimes chili peppers are green, sometimes they are red; they are never hot; they are never chilly; they are not even *pepper*. But, they are antioxidant and they are anti-inflammatory. What are they?

The chili pepper is the fruit of plants from the genus *Capsicum*, members of the nightshade family. The substances that give chili peppers their intense taste or sensation when they are applied topically are capsaicin (8-methyl-N-vanillyl-6-nonenamide) and several related compounds collectively called capsaicinoids. Chili peppers originated in the Americas but cultivars are grown across the world and are used as spices in foods and for medicine.

Capsaicinoids bind with pain receptors in the mouth and throat that are responsible for sensing heat. Once activated, these receptors send a message to the brain that the person has consumed something hot. The brain responds to the burning sensation by raising the heart rate, increasing perspiration, and releasing endorphins.

The sensation of heat from consuming chili peppers was historically measured in *Scoville heat units* (SHU), based on the dilution of an amount of chili extract added to sugar syrup before its heat becomes undetectable to a panel of tasters: the more it has to be diluted to be undetectable, the more powerful the variety and therefore the higher the SHU rating.

Chili peppers contain capsaicin, a potent inhibitor of *substance P*, a neuropeptide associated with inflammatory processes and more. A neuropeptide is a compound that acts as a neurotransmitter conveying information within the nervous system. The hotter the chili pepper, the more capsaicin it contains.

8.8.1 SUBSTANCE P IS ALSO IMPLICATED IN DEPRESSION

Experimental studies of mood disorders have largely focused on the role of well-established neurotransmitters such as serotonin, noradrenaline, and gamma-amino-butyric acid (GABA). But the neuropeptide substance P and its receptor (neurokinin-1 receptor, NK1R) have also been implicated in depression. In fact, inflammation has likewise been strongly implicated in major depressive disorder (Miller et al. 2009).

There now is evidence for the regulatory role of the NK1R system in mood disorder, and that role may be mediated by the serotonin system. Future studies may unravel the interaction between the NK1R system and various neurotransmitter pathways in greater detail and address the specific role(s) of this system in different brain regions (Santarelli et al. 2002). In fact, in another study published in the same journal as the one cited above, *The Journal of Clinical Psychiatry*, reported in 2002 that recent studies employing pharmacologic inactivation of the NK1 receptors for substance P demonstrate its important role in regulating mood and suggest that inhibition of this mechanism may be a useful approach to treatment of depression and associated anxiety (Mantyh 2002).

8.8.2 *CAPSICUM BACCATUM* IS ANTI-INFLAMMATORY

A study appearing in *The Journal of Pharmacy and Pharmacology*, in 2008, aimed to evaluate the effects of the *Capsicum baccatum* cultivar juice in an animal model of acute inflammation induced by two types of abdominal inflammatory substances. The authors report that this is the first demonstration of the anti-inflammatory effect of *C. baccatum* juice and that the data suggest that this effect may be induced by capsaicin. Moreover, the anti-inflammatory effect induced by red pepper may be through inhibition of pro-inflammatory cytokine production at the inflammatory site (Spiller et al. 2008).

Likewise, a study published in the journal *Food Chemistry* in 1996 was conducted to determine the antioxidant vitamin content of paprika during ripening, processing, and storage. The most biologically effective antioxidant vitamins, such as ascorbic acid, tocopherols, and carotenoids, were separated, identified, and evaluated in different samples.

The rate of synthesis of the three antioxidants increased after the onset of ripening. As ripening progressed, antioxidant vitamins tended to increase proportionally except that ascorbic acid reached a maximum level at the color break II stage and then declined. During drying and storage, there was a dramatic decrease in the concentration of tocopherol and ascorbic acid as a result of active antioxidation activity, while carotenoid content decreased at a lower rate (Daood et al. 1996).

Note: The types and levels of carotenoids differ between different chili pepper fruits, and are also influenced by environmental conditions. The yellow-orange colors of chili pepper fruits are mainly due to the accumulation of alpha- and beta-carotene, zeaxanthin, lutein, and beta-cryptoxanthin. Carotenoids such as capsanthin, capsorubin, and capsanthin-5,6-epoxide confer the red colors (del Rocío Gómez-García and Ochoa-Alejo 2013). Many websites provide recipes for meals incorporating chili.

A Cautionary Note: Capsicum and paprika are generally recognized as safe for use in food by the US Food and Drug Administration (No authors listed 2007). However, a clinical report in the *International Journal of Emergency Medicine*, in 2012, concerned the case of a previously healthy young man who reported severe chest pain after using cayenne pepper pills for slimming. He was diagnosed with extensive inferior myocardial infarction which was confirmed by electrocardiography combined with a bedside echocardiogram. The patient denied using illicit substances and had no risk factors for coronary artery disease. His medication history revealed that he had recently started taking cayenne pepper pills for slimming. A subsequent coronary angiogram revealed normal coronary arteries, suggesting that the mechanism was vasospasm. The authors postulated that the patient developed acute coronary vasospasm and a myocardial infarction in the presence of stimulating compounds. This case highlights the unlikely but nevertheless possible danger of capsaicin, even when used by otherwise healthy individuals (Sogut et al. 2012).

8.9 CINNAMON

Cinnamon belonging to the Lauracea family is a popular spice often used as a flavoring agent in baked goods. It is now known that it has beneficial antioxidant and anti-inflammatory properties. It is considered by many as an adjunct in complementary and alternative medicine (Kawatra and Rajagopalan 2015).

Cinnamon is exported mainly from Indonesia, China, Vietnam, and Sri Lanka as quills that are made by peeling the bark and then rolling it into pipes.

There are four types of cinnamon:

- True cinnamon or Ceylon cinnamon (*Cinnamomum zeylanicum*)
- Indonesian cinnamon (*Cinnamomum burmanni*)
- Vietnamese cinnamon (*Cinnamomum loureiroi*)
- Cassia* cinnamon or Chinese cinnamon (*Cinnamomum aromaticum*)

The authors of a 2011 report in the journal *Critical Reviews in Food Science and Nutrition*, are from the Central Food Technological Research Institute, Mysore, India. They inform us that there are several hundred different species of *Cinnamomum* distributed in Asia and Australia. *C. zeylanicum*, a common source of cinnamon bark and leaf oils, is native to Sri Lanka, although most oil now comes from cultivated areas.

C. zeylanicum is a spice with wide applications in flavoring, perfumery, beverages, and medicines. Volatile oils from different parts of the cinnamon plant such as the leaves, bark, fruit, root bark, flowers, and buds have been isolated by conventional laboratory and industrial methods and the chemical compositions of more than 80 compounds have been identified from different parts of cinnamon. The leaf oil has a major component called eugenol. Cinnamaldehyde and camphor have been reported to be the major components of volatile oils from stem bark and root bark, respectively. Trans-cinnamyl acetate was found to be the major compound in fruit, flowers, and fruit stalks.

Chronic inflammation contributes to many age-related diseases. These volatile oils were found to exhibit antioxidant, anti-inflammatory, antimicrobial, and antidiabetic activities. *C. zeylanicum* bark and fruit were found to contain proanthocyandins (Jayaprakasha and Rao 2011).

8.9.1 CINNAMON IS ANTIOXIDANT

The antioxidant property of cinnamon is largely due to the eugenol component which inhibits lipid peroxidation: the oxygen radical absorbance capacity (ORAC) value of cinnamon is 131,420, among the highest for common foods. A significant relationship was found between antioxidant capacity and total phenolic content, indicating

---

* *Cinnamomum cassia*, also called Chinese cassia or Chinese cinnamon, is the most common type of cinnamon used as a spice in the United States. Due to a blood anticoagulant constituent, coumarin, that could damage the liver, European health agencies have warned against consuming high amounts of cassia. A report appearing in the journal *Food and Chemical Toxicology*, in 1999, informs us that ordinary consumption is considered safe (Lake 1999).

that phenolic compounds are major contributors to the antioxidant properties of these plants (Dudonne et al. 2009; Mathew and Abraham 2006; Su et al. 2007).

8.9.2 CINNAMON IS ANTI-INFLAMMATORY

Sri Lankan cinnamon (*C. zeylanicum*) has been found to be one of the most potent anti-inflammatory foods out of 115 tested by the authors of a study published in the journal *Food & Function*, in 2015. Because the exact nature of the anti-inflammatory compounds and their distribution in the two major cinnamon species used for human consumption is limited, the aim of this investigation was to determine the anti-inflammatory activity of *C. zeylanicum* and *Cinnamomum cassia* and define their main compounds.

When extracts were tested in macrophages, most of the anti-inflammatory activity, measured by down-regulation of nitric oxide (NO), was observed in the organic extracts. The most abundant compounds in these extracts were E-cinnamaldehyde and o-methoxycinnamaldehyde. The highest concentration of E-cinnamaldehyde was found in the *C. zeylanicum* and *C. cassia* extracts. When these and other constituents were tested for their anti-inflammatory activity in macrophages, the most potent compounds were E-cinnamaldehyde and o-methoxycinnamaldehyde. The authors concluded that these could be useful in the treatment of age-related inflammatory conditions (Gunawardena et al. 2015).

According to a report published in the journal *BMC Complementary and Alternative Medicine*, in 2013, the beneficial health effects of "true" cinnamon (*C. zeylanicum*) were: (a) anti-microbial, (b) lowering of blood glucose, blood pressure, and serum cholesterol, (c) antioxidant and free-radical scavenging activity, and (d) anti-inflammatory activity (Ranasinghe et al. 2013).

8.9.3 CINNAMON AND TYPE 2 DIABETES

Cinnamon has often been cited in connection with glycemic control. Glycemic control is complex and rests on many factors a good number of them being medical issues involving also those in metabolic syndrome. The following studies reporting glycemic control with cinnamon are essentially generalizations that do not take into account individual medical considerations. This is, therefore, a reminder that information about the potential palliative value of any functional food, or beverage, in connection with a medical disorder, is not suggested as an alternative to competent conventional medical treatment. Besides, although reports of the efficacy of cinnamon in glycemic control are, by and large, positive, nevertheless there are also conflicting reports in the medical literature.

The authors of a report in the *Annals of Family Medicine*, in 2013, tell us that cinnamon has been studied in clinical trials for its glycemic-lowering effects, but studies have been small and show conflicting results. Therefore, the authors undertook a systematic review of meta-analyses evaluating the effects of cinnamon on glycemia and lipid levels.

They searched Embase and the Cochrane Central Register of Controlled Trials (CENTRAL) through February 2012. The trials evaluated cinnamon in patients with type 2 diabetes and reported at least one of the following: glycated hemoglobin (A1c), fasting plasma glucose, total cholesterol, low-density lipoprotein cholesterol (LDL-C), high-density lipoprotein cholesterol (HDL-C), or triglycerides.

The authors report that cinnamon doses ranging from 120 mg/day to 6 g/day for 4–18 weeks significantly reduced levels of fasting plasma glucose, total cholesterol, LDL-C, and triglycerides. Cinnamon also raised levels of HDL-C. No significant effect on hemoglobin A1c levels was observed. However, it was concluded that the high degree of heterogeneity of the data may limit the applicability of these results to patient care because the preferred dose and duration of therapy are often unclear (Allen et al. 2013).

Another meta-analysis reported in the *Journal of Medical Foods*, in 2011, found that cinnamon intake, either as whole cinnamon or as cinnamon extract, results in a significant lowering of fasting blood sugar, while intake of cinnamon extract only also lowered fasting blood sugar in people with type 2 diabetes or prediabetes (Davis and Yokoyama 2011).

Another review of several clinical trials on the effectiveness of cinnamon in type 2 diabetes was published in the journal *Pharmacotherapy* in 2007. It concluded that cinnamon has a possible modest effect in lowering plasma glucose levels in patients with poorly controlled type 2 diabetes. The authors stated that "clinicians are strongly urged to refrain from recommending cinnamon supplementation in place of the proven standard of care, which includes lifestyle modifications, oral antidiabetic agents, and insulin therapy" (Pham et al. 2007).

Entering "cinnamon and type 2 diabetes" into PubMed results in more than 100 citations. The considerable scientific interest in that topic. It may be due in large measure to the fact that current interventions in glycemic control in type 2 diabetes seem to leave much to be desired. The problem is that Type 2 diabetes is a health hazard of epidemic proportions. It would be good to be able to say that cinnamon is a successful functional food and an effective adjunct to alternative medicine.

It is difficult to know why there is inconsistency in the outcome of studies of the effectiveness of cinnamon in glycemic control in type 2 diabetes. There are many possibilities: varieties differ in type and concentration of effective constituents. The same variety has different concentration of constituents depending on the geographic regions in the world where it is cultivated. However, we know of no data that would shed light on this problem. For that reason, and because apparently valid clinical studies support the role of cinnamon in glycemic control, we present both sides of the picture.

Investigators from the Netherlands reported in the *Journal of Nutrition* in 2006 that they found that the blood lipid profile of fasting subjects did not change after cinnamon supplementation. They therefore concluded that cinnamon (*C. cassia*) supplementation with 1.5 g/day does not improve whole-body insulin sensitivity or oral glucose tolerance, nor did it affect blood lipid profile in postmenopausal patients with type 2 diabetes. They concluded that "more research on the proposed health benefits of cinnamon supplementation is warranted before health claims should be made." (Vanschoonbeek et al. 2006) Another study likewise from a diabetes clinic in The Netherlands appearing in the journal *Nederlands Tijdschrift voor Geneeskunde*, in 2007, concluded that no evidence supports recommending cinnamon for improvement of glycemic control (Kleefstra et al. 2007).

8.9.4 SAFETY OF CINNAMON

Finally, as noted above, cassia cinnamon contains relatively high levels of coumarins that can be toxic in high doses. A daily intake of more than 0.1 mg/kg body weight can have a conspicuous effect on the blood coagulation profile if one is also on anticoagulant drugs such as warfarin. (Coumarin can also be highly toxic to the liver and its addition to food products is prohibited.) However, due to the lack of awareness regarding the standard limits of cinnamon in these products, it is probably advisable for anyone with liver disorders to avoid cinnamon.

8.10 EDIBLE SEAWEED, A SEA VEGETABLE

Edible seaweed is included in this limited list of functional foods because it contains iodine which is essential for healthy metabolic function. However, diet is the sole source and health authorities report that there is a significant worldwide iodine deficiency (Li and Eastman 2012). In the developed world, iodine deficiency has increased more than fourfold over the past 40 years with nearly 74% of normal "healthy" adults possibly no longer consuming enough iodine (http://www.lifeextension.com/magazine/2011/10/the-silent-epidemic-of-iodine-deficiency/Page-01).

In 1922, David Cowie, chairman of the Pediatrics Department at the University of Michigan, proposed that the US adopt salt iodinization to eliminate simple goiter (Markel 1987). Dr. Cowie was instrumental in the history of the US iodine supplementation effort.

In the United States, salt is iodized usually with potassium iodide at 100 parts per million (76 mg of iodine per 1 kg of salt). However, approximately 70% of ingested salt now comes from processed food that is typically not iodinized in the United States. Iodine deficiency is one of the most important public health issues globally, with an estimated 2.2 billion people living in iodine-deficient areas: the oceans are the main repositories of iodine and very little is found in the soil in most of the inhabited world.

Although the International Council for the Control of Iodine Deficiency Disorders (ICCIDD) Global Network estimates that the proportion of US households with access to iodized salt now exceeds 90%, data regarding actual usage are limited and the contribution of iodinized salt to the overall iodine sufficiency of the US population is uncertain. This is particularly the case as there is a trend to reduce table salt intake consistent with the rising concerns about "sodium" in the diet and hypertension and cardiovascular and heart disease.

In fact, the *Harvard Health Letter* (Jun 21, 2011) seemingly supported that trend in an article titled, "Cut salt—it won't affect your iodine intake," stating that iodinized salt provided only a small fraction of daily iodine intake (No authors listed 2011).

While iodine deficiency has many implications for serious medical disorders and poor cognitive function, our concern here is dietary deficiency that sets the stage for chronic inflammation and an adverse serum lipid profile.

"Sea-vegetables" are included here as a dietary source of iodine where it is suspected that the typical diet supplies insufficient amounts. However, it is not intended to propose self-treatment for any thyroid condition related to iodine. Thyroid disease can be a serious medical problem which needs to be addressed by competent medical means. In fact, even subclinical hypothyroidism (elevated *thyroid-stimulating hormone,* TSH) may be a mild form of thyroid failure that needs to be treated medically, with all indications suggesting it will worsen in the long term (McDermott and Ridgway 2011).

8.10.1 THE BARNES TEST

Barring medical evidence of even minimal thyroid dysfunction, how can one tell if dietary intake of iodine is adequate? For one thing, a routine medical TSH test can readily reveal thyroid deficiency. Furthermore, if it is simply a matter that dietary intake of iodine is inadequate, the basal metabolic rate will be lower than normal. Basal metabolic rate is the rate at which the body uses energy while at rest to keep vital functions going, such as breathing and keeping warm.

Assuming that one is not on medication(s) that would directly affect these measures, a consistently low body temperature (below 98.0°F) and pulse rate below 65 may be an indication of low thyroid function. The Barnes basal temperature test is a simple, do-it-at-home, self-test. It is reasonably accurate and requires only a digital thermometer.

- When awakening in the morning, and before rising, note the basal body temperature (BBT) and make a record of it.
- Repeat this procedure each morning for 5 days. Keep in mind that a woman's body temperature varies with the different phases of the menstrual cycle. The most accurate/reliable BBT temperature can be obtained on the second and third days of the menstrual cycle.
- If the basal temperature is consistently below 98.0°F one may have hypothyroidism and should consult a physician.

The healthy adult body should contain about 15–20 mg of iodine, 70–80% of which is stored in the thyroid gland. The daily intake requirement for adults is about 150 mg. The body conserves only about 10–20% of iodine consumed in the daily diet, with the rest excreted from the body. Also, supplementing iodine is not invariably medically sound as there may be contraindications. But assuming safe supplementation, success should be seen in just a few days as normalizing BBT.

Supplementing the diet with iodine has been found to be effective where the cause is iodine deficiency, but one needs to be careful not to take too much of it or too quickly as that is not good for the thyroid: too much iodine can result in hyperthyroidism. In some instances, also supplementing the diet with tyrosine can be helpful. Here again, professional medical or nutritionist advice is recommended.

For most people, iodine intake from usual foods and supplements is unlikely to exceed the tolerable upper intake level (1100 µg/day). The Institute of Medicine recommends a daily iodine intake of 150 µg/day for non-pregnant adults, 220 µg/day for pregnant women, and 290 μg/day during lactation (https://www.cdc.gov/nutritionreport/99-02/pdf/nr_ch4a.pdf) (No authors listed 2001).

8.10.2 KELP IS ON THE WAY

Different varieties of edible seaweed/sea vegetables are sources of iodine. The better-known varieties are:

- Kelps, large seaweeds (algae) belonging to the brown algae Phaeophyceae class in the order Laminariales. They typically have a long, tough stalk with a broad frond divided into strips. Some kinds grow to a very large size and form underwater "forests" that support a large population of animals. The Japanese version is:
- Kombu or haidai (*Laminaria japonica*):
- Nori or purple laver (*Porphyra* spp.).
- Wakame or quandai-cai (*Undaria pinnatifida*).
- Dulse (*Palmaria palmata*).

Seaweed, such as kelp, nori, kombu, and wakame, is one of the best food sources of iodine, but it is highly variable in its content. It is used extensively as a food in coastal cuisines around the world and is a rich source of iodine, an essential component of the thyroid hormones thyroxine (T4) and triiodothyronine (T3).

Iodine in food and iodized salt is present in several chemical forms including sodium and potassium salts, inorganic iodine (I2), iodate, and iodide, the reduced form of iodine. Iodine rarely occurs as the element, but rather as a salt and so is referred to as iodide and not iodine. Iodide is quickly and almost completely absorbed in the stomach and duodenum. Iodate is reduced in the gastrointestinal tract and absorbed as iodide. When iodide enters the circulation, the thyroid gland concentrates it in appropriate amounts for thyroid hormone synthesis with most of the remaining amount excreted in the urine.

8.10.3 IODINE CONTENT OF DIFFERENT VARIETIES OF SEAWEED

A report in the *Journal of Food and Drug Analysis*, in 2014, lists the following Asian seaweed iodine concentrations:

- Nori: 29.3–45.8 mg/kg
- Wakame: 93.9–185.1 mg/kg
- Kombu: 241–4921 mg/kg (Yeh et al. 2014)

The iodine concentration in samples of kelp from British Columbia, Canada, was reported in the journal *Thyroid*, in 2004, to range between 1259 and 1513 μg/g. The authors of that report also caution that iodine is water-soluble in cooking and may vaporize in humid storage conditions making the average iodine content of prepared foods difficult to estimate. Also, it is possible that some Asian seaweed dishes may exceed the tolerable upper iodine intake level of 1100 μg/day (Teas et al. 2004).

Iodine can also be supplied by commercially available kelp supplements that list the iodine content per capsule or pill.

8.10.4 HEALTH RISKS OF EXCESSIVE IODINE INTAKE

High intakes of iodine can cause some of the same symptoms as iodine deficiency, including goiter, elevated TSH levels, and hypothyroidism, because excess iodine in susceptible individuals inhibits thyroid hormone synthesis and thereby increases TSH stimulation, which can produce goiter. Iodine-induced hyperthyroidism can also result from high iodine intakes, usually when iodine is administered to treat iodine deficiency.

Studies have also shown that excessive iodine intakes can cause thyroiditis and thyroid papillary cancer. Cases of acute iodine poisoning are rare and usually caused by doses weighing many grams. Acute poisoning symptoms include burning of the mouth, throat, and stomach, fever, abdominal pain, nausea, vomiting, diarrhea, weak pulse, and coma.

Some people, such as those with autoimmune thyroid disease and iodine deficiency, may experience adverse effects with iodine intakes considered safe for the general population.

The Food and Nutrition Board (FNB) set iodine upper intake levels (ULs) from food and supplements (see Table 8.1). In most people, iodine intake from foods and supplements is unlikely to exceed the UL. Long-term intake above the UL raises the risk of adverse health effects. The ULs do not apply to individuals receiving iodine for medical treatment under the care of a physician (Institute of Medicine, Food and Nutrition Board 2001).

8.10.5 INTERACTION WITH MEDICATIONS

Iodine supplements have the potential to interact with several types of medications. A few examples are provided below. Individuals taking these medications on a regular basis should discuss their iodine intakes with their healthcare providers. There are other conditions and medical consultation is advised.

8.10.5.1 Anti-Thyroid Medications

Anti-thyroid medications, such as methimazole (Tapazole®), are used to treat hyperthyroidism. Taking high doses of iodine with anti-thyroid medications can have an additive effect and could cause medical problems.

TABLE 8.1
Tolerable Upper Intake Levels (ULs) for Iodine

Age	Male	Female	Pregnancy	Lactation
14–18 years	900 μg	900 μg	900 μg	900 μg
19+ years	1100 μg	1100 μg	1100 μg	1100 g

Source: https://ods.od.nih.gov/factsheets/Iodine-HealthProfessional/.

8.10.5.2 Angiotensin-Converting Enzyme (ACE) Inhibitors

Angiotensin-converting enzyme (ACE) inhibitors, such as benazepril (Lotensin®), lisinopril (Prinivil® and Zestril®), and fosinopril (Monopril®), are used primarily to treat high blood pressure. Taking potassium iodide with ACE inhibitors can increase the risk of hyperkalemia (elevated blood levels of potassium).

8.10.5.3 Potassium-Sparing Diuretics

Taking potassium iodide with potassium-sparing diuretics, such as spironolactone (Aldactone®) and amiloride (Midamor®), can increase the risk of hyperkalemia (see http://naturaldatabase.therapeuticresearch.com/nd/Search.aspx?pt=100 &id=35&AspxAutoDetectCookieSupport=1 and https://ods.od.nih.gov/factsheets/ Iodine-HealthProfessional/).

8.11   MASTIC: *PISTACIA LENTISCUS* VAR. *CHIA*

Then [his brothers] sat down to eat; and looking up, they saw a caravan of Ishmaelites coming from Gilead with their camels carrying gum, balm and resin, on their way to carry it down to Egypt. (Genesis 37:25–27)

Biblical scholars have suggested that "balm" is a pseudonym for *laudanum*, and that "resin" is terebinth (*Pistacia therebinthus* or *atlantica*), probably used to extend the shelf-life of wine, while *gum* may be a pseudonym for lentisc (also called as lentisk) or mastic (*Pistacia lentiscus*) as it is now known. Mastic is a gummy resinous sap that seeps from a small bush-like tree that thrives on the Mediterranean Greek island of Chios where it is called the "Schinos tree."

In Biblical times, mastic was considered a soothing, inflammation-reducing "packing" for broken and infected teeth: anthropological evidence from Egyptian mummified human remains points to the common occurrence of teeth ground down by sand, teeth chipped and broken, and numerous instances of jawbone erosion due to dental-root abscesses. A mastic bead will soften in the mouth but will not readily dissolve in saliva, so it is quite easy to fit into a crack in a tooth. What is more, it was more recently shown to be bactericidal.

Mastic gum featured prominently in ancient Hebrew remedies. It was widely chewed to reduce bad breath (halitosis) and is, even to this day, incorporated in a breath-freshening chewing gum brand-named "Elma" (sugar-free) sold principally in Greece, with limited availability in the US (see for instance http://www.greekshops.com/ Food__ Cookware__Beauty/Snacks_and_Desserts/ELMA_Mastic_Gum_from_Chios_w_ sugar__Mastixa_Xiou.html?pdi=GMXS&ug=28).

A clear indication of its traditional importance, chewing mastic gum for relief of bad breath is permitted on the Jewish Sabbath.

Roman legion physicians used it to treat gastric distress. In the first century CE, Dioscorides, a Greek battlefield physician who served with the Roman army, wrote *De Materia Medica* that listed mastic gum from the tree *P. lentiscus* as one of the most valuable substances for the treatment of gastric distress and indigestion.

Today, Chios mastic is a known spice in Eastern Mediterranean cuisine. In Greece, it is used in liqueurs such as Chios Mastiha, beverages, chewing gum, sweets, desserts, breads, and cheese. One of the earliest uses of mastic was as chewing gum, and mastic-flavored chewing gum is still sold in Syria, Lebanon, Turkey, and Greece. In Egypt, mastic is used in vegetable preserves, in jams that have a gummy consistency, in soups, and in the preparation of meats. In Morocco, mastic is used in the preparation of smoked foods. In Turkey, it is widely used in desserts such as Turkish delight, in puddings, and in soft drinks. It is also added to Turkish coffee on the Aegean coast.

That said, inclusion of Chios mastic in this selection of functional foods is, however, based on its antioxidant capacity, and its bactericidal and anti-inflammatory activity.

Mastic has remarkable palliative properties. Its bactericidal activity targets *H. pylori* bacteria implicated in peptic ulcers, and the bacteria that cause periodontal disease. To the extent that it reduces *H. pylori* in the stomach, it has also been shown to help alleviate iron deficiency-anemia caused by the bacterial iron consumption.

8.11.1 Mastic Is Anti-inflammatory

First and foremost for our purpose, mastic is anti-inflammatory. A study published in the *Nutrition Journal*, in 2010, reported that Chios mastic gum reduces reactive oxygen species (ROS), specifically, hydrogen peroxide (H_2O_2). This antioxidant property was said by the authors to explain its anti-inflammatory activity (Triantafyllou et al. 2010).

One explanation for the role of inflammation in the development of atherosclerosis is that typically, immune system cells (leukocytes) adhere to blood vessel endothelium, and from there migrate into the blood vessel wall where they become attached. Attachment requires a type of molecular glue termed "endothelial adhesion molecules."

A study published in the journal *Experimental Biology and Medicine*, in 2009, examined the effect of Chios mastic gum neutral extract and a phytosterol anti-inflammatory, tirucallol, on (a) the expression of adhesion, and (b) the attachment of monocytes (large white immune system cells) in human aortic endothelial cells (HAEC).

Both Chios mastic gum extract and tirucallol significantly inhibit adhesion and binding to HAEC. This study extends existing data regarding the cardio-protective effect of Chios mastic gum and its promotion of healthy endothelial function (Loizou et al. 2009). A study published in the *European Review for Medical and Pharmacological Science*, in 2010, reported that mastic (*P. lentiscus*) effectively treated skin inflammation in rats. The inflammation was caused by a laboratory irritant procedure (Mahmoudi et al. 2010) .

8.11.2 A Mediterranean Spice That Targets *H. pylori*

In 1984, three Iraqi physicians, Drs. J. Al-Habbal, A. Al-Habbal, and F. Huwez, attempted unsuccessfully to treat a 65-year-old woman for gastritis and duodenal ulcers with conventional anti-ulcer drugs. The patient was subsequently prescribed mastic by a local traditional healer and experienced rapid relief of her symptoms and healing of her ulcers.

The high reported incidence of active duodenal ulcers in the Arbil region of Iraq among patients with gastritis, and the failure of many of them to respond to currently used anti-ulcer therapy, as well as the side effects of those treatments, encouraged the physicians to conduct a conventional clinical trial of mastic and a comparison placebo, in patients with a proven duodenal ulcer. Neither the patients nor the investigators knew who in the trial was receiving the treatment and who was receiving an inert comparison placebo until the trial was over.

One group of patients received a daily dose of 1 g of mastic for 2 weeks, while the placebo group received a daily dose of 1 g of lactose.

The authors reported that 80% of the patients receiving the mastic experienced symptom relief, versus 50% on placebo. In addition, 70% of the patients on mastic experienced healing as proven by endoscopic examination (an endoscope is a tubular instrument with which one can examine internal organs). Only 22% of the patients receiving lactose saw any improvement.

The authors reported that mastic, composed of about 90% resins, 2% volatile oils, and a "bitter principle," was well tolerated by the patients and seemed to have no discernible adverse side effects (Al-Habbal et al. 1984). They made no attempt to explain how any of these constituents led to symptom relief and healing.

Then, in 1986, two of the authors followed the above research with case reports of mastic used for the treatment of gastric ulcers. Mastic powder was given for 4 weeks in doses of 1 g twice daily, with one dose before breakfast and the other at bedtime. Routine laboratory and endoscopic follow-up examinations were performed every 2 weeks. Complete symptomatic relief was found in all patients including one who had double gastric ulcers.

In their comments, the authors reported that the amount of mastic administered to the patients did not exceed the quantities commonly found in chewing gum, breath sweetener, or food flavorings. Treatment was again reported to be safe and no adverse side effects were noted (Huwez and Al-Habbal 1986).

One of the original investigators, Dr. Huwez, and his colleagues, then reported in 1998 in *The New England Journal of Medicine* in an article titled "Mastic gum kills *Helicobacter pylori*" that it can cure peptic ulcers very rapidly even at doses as low as 1 g per day for 2 weeks.

They continue:

These results suggest that mastic has definite antibacterial activity against *Helicobacter pylori*. This activity may at least partly explain the anti-peptic-ulcer properties of mastic. Examination of the anti-*H. pylori* effect of the various constituents of mastic, which have been recently identified, may pinpoint the active ingredient. Mastic is cheap and widely available in Third World countries; therefore, our data should have important implications for the management of peptic ulcers in developing countries. (Huwez et al. 1998:1946)

In 2001, the *Journal of Chemotherapy* confirmed earlier findings by Huwez and colleagues that mastic is bactericidal and targets *H. pylori* (also *Staphylococcus aureus* and even *Escherichia coli*) (Marone et al. 2001). And, in 2010, this was confirmed again in the journal *Phytomedicine*, with the authors concluding that "Mastic gum has bactericidal activity on *H. pylori* in vivo" (in vivo here means "in patients") (Dabos et al. 2001). However, some investigators reported that they could not verify the antimicrobial activity of mastic against *H. pylori* (Bebb et al. 2003).

Knowledge of the chemical constituents of mastic shed little light on its bactericidal action against *H. pylori* except for the flavonoids, catechin tannins, and polymeric proanthocyanidins (Sanz et al. 1992; Papageorgiou et al. 1997; Magiatis et al. 1995).

A detailed description of the chemical composition of the essential oils of mastic (*P. lentiscus* var. *chia*) appeared in the journal *Planta Medica* in 1999 (Magiatis et al. 1999). However, although it documents its bactericidal and fungicidal activity in connection with a number of pathogens such as the bacteria *Staphylococcus aureus* (ATCC 2593), *Staphylococcus epidermidis* (ATCC 12228), *Escherichia coli* (ATCC 25922), *Enterobacter cloacae* (ATCC 13047), *Klebsiella pneumoniae* (ATCC 13883), and *Pseudomonas aeruginosa* (ATCC 227853), and the fungi *Candida albicans*, *Candida tropicalis*, and *Torulopsis glabrata*, the report makes no mention of *H. pylori*.

8.11.3   MASTIC LOWERS OXIDATIVE STRESS

A report in the *Nutrition Journal*, in 2011, examined the molecular mechanisms of the anti-inflammatory activity of mastic. It was found that mastic reduced oxidative stress through inhibition of protein kinase C (PKC). PKC controls the function of proteins through its effects on amino acid residues of protein metabolism, thereby also affecting lipids. It is implicated in endothelium dysfunction, diabetes, and many more metabolic complications (Triantafyllou et al. 2011).

8.11.4   MASTIC TARGETS THE BACTERIA THAT CAUSE PERIODONTITIS

A study of the antibacterial effects of mastic chewing gum against *Streptococcus mutans*, among the usual suspects in the mouth, was published in the journal *Archives of Oral Biology*, in 2006. The authors concluded mastic gum had significant antibacterial activity against *S. mutans* and may be a useful adjunct in the prevention of caries (cavities) (Aksoy et al. 2006).

A clinical study of the "anti-plaque effects of mastic chewing gum in the oral cavity" was published in the *Journal of Periodontology* in 2003. The authors found that the total number of bacterial colonies was significantly reduced during 4 hours of chewing mastic gum compared to the comparison placebo gum. The mastic group showed a significantly reduced plaque and gingival index compared to the placebo group: "These results suggest that mastic chewing gum is a useful anti-plaque agent in reducing the bacterial growth in saliva and plaque formation on teeth." (Takahashi et al. 2003)

A number of mastic chewing gum products are available online. The authors cannot recommend any one product because they cannot evaluate the nature, purity, or safety of the constituents, nor the sanitary conditions of the manufacturing, packaging, and shipping methods. It stands to reason, however, that anyone who wishes to use such a product would choose sugar-free.

8.11.5 Mastic Protects the Heart

The triterpenic compounds of Chios mastic gum have been associated with cardio-vascular protection, mainly through increasing the antioxidant defense system and effectively lowering levels of serum cholesterol. In a study published in the journal *Experimental Biology and Medicine* in 2009, it was found that mastic inhibited human aortic endothelial cell (HAEC) adhesion. This study was said to extend understanding of the cardio-protective effect of Chios mastic gum, and expands knowledge of phytosterols with potent anti-atherosclerosis activity and the beneficial effects of mastic on endothelial function (Loizou et al. 2009).

8.11.6 Anemia: *H. pylori* Is an Iron Glutton

In 2013, an article published in the *World Journal of Gastroenterology* confirmed previous reports that in most cases of *H. pylori* infection, iron-refractory or iron-dependent anemia of unknown origin is due to the infection (Monzón et al. 2013).

Many authorities believe that iron-deficiency anemia in gastric disease derives from loss of blood. That may be the case with some bleeding ulcers, but the most common cause of anemia is the use by *H. pylori* bacteria of significant amounts of iron in the stomach, thus depriving red blood cells of the iron they need to form hemoglobin. Most nutrients are "sequestered" during digestion in the stomach so that the host gets preferential access to them. But *H. pylori* manage to get there first, as it were (Pich and Merrell 2013). However, red blood cells must be replaced regularly, and their number is determined by the availability of iron.

Mastic can be consumed in many forms: raw pearls can be chewed, there is mastic chewing gum (sugar free); it can be purchased in nutraceutical capsules available at most pharmacies and health foods stores, and it is an ingredient in many recipes.

8.11.6.1 Serum Ferritin

While a red blood cell count is the conventional way of assessing iron deficiency anemia, serum ferritin is a better marker of total body iron. Ferritin is an iron–protein complex which regulates iron storage and transport from the digestive system to plasma. In a study conducted in Denmark, and published in the journal *Gastroenterology* in 1998, serum ferritin, hemoglobin, and *H. pylori* antibodies were assessed in about 3000 adults. Serum ferritin levels were considerably lower in men who tested positive for *H. pylori*. The authors concluded that *H. pylori* infection interferes with iron metabolism (Milman et al. 1998).

Clearly, eradicating *H. pylori* may confer many health benefits. The question is, as always, is it invariably a good idea? Some authorities hold that it may not be beneficial in the non-infected or the non-symptomatic, and that *H. pylori* may serve an important symbiotic function in the stomach (Sachs and Scott 2012). The relationship with gastroesophageal reflux disease (GERD) is even more complex and controversial.

Mastic gum in capsule form is available at most pharmacies and health foods stores, and online.

8.12 ELDERBERRY (*SAMBUCUS NIGRA CANADENSIS*)

Sambucus is a genus of flowering plants of in the family Adoxaceae. The various species are commonly called elder or elderberry. The fruits of common elderberry are a kind of berry called a drupe. Only the blue or purple fruits of elderberry are edible. The active alkaloids in elderberry plants are hydrocyanic acid and sambucine: both will cause nausea, so care should be observed with this plant. The red berries of other species are toxic and should not be consumed.

Elderberries are very rich in vitamin C, vitamin A, vitamin B complex, and the minerals calcium, copper, iron, potassium, phosphorus, and magnesium. Just 1 cup of elderberries is high in fiber and antioxidant bioflavonoids including quercitin, rutin, and anthocyanins, energy producing carbohydrates, amino acids, and protein. They have no cholesterol and are very low in fat and calories.

At the Bundesforschungsanstalt (Federal Research Center) for food in Karlsruhe, Germany, scientists conducting studies on elderberry showed that elderberry anthocyanins enhance immune function by boosting the production of cytokines. These unique proteins act as messengers in the immune system to help regulate immune response, thus helping to defend the body against disease. Further research indicated that anthocyanins found in elderberries possess appreciably more antioxidant capacity than either vitamin E or vitamin C.

Studies at the University of Graz in Austria found that elderberry extract reduces oxidation of low-density lipoprotein (LDL) cholesterol, thus preventing atherosclerosis and eventually, cardiovascular and heart disease (Murkovic et al. 2004).

A Cautionary Note: Most species of *Sambucus* berries are edible when picked ripe and then cooked, and both the skin and pulp can be eaten. However, most uncooked berries and other parts of plants from this genus are poisonous. *S. nigra* is the variety of elderberry that is most often used for health benefits as it is the only variety considered to be non-toxic even when not cooked; nevertheless, it is still recommended that the berries be cooked at least a little to enhance their taste and digestibility.

8.12.1 ELDERBERRY IS ANTIOXIDANT AND REDUCES INFLAMMATION AND OXIDATIVE STRESS

The objective of a study published in the journal *Food & Function*, in 2015, was to determine whether an anthocyanin-rich black elderberry extract (*S. nigra*) containing 13% anthocyanins would protect against inflammation-related impairments in HDL function and atherosclerosis in a mouse model of hyperlipidemia and HDL dysfunction. Mice were fed a diet supplemented with 1.25% (w/w) black elderberry extract or a comparison control diet for 6 weeks. The black elderberry extract was rich in cyanidin 3-sambubioside (~9.8% w/w) and cyanidin 3-glucoside (~3.8% w/w).

After 6 weeks, serum lipids did not differ significantly between groups, while fasting glucose was reduced in black elderberry extract-fed mice. Hepatic and intestinal mRNA changes in mice fed black elderberry extract were consistent with an improvement in HDL function and a reduction in hepatic cholesterol levels. Notably, there were significant reductions in total cholesterol content of the aorta in mice fed black elderberry extract, indicating less atherosclerosis progression. This study suggests that black elderberry may have the potential to influence HDL dysfunction associated with chronic inflammation (Farrell et al. 2015).

The objective of a study published in the journal *Free Radical Biology & Medicine*, in 2000, was to determine whether endothelial cells could incorporate anthocyanins, and to examine the potential benefits of anthocyanins in protection from various oxidative stressors. Elderberry extract contains four anthocyanins, and they were incorporated into the plasma membrane and plasma of endothelial cells for 4 hours of standard incubation.

The enrichment of endothelial cells with elderberry anthocyanins conferred significant protective effects against hydrogen peroxide. These results show for the first time that vascular endothelial cells can incorporate anthocyanins into their membrane and cytoplasm, conferring significant protective effects against oxidative stress. These findings may have important implications for preserving endothelial cell function and preventing the initiation of changes, such as atherosclerosis, associated with vascular disease.

8.12.2 ACUTE INFLAMMATION VERSUS CHRONIC INFLAMMATION

As previously noted, all forms of inflammation leave an indelible mark. The damage that oxidative stress causes our cells even by immune defense that successfully eradicated an infection may result in shorter telomeres. Until now, the antioxidant characteristics of functional foods were examined in the presence of chronic inflammation. *Sambucus* may actually be helpful in some forms of acute inflammation.

A study published in the journal *BMC Complementary and Alternative Medicine*, in 2011, reported for the first time that a standardized elderberry liquid extract possesses antimicrobial activity against both the Gram-positive bacteria *Streptococcus pyogenes* and group C and G *Streptococci*, and the Gram-negative bacterium *Branhamella catarrhalis* in liquid cultures. The liquid extract also displays an inhibitory effect on the propagation of human pathogenic influenza viruses (Krawitz et al. 2011).

Sambucus nigra L. products based on a standardized black elderberry extract are natural remedies available to the consumer that have antiviral properties, especially against different strains of influenza virus. As reported in the journal *European Cytokine Network* in 2001, one such product, Sambucol, was shown to be effective in vitro against 10 strains of influenza virus. Sambucol was developed at the Immunology Laboratory for Tumor Diagnosis, Department of Oncology, Hadassah University Hospital, Jerusalem, Israel, and is available without prescription at www.sambucolusa.com.

In one clinical study, Sambucol is reported to have reduced the duration of flu symptoms to 3–4 days. Convalescent phase serum showed a higher level of antibodies to influenza virus in a Sambucol group than in the comparison group. A follow-up study aimed to assess the effectiveness of Sambucol products on the healthy immune system, namely, its effect on cytokine production.

The production of inflammatory cytokines was tested using monocytes from 12 healthy participants. Adherent monocytes were separated from lymphocytes and incubated with different product preparations. The production of inflammatory cytokines was significantly increased, mostly by the Sambucol black elderberry extract as compared to a known monocyte activator.

The authors concluded that in addition to its antiviral properties, the elderberry extract and its formulations activate the healthy immune system by increasing inflammatory cytokine production. Therefore, it promotes immune system activation during the inflammatory process in healthy individuals or in patients with various diseases.

Previous sections showed functional foods sometimes in the form of spice or berries or their extracts. However, in a sense, the Proactive Nutrition Program is, in fact, functional foods due to the antioxidant-rich constituents.

8.13 TURMERIC

Turmeric (*Curcuma longa*) is a rhizomatous herbaceous perennial plant of the ginger family, Zingiberaceae. A spice that comes from the turmeric plant contains curcumin commonly used in Asian food. Turmeric is the main spice in curry. It has a warm, bitter taste and is frequently used to flavor or color curry powders, mustards, butters, and cheeses.

8.13.1 CURCUMIN IS ANTIOXIDANT AND ANTI-INFLAMMATORY

According to a report published in the journal *Advances in Experimental Medicine and Biology*, in 2007, the anti-inflammatory effect of curcumin (diferuloylmethane) is probably due to its ability to inhibit important enzymes that mediate inflammatory processes (Menon and Sudheer 2007).

There are a considerable number of experimental studies on the effects of curcumin on inflammatory conditions, including oxidative stress, atherosclerosis, diabetes, and more. For the most part, these studies show encouraging positive outcomes of curcumin treatment. However, due to the nature of the experimental procedures, they are almost invariably performed on animal models. The beneficial effects of curcumin are, therefore, extrapolated from those studies.

A study published in the *Medical Science Monitor,* in 2007, aimed to determine the protective effect of curcumin against oxidative stress in chemically stressed rats. Diabetes was induced in the rats who were then fed either only the AIN-93 (standard rodent formulation) diet or the AIN-93 diet containing 0.002%, 0.01%, or 0.5% curcumin for 8 weeks. The levels of oxidative stress and antioxidant enzymes were then determined in various tissues.

Hyperglycemia resulted in increased lipid peroxidation and protein components in red blood cells and other tissues and altered antioxidant enzyme activities. Curcumin controlled oxidative stress in the diabetic rats by inhibiting the increase in TBARS (see Chapter 3 on antioxidants) and protein components and reversing altered antioxidant enzyme activities without altering the hyperglycemic state in most of the tissues. The authors concluded that curcumin appears to be beneficial in preventing diabetes-induced oxidative stress in rats despite unaltered diabetic (hyperglycemic) status (Suryanarayana et al. 2007).

According to a report in the journal *Trends in Pharmacological Sciences*, appearing in 2009, curcumin mediates its anti-inflammatory effects through the downregulation of inflammatory transcription factors (such as nuclear factor kappaB), enzymes (such as cyclooxygenase 2 and 5 lipoxygenase), and cytokines (such as tumor necrosis factor, interleukin 1, and interleukin 6) (Aggarwal and Sung 2009).

A study on human volunteers, published in the *Indian Journal of Physiology and Pharmacology*, in 1992, aimed to assess effects of curcumin administration on the serum levels of cholesterol and lipid peroxides in healthy volunteers given 500 mg of curcumin per day for 7 days. A significant decrease (33%) in the serum lipid peroxides, an increase in HDL cholesterol (29%), and a decrease in total serum cholesterol (11.63%) were noted (Soni and Kuttan 1992).

8.13.2 Is it Safe to Consume Curcumin

A study on the dosage safety of curcumin was reported in the journal *BMC Complementary and Alternative Medicine*, in 2006. It detailed a dose-escalation study to determine the maximum tolerable dose and safety of a single oral dose of curcumin in healthy volunteers. Subjects were given increasing doses of curcumin ranging from 500 to 12,000 mg, and safety was assessed for 72 hours after administration. Of the participants who completed the trial, seven experienced minimal toxicity that did not appear to be dose-related including diarrhea, headache, rash, and yellow stool (Lao et al. 2006).

In another study with human participants, curcumin at doses ranging from 0.45 to 3.6 g/day for 1–4 months was associated with nausea and diarrhea and caused an increase in serum alkaline phosphatase and lactate dehydrogenase (Sharma et al. 2004).

However, in one study patients with advanced pancreatic cancer receiving curcumin (8 g/day) in combination with gemcitabine reported intractable abdominal pain after a few days to 2 weeks of curcumin intake. Thus, more studies are required to evaluate the long-term toxicity associated with curcumin before it can be recommended for human use (Epelbaum et al. 2010).

8.14 SUPPLEMENTS

Functional foods are foods, whereas supplements are not foods. Here is a small number of supplements that can play a major role in combating both acute and chronic inflammation. The citation here is limited to the assertion that the supplement is effective against acute or chronic inflammation that may abbreviate telomeres.

8.14.1 Zinc Is Antioxidant, Anti-inflammatory, and Protects Telomeres

Zinc is an essential micronutrient required for many cellular processes, especially for the normal development and functioning of the immune system. Zinc deficiency causes significant impairment in both adaptive and innate immune responses, and promotes systemic inflammation. National surveys indicate that a significant number of the elderly population has inadequate zinc intake, and a decline in zinc status is observed with age.

Both zinc deficiency and the aging process are characterized by impaired immune responses and systemic low grade chronic inflammation. It has been suggested that age-related zinc deficiency may be an important contributor to chronic inflammation during the aging process.

A review appearing in the journal *Molecular Nutrition & Food Research* in 2012 emphasizes the effects of zinc status on aging, and particularly the role of zinc deficiency in age-related immune dysfunction and chronic inflammation (Wong and Ho 2012).

The following additional references also support the role of zinc as an antioxidant and anti-inflammatory which protects telomeres (Cipriano et al. 2009; Prasad 2014; Vasto et al. 2006).

8.14.2 Magnesium Is Anti-inflammatory and Protects Telomeres

A review appearing in the journal *BioMedicine* (Taipei) in 2016 details the relationship between magnesium (Mg) deficiency and oxidative stress. Magnesium deficiency is associated with higher levels of oxidative stress markers including lipid, protein, and DNA oxidative modification products (noted earlier), and weakened antioxidant defense. These may account for systemic reactions such as inflammation and endothelial dysfunction, as well as changes at the cellular level, such as mitochondrial dysfunction and excessive fatty acid production (Zheltova et al. 2016).

The following additional references also support the role of magnesium as an antioxidant and anti-inflammatory which protects telomeres (Dibaba et al. 2014; Killilea and Maier 2008; Shah et al. 2014).

8.14.3 Niacin Reduces Oxidative Stress

A clinical study published in the journal *Arteriosclerosis, Thrombosis and Vascular Biology* in 2010 aimed to determine whether niacin could inhibit vascular inflammation and improve endothelial function independent of changes in plasma lipid and lipoprotein levels.

New Zealand white rabbits received normal chow or chow supplemented with 0.6% or 1.2% (wt/wt) niacin. This regimen had no effect on plasma cholesterol, triglyceride, or high-density lipoprotein levels. Acute vascular inflammation and endothelial dysfunction were then induced in the animals with carotid artery constriction.

The endothelial expression of vascular cell adhesion molecules and intercellular adhesion molecules was markedly decreased in the niacin-supplemented animals compared with controls 24 hours after constriction. Niacin also enhanced endothelial-dependent vasorelaxation and cGMP production, and increased vascular reduced glutathione content.

The authors concluded that niacin inhibits vascular inflammation and protects against endothelial dysfunction, independent of changes in plasma lipid levels (Wu et al. 2010).

Note: Statins lower cholesterol, but the results of this study underscore the danger of lipid peroxidation, not serum levels. Protecting endothelium function seems to rest more on reducing ROS than on reducing serum levels. Thus, research suggests that antioxidants may prove to be more helpful than statins in averting atherosclerosis and its sequelae (see also the study cited below).

Based on a study on the effects of niacin on cultured human aortic endothelial cells (HAEC), published in the journal *Atherosclerosis* in 2008, the authors concluded that niacin reduces vascular inflammation by decreasing endothelial ROS production and subsequent LDL oxidation and inflammatory cytokine production. These are major factors in atherogenesis. Their initial data support the novel concept that niacin has vascular anti-inflammatory and potentially anti-atherosclerotic properties independent of its effects on lipid regulation (Ganji et al. 2008; see also Canner et al. 1986; Guyton 1998; Matuoka et al. 2001; Surjana et al. 2010).

8.15 TAURINE

Taurine is antioxidant and anti-inflammatory, and protects muscles, eyes, and nerves. It is a sulfur-containing amino acid widely distributed in tissues. It is a major constituent of bile and therefore important in the metabolism of fats. One of the most abundant amino acids in the brain, retina, muscle tissue, and organs throughout the body, it is however one of the few amino acids not incorporated into proteins (Ripps and Shen 2012).

8.15.1 TAURINE HELPS MAINTAIN MUSCLES IN AGING

Aging generally entails chronic low-grade inflammation, increased oxidative stress, and reduced regenerative capacity. Therefore, it leads also to alterations in the form and function of skeletal muscle, thus promoting sarcopenia. This condition is characterized by an age-related gradual loss of muscle mass and function due to insufficiency protein synthesis and degradation. Changes in the quantity and the quality of dietary proteins, as well as the intake of specific amino acids, can counteract some of the adverse processes that can lead to sarcopenia.

A review appearing in the journal *Current Protein & Peptide Science* in 2016 summarized the effects of taurine on specific muscle targets and emphasized its role in regulating the maintenance of muscle homeostasis. The review further proposed the potential use of taurine as a therapeutic molecule for the amelioration of skeletal muscle function and performance severely compromised during aging (Scicchitano and Sica 2016).

While taurine regulates oxidative stress, it is neither a classical free radical scavenger nor a regulator of the antioxidative defenses. Consequently, its antioxidant mechanism is not known.

In a study published in the journal *Amino Acids* in 2012, a taurine antagonist and taurine transport inhibitor was used to examine the mechanism underlying antioxidant activity. Isolated heart muscle cells were exposed to medium containing beta-alanine for a period of 48 hours. This led to a 45% decrease in taurine content and an increase in mitochondrial oxidative stress, as shown by enhanced superoxide generation and the oxidation of glutathione.

Co-administration of taurine with beta-alanine largely prevents the mitochondrial effects of beta-alanine. Thus, taurine serves as a regulator of mitochondrial protein formation, thereby protecting the mitochondria from excessive superoxide generation (Jong et al. 2012).

8.15.2 TAURINE HAS BENEFICIAL EFFECTS IN TYPE 1 AND TYPE 2 DIABETES

The unifying hypothesis of diabetes holds that reactive oxygen species (ROS) generated in the mitochondria of glucose-treated cells promote reactions leading to the development of diabetic complications. Although this hypothesis attributes the generation of oxidants solely to impaired glucose and fatty acid metabolism, diabetes is also associated with a decline in the availability of the endogenous antioxidant taurine. This points to the possibility that changes in taurine status might also contribute to the severity of oxidant-mediated damage. Although taurine is incapable of directly scavenging the classic ROS, such as superoxide anion, hydroxyl radical, and hydrogen peroxide, there are numerous studies suggesting that it is an effective inhibitor of ROS generation (Ito et al. 2012; Schaffer et al. 2009; Sirdah 2015; See also: El Idrissi et al. 2009).

8.16 FINAL NOTE

We described selected important functional foods and supplements here and supported their anti-inflammatory and antioxidant benefits with scientific data. The selection is by no means comprehensive but is intended to give an overview of how such dietary constituents are scientifically validated.

Most sources of information about such matters of necessity omit the validation studies, thus leaving them open to the accusation either that they are an "expert opinion," or that the data are equivocal. This is an unfortunate disservice to the consumer public—one that we went to some effort to correct here.

REFERENCES

Aggarwal, B. B., and B. Sung. 2009. Pharmacological basis for the role of curcumin in chronic diseases: An age-old spice with modern targets. *Trends in Pharmacological Sciences*, 30(2):85–94.

Aksoy, A., N. Duran, and F. Koksal. 2006. In vitro and in vivo antimicrobial effects of mastic chewing gum against Streptococcus mutans and mutans streptococci. *Archives of Oral Biology*, 51(6):476–481.

Al-Fawaeir, A., and M. B. Abu Zaid. 2013. Serum levels of high-sensitivity C-reactive protein (hs-CRP) in Helicobacter pylori infected patients. *Journal of Investigational Biochemistry*, 2(1):32–36.

Al-Habbal, M. J., Z. Al-Habbal, and F. U. Huwez. 1984. A double-blind controlled clinical trial of mastic and placebo in the treatment of duodenal ulcer. *Clinical & Experimental Pharmacology & Physiology*, 11:541–544.

Allen, R. W., E. Schwartzman, W. I. Baker, et al. 2013. Cinnamon use in type 2 diabetes: An updated systematic review and meta-analysis. *Annals of Family Medicine*, 11(5):452–459.

Anderson, R. A., and M. M. Polansky. 2002. Tea enhances insulin activity. *Journal of Agricultural & Food Chemistry*, 50(24):7182–7186.

Aulinas, A., M.-R. Ramírez, M.-R. Barahona, et al. 2015. Dyslipidemia and chronic inflammation markers are correlated with telomere length shortening in Cushing's syndrome. *PLoS One*, 10(3):e0120185.

Bansal, T., A. Pandey, D. Deepa, et al. 2014. C-reactive protein (CRP) and its association with periodontal disease: A brief review. *Journal of Clinical & Diagnostic Research*, 8(7):ZE21–ZE24.

Bebb, J. R., N. Bailey-Flitter, D. Ala'Aldeen, et al. 2003. Mastic gum has no effect on Helicobacter pylori load in vivo. *Journal of Antimicrobial Chemotherapy*, 52(3):522–523.

Bode, A. M., and Z. Dong. 2011. The amazing and mighty ginger, Chapter 7. In Benzie, I. F. F., and S. Wachtel-Galor, editors. *Herbal Medicine: Biomolecular and Clinical Aspects*. 2nd edition. Boca Raton,FL: CRC Press/Taylor & Francis.

Canner, P. L., K. G. Berge, N. K. Wenger et al. 1986. Fifteen year mortality in Coronary Drug Project patients: Long-term benefit with niacin. *Journal of the American College of Cardiology*, 8(6):1245–1255.

Castellon, X., and V. Bogdanova. 2016. Chronic inflammatory diseases and endothelial dysfunction. *Aging & Disease*, 7(1):81–89.

Charrier, M. J., G. P. Savage, and L. Vanhanen. 2002. Oxalate content and calcium binding capacity of tea and herbal teas. *Asia Pacific Journal of Clinical Nutrition*, 11(4):298–301.

Chow, H. H., Y. Cai, I. A. Hakim, et al. 2003. Pharmacokinetics and safety of green tea polyphenols after multiple-dose administration of epigallocatechin gallate and polyphenon E in healthy individuals. *Clinical Cancer Research*, 9(9):3312–3319.

Cipriano, C., S. Tesei, M. Malavolta et al. 2009. Accumulation of cells with short telomeres is associated with impaired zinc homeostasis and inflammation in old hypertensive participants. *Journal of Gerontology. Series A, Biological Science & Medical Science*, 64(7):745–751.

Dabos, K. J., E. Sfika, L. J. Vlatta, et al. 2001. The effect of mastic gum on Helicobacter pylori: A randomized pilot study. *Phytomedicine*, 17(3–4):296–299.

Daood, H. G., M. Vinkler, F. Markus, et al. 1996. Antioxidant vitamin content of spice red pepper (paprika) as affected by technological and varietal factors. *Food Chemistry*, 55(4):365–372.

Davis, P. A., and W. Yokoyama. 2011. Cinnamon intake lowers fasting blood glucose: Meta-analysis. *Journal of Medical Foods*, 14(9):884–889.

del Rocío Gómez-García, M., and N. Ochoa-Alejo. 2013. Biochemistry and molecular biology of carotenoid biosynthesis in chili peppers (*Capsicum* spp.). *International Journal of Molecular Sciences*, 14(9):19025–19053.

Devaraj, S., U. Singh, and I. Jialal. 2009. Human C-reactive protein and the metabolic syndrome. *Current Opinion in Lipidology*, 20(3):182–189.

Dibaba, D. T., P. Xun, and K. He. 2014. Dietary magnesium intake is inversely associated with serum C-reactive protein levels: Meta-analysis and systematic review. *European Journal of Clinical Nutrition*, 68(4):510–516.

Dudonne, S., X. Vitrac, P. Vouitiere, et al. 2009. Comparative study of antioxidant properties and total phenolic content of 30 plant extracts of industrial interest using DPPH, ABTS, FRAP, SOD, and ORAC assays. *Journal of Agricultural & Food Chemistry*, 57:1768–1774.

El Idrissi A., L. Boukarrou, K. Splavnyk, et al. 2009. Functional implication of taurine in aging. *Advances in Experimental Medicine & Biology*, 643:199–206.

Epelbaum, R., M. Schaffer, B. Vizel, et al. 2010. Curcumin and gemcitabine in patients with advanced pancreatic cancer. *Nutrition & Cancer*, 62(8):1137–1141.

Farrell, N., G. Norris, S. S. Lee, et al. 2015. Anthocyanin-rich black elderberry extract improves markers of HDL function and reduces aortic cholesterol in hyperlipidemic mice. *Food & Function*, 6(4):1278–1287.

Festa, A., R. D'Agostino, G. Howard, et al. 2000. Chronic subclinical inflammation as part of the insulin resistance syndrome. The Insulin Resistance Atherosclerosis Study (IRAS). *Circulation*, 102(1):42-47. doi: http://dx.doi.org/10.1161/01.

Franceschi, C. 2007. Inflammaging as a major characteristic of old people: Can it be prevented or cured? *Nutrition Reviews*, 65(12 Pt 2):S173–S176.

Franceschi, C., M. Bonafè, S. Valensin, et al. 2000. Inflamm-aging. An evolutionary perspective on immunosenescence. *Annals of the New York Academy of Sciences*, 908:244–254.

Gan, W. Q., S. F. P. Man, A. Senthilselvan, et al. 2004. Association between chronic obstructive pulmonary disease and systemic inflammation: A systematic review and a meta-analysis. *Thorax*, 59:574–580.

Ganji, S. H., S. Qin, L. Zhang, et al. 2008. Niacin inhibits vascular oxidative stress, redox-sensitive genes, and monocyte adhesion to human aortic endothelial cells. *Atherosclerosis*, 202(1):68–75.

Grzanna, R., L. Lindmark, and C. G. Frondoza. 2005. Ginger—An herbal medicinal product with broad anti-inflammatory actions. *Journal of Medicinal Foods*, 8(2):125–132.

Guarner, V., and M. E. Rubio-Ruiz. 2015. Low-grade systemic inflammation connects aging, metabolic syndrome and cardiovascular disease. *Interdisciplinary Topics in Gerontology*, 40:99–106.

Gunawardena, D., N. Karunaweera, S. Lee, et al. 2015. Anti-inflammatory activity of cinnamon (C. zeylanicum and C. cassia) extracts—Identification of E-cinnamaldehyde and o-methoxy cinnamaldehyde as the most potent bioactive compounds. *Food & Function*, 6(3):910–919.

Guyton, J. R. 1998. Effect of niacin on atherosclerotic cardiovascular disease. *American Journal of Cardiology*, 82(12A):18U–23U; discussion 39U-41U.

Haniadka, R., E. Saldanha, V. Sunita, et al. 2013. A review of the gastroprotective effects of ginger (Zingiber officinale Roscoe). *Food & Function*, 4(6):845–855.

Harman, D. 1992. Free radical theory of aging. *Mutation Research*, 275(3–6):257–266.

Hininger-Favier, I., R. Benaraba, S. Coves, et al. 2009. Green tea extract decreases oxidative stress and improves insulin sensitivity in an animal model of insulin resistance, the fructose-fed rat. *Journal of the American College of Nutrition*, 28(4):355–561.

Huwez, F. U., and M. J. Al-Habbal. 1986. Mastic in treatment of benign gastric ulcer. *Gastroenterologica Japonica*, 21:273–274.

Huwez, F. U., D. Thirlwell, A. Cockayne, et al. 1998. Mastic gum kills *Helicobacter pylori*. *The New England Journal of Medicine*, 339(26):1946.

Institute of Medicine, Food and Nutrition Board 2001. *Dietary Reference Intakes: Vitamin A, Vitamin K, Arsenic, Boron, Chromium, Copper, Iodine, Iron, Manganese, Molybdenum, Nickel, Silicon, Vanadium, and Zinc.* Washington, DC: National Academy Press.

Ito, T., S. W. Schaffer, and J. Azuma. 2012. The potential usefulness of taurine on diabetes mellitus and its complications. *Amino Acids*, 42(5):1529–1539.

Jayaprakasha, G. K., and L. J. Rao. 2011. Chemistry, biogenesis, and biological activities of Cinnamomum zeylanicum. *Critical Review in Food Science & Nutrition*, 51(6):547–562.

Jong, C. J, J. Azuma, and S. Schaffer. 2012. Mechanism underlying the antioxidant activity of taurine: Prevention of mitochondrial oxidant production. *Amino Acids*, 42(6):2223–2232.

Jurk, D., C. Wilson, J. F. Passos, et al. 2014. Chronic inflammation induces telomere dysfunction and accelerates ageing in mice. *Nature Communications*, 2:4172.

Kawatra, P., and R. Rajagopalan. 2015. Cinnamon: Mystic powers of a minute ingredient. *Pharmacognosy Research*, 7(Suppl 1):S1–S6.

Khandouzi, N., F. Shidfar, A. Rajab, et al. 2015. The effects of ginger on fasting blood sugar, hemoglobin A1c, apolipoprotein B, apolipoprotein a-I and malondialdehyde in type 2 diabetic patients. *Iranian Journal of Pharmaceutical Research*, 14(1):131–140.

Killilea, D. W., and J. A. M. Maier. 2008. A connection between magnesium deficiency and aging: New insights from cellular studies. *Magnesium Research*, 21(2):77–82.

Kleefstra, N., S. J. Logtenberg, S. T. Houweling, et al. 2007. Cinnamon: Not suitable for the treatment of diabetes mellitus. [Article in Dutch] *Nederlands Tijdschrift voor Geneeskunde*, (51):–2837.

Krawitz, C., M. Abu Mraheil, M. Stein, et al. 2011. Inhibitory activity of a standardized elderberry liquid extract against clinically-relevant human respiratory bacterial pathogens and influenza A and B viruses. *BMC Complementary & Alternative Medicine*, 11:16.

Kuniyasu, H., Y. Kitadai, H. Mieno, et al. 2003. Helicobactor pylori infection is closely associated with telomere reduction in gastric mucosa. *Oncology*, 65:275–282.

Lake, B. G. 1999. Coumarin metabolism, toxicity and carcinogenicity: Relevance for human risk assessment. *Food & Chemical Toxicology*, 37(4):423–453.

Langley-Evans, S. C. 2000. Antioxidant potential of green and black tea determined using the ferric reducing power (FRAP) assay. *International Journal of Food Science & Nutrition*, 51(3):181–188.

Lao, C. D., M. T. Ruffin, D. Normolle, et al. 2006. Dose escalation of a curcuminoid formulation. *BMC Complementary & Alternative Medicine*, 6:10. doi:10.1186/1472-6882-6-10

Li, M., and C. G. Eastman. 2012. The changing epidemiology of iodine deficiency. *Nature Reviews Endocrinology*, 8(7):434–440. doi: 10.1038/nrendo .2012.43

Lin, Y. S., Y. J. Tsai, J. S. Tsay, et al. 2003. Factors affecting the levels of tea polyphenols and caffeine in tea leaves. *Journal of Agricultural & Food Chemistry*, 51(7):1864–1873.

Liu, K., R. Zhou, B. Wang, et al. 2013. Effect of green tea on glucose control and insulin sensitivity: A meta-analysis of 17 randomized controlled trials. *American Journal of Clinical Nutrition*, 98(2):340–348.

Loizou, S., S. Paraschos, S. Mitakou, et al. 2009. Chios mastic gum extract and isolated phytosterol tirucallol exhibit anti-inflammatory activity in human aortic endothelial cells. *Experimental Biology & Medicine (Maywood)*, 234(5):553–561.

Lorenz, M., J. Urban, U. Engelhardt, et al. 2009. Green and black tea are equally potent stimuli of NO production and vasodilation: New insights into tea ingredients involved. *Basic Research in Cardiology*, 104(1):100–110.

Magiatis, P., E. Melliou, A.-L. Skaltsounis, et al. 1999. Chemical composition and antimicrobial activity of the essential oils of *lentiscus* var. chia. *Planta Medica*, 65:749–752.

Mahluji, S., A. Ostadrahimi, M. Mobasseri, et al. 2013. Anti-inflammatory effects of zingiber officinale in type 2 diabetic patients. *Advanced Pharmaceutical Bulletin*, 3(2):273–276.

Mahmoudi, M., M. A. Ebrahimzadeh, S. F. Nabavi, et al. 2010. Anti-inflammatory and antioxidant activities of gum mastic. *European Review for Medical & Pharmacological Science*, 14(9):765–769.

Mantyh, P. W. 2002. Neurobiology of substance P and the NK1 receptor. *The Journal of Clinical Psychiatry*, 63 Suppl 11:6–10.

Markel, H. 1987. "When it rains it pours": Endemic goiter, iodized salt, and David Murray Cowie, MD. *American Journal of Public Health*, 77(2):219–229.

Marone, P., L. Bobo, E. Leone, et al. 2001. Bactericidal activity of mastic gum against *Helicobacter pylori*. *Journal of Chemotherapy*, 13(6):611–614.

Masi, S., K. D. Salpea, K.-W, Li, et al. 2011. Oxidative stress, chronic inflammation, and telomere length in patients with periodontitis. *Free Radical Biology and Medicine*, 50(6):730–735.

Mathew, S., and E. Abraham. 2006. Studies on the antioxidant activities of cinnamon (Cinnamomum verum) bark extracts, through various in vitro models. *Food Chemistry*, 94(4):520–528.

Matuoka, K., K. Y. Chen, and T. Takenawa. 2001. Rapid reversion of aging phenotypes by nicotinamide through possible modulation of histone acetylation. *Cellular & Molecular Life Science*, 58(14):2108–2116.

McDermott, M. T., and E. C. Ridgway. 2011. Subclinical hypothyroidism is mild thyroid failure and should be treated. *The Journal of Clinical Endocrinology & Metabolism*, 86(10):4585–4590.

Menon, V. P., and A. R. Sudheer. 2007. Antioxidant and anti-inflammatory properties of curcumin. *Advances in Experimental Medicine & Biology*, 595:105–125.

Mikutis, G., H. Karaköse, R. Jaiswal, et al. 2013a. Green tea catechins and cardiovascular health: An update. *Current Medicinal Chemistry*, 15(18):1840–1850.

Mikutis, G., H. Karaköse, R. Jaiswal, et al. 2013b. Phenolic promiscuity in the cell nucleus— Epigallocatechingallate (EGCG) and theaflavin-3,3'-digallate from green and black tea bind to model cell nuclear structures including histone proteins, double stranded DNA and telomeric quadruplex DNA. *Food & Function*, 4(2):328–337.

Miller, A. H., V. Maletic, and C. L. Raison. 2009. Inflammation and its discontents: The role of cytokines in the pathophysiology of major depression. *Biological Psychiatry*, 65(9):732–741.

Milman, N., S. Rosenstock, L. Andersen, et al. 1998. Serum ferritin, hemoglobin, and Helicobacter pylori infection: A seroepidemiologic survey comprising 2794 Danish adults. *Gastroenterology*, 115:749–774.

Minghetti. P., S. Sosa, F. Cilurzo, et al. 2007. Evaluation of the topical anti-inflammatory activity of ginger dry extracts from solutions and plasters. *Planta Medica*, 73(15):1525–1530.

Monzón, H., M. Forné, M. Esteve, et al. 2013. Helicobacter pylori infection as a cause of iron deficiency anaemia of unknown origin. *World Journal of Gastroenterology*, 19(26):4166–4171.

Mozaffari-Khosravi, H., B. Talaei, B. A. Jalali, et al. 2014. The effect of ginger powder supplementation on insulin resistance and glycemic indices in patients with type 2 diabetes: A randomized, double-blind, placebo-controlled trial. *Complementary Therapies in Medicine*, 22(1):9–16.

Murkovic, M., P. M. Abuja, A. R. Bergmann, et al. 2004. Effects of elderberry juice on fasting and postprandial serum lipids and low-density lipoprotein oxidation in healthy volunteers: A randomized, double-blind, placebo-controlled study. *European Journal of Clinical Nutrition*, 58:244–249.

Naderi, Z., H. Mozaffari-Khosravi, A. Dehghan, et al. 2015. Effect of ginger powder supplementation on nitric oxide and C-reactive protein in elderly knee osteoarthritis patients: A 12-week double-blind randomized placebo-controlled clinical trial. *Journal of Traditional and Complementary Medicine*, 6(3):199–203. doi:10.1016/j. jtcme.2014.12.007

No authors listed. 2007. Final report on the safety assessment of capsicum annuum extract, capsicum annuum fruit extract, capsicum annuum resin, capsicum annuum fruit powder, capsicum frutescens fruit, capsicum frutescens fruit extract, capsicum frutescens resin, and capsaicin. *International Journal of Toxicology*, 26 Suppl 1:3–106.

No authors listed. 2011. Cut salt—It won't affect your iodine intake. Iodized salt provided only a small fraction of daily iodine intake. *The Harvard Health Letter*, 21(10):1.

O'Donovan, O., M. S. Pantell, E. Puterman, et al. 2011. Cumulative inflammatory load is associated with short leukocyte telomere length in the health, aging and body composition study. *PLoS One*, 6(5):e19687. http://dx.doi.org/10.1371/ journal.pone.0019687.

Papageorgiou, V. P., M. N. Bakola-Christianopoulou, K. K. Apazidou, et al. 1997. Gas chromatographic-mass spectroscopic analysis of the acidic triterpenic fraction of mastic gum. *Journal of Chromatography A*, 769:263–273.

Park, M., J. Bae, and D. S. Lee. 2008. Antibacterial activity of [10]-gingerol and [12]-gingerol isolated from ginger rhizome against periodontal bacteria. *Research*, 22(11):1446–1449.

Pham, A. Q., H. Kourlas, D. Q. Pham. 2007. Cinnamon supplementation in patients with type 2 diabetes mellitus. *Pharmacotherapy*, 27(4):595–599.

Pich, O. Q., and D. S. Merrell. 2013. Iron sources in the stomach, iron utilization mechanisms of H. pylori & association of H. pylori infection with iron-deficient anemia. *Future Microbiology*, 8(6):725–738.

Portnoi, G., L. A. Chng, L. Karimi-Tabesh, et al. 2003a. Prospective comparative study of the safety and effectiveness of ginger for the treatment of nausea and vomiting in pregnancy. *American Journal of Obstetrics & Gynecology*, 189(5):1374–1377.

Portnoi, G., L. A. Chng, L. Karimi-Tabesh, et al. 2003b. Cytotoxic components from the dried rhizomes of Zingiber officinale Roscoe. *Archives of Pharmacal Research*, 31(4):415–418.

Prasad, A. S. 2014. Zinc is an antioxidant and anti-inflammatory agent: Its role in human health. *Frontiers in Nutrition*, 1:14.

Ranasinghe, P., S. Pigera, G. A. S. Premakumara, et al. 2013. Medicinal properties of: A systematic review. *BMC Complementary & Alternative Medicine*, 13:275.

Ridker, P. M. 2003. Clinical application of C-reactive protein for cardiovascular disease detection and prevention. *Circulation*, 107(3):363–369. http://dx.doi.org/10.1161/01.CIR.0000053730.47739.3C.

Ripps, H., and W, Shen. 2012. Review: Taurine: A "very essential" amino acid. *Molecular Vision*, 18:2673–2686.

Sachs, G., and D. R. Scott. 2012. Helicobacter pylori: Eradication or preservation. *F1000 Medical Reports*, 4:7.

Sadr, M., S. M. H. N. Mugahi, G. Hassanzadeh, et al. 2015. Telomere shortening in blood leukocytes of patients with chronic obstructive pulmonary disease. *Tanaffos*, 14(1):10–16.

Salzano, S., P. Checconi. E.-M. Hanschmann, et al. 2014. Linkage of inflammation and oxidative stress via release of glutathionylated peroxiredoxin-2, which acts as a danger signal. *Proceedings of the National Academy of Sciences USA*, 111(33):12157–12162.

Santarelli, L., G. Gobbi, P. Blier, et al. 2002. Behavioral and physiologic effects of genetic or pharmacologic inactivation of the substance P receptor (NK1). *The Journal of Clinical Psychiatry*, 63 Suppl 11:11–17.

Sanz, M. J., M. C. Terencio, and M. Paya. 1992. Isolation and hypotensive activity of a polymeric procyanidin fraction from *Pistacia lentiscus*. *Pharmazie*, 47:466–467.

Sarma, D. N.,M. L. Barrett, M. L. Chavez, et al. 2008. Safety of green tea extracts: A systematic review by the US Pharmacopeia. *Drug Safety*, 31(6):469–484.

Schaffer, S. W., J. Azuma, and M. Mozaffari. 2009. Role of antioxidant activity of taurine in diabetes. *Canadian Journal of Physiology & Pharmacology*, 87(2):91–99.

Scicchitano, B. M., and G. Sica. 2016. The beneficial effects of taurine to counteract sarcopenia. *Current Protein & Peptide Science* PMID:27875962, [Epub ahead of print].

Semwal, R., B., D. K. Semwal, S. Combrinck, et al. 2015. Gingerols and shogaols: Important nutraceutical principles from ginger. *Phytochemistry*, 117:554–568.

Serafini, M., A. Ghiselli, and A. Ferro-Luzzi. 1996. In vivo antioxidant effect of green and black tea in man. *European Journal of Clinical Nutrition*, 50(1):28–32.

Shah, N. C., G. J. Shah, Z. Li et al. 2014. Short-term magnesium deficiency downregulates telomerase, upregulates neutral sphingomyelinase and induces oxidative DNA damage in cardiovascular tissues: Relevance to atherogenesis, cardiovascular diseases and aging. *International Journal of Clinical & Experimental Medicine*, 7(3):497–514.

Sharma, R. A., S. A. Euden, S. L. Platton, et al. 2004. Phase I clinical trial of oral curcumIn: Biomarkers of systemic activity and compliance. *Clinical Cancer Research*, 10(20):6847–6854.

Sheng, R., Z. L. Gu, M. L. Xie. 2013. Epigallocatechin gallate, the major component of polyphenols in green tea, inhibits telomere attrition mediated cardiomyocyte apoptosis in cardiac hypertrophy. *Journal of Cardiology*, 162(3):199–209.

Sirdah, M. M. 2015. Protective and therapeutic effectiveness of taurine in diabetes mellitus: A rationale for antioxidant supplementation. *Diabetes & metabolic syndrome*, 9(1):55–64.

Sogut, O., H. Kaya, M. T. Gokdemir, et al. 2012. Acute myocardial infarction and coronary vasospasm associated with the ingestion of cayenne pepper pills in a 25-year-old male. *International Journal of Emergency Medicine*, 5:5.

Soni, K. B., and R. Kuttan. 1992. Effect of oral curcumin administration on serum peroxides and cholesterol levels in human volunteers. *Indian Journal of Physiology & Pharmacology*, 36(4):273–275.

Spiller, F., M. K. Alves, S. M. Vieira, et al. 2008. Anti-inflammatory effects of red pepper (*Capsicum baccatum*) on carrageenan- and antigen-induced inflammation. *The Journal of Pharmacy & Pharmacology*, 60(4):473–478.

Spranger, J., A. M. Kroke, Möhlig, et al. 2003. Inflammatory cytokines and the risk to develop type 2 diabetes. *Diabetes*, 52(3):812–817.

Steyers, C. M., 3rd, and F. J. Miller, Jr. 2014. Endothelial dysfunction in chronic inflammatory diseases. *International Journal of Molecular Science*, 15(7):11324–11349.

Su, L., J.-J. Yin, D. Charles, et al. 2007. Total phenolic contents, chelating capacities, and radical-scavenging properties of black peppercorn, nutmeg, rosehip, cinnamon and oregano leaf. *Food Chemistry*, 100(3):990–997.

Surjana, D., G. M. Halliday, and D. L. Damian. 2010. Role of nicotinamide in DNA damage, mutagenesis, and DNA repair. *Journal of Nucleic Acids*, 2010:157591.

Suryanarayana, P., A. Satyanarayana, N. Balakrishna, et al. 2007. Effect of turmeric and curcumin on oxidative stress and antioxidant enzymes in streptozotocin-induced diabetic rat. *Medical Science Monitor*, 13(12):BR286–BR292.

Takahashi, K., M. Fukazawa, H. Motohira, et al. 2003. A pilot study on antiplaque effects of mastic chewing gum in the oral cavity. *Journal of Periodontology*, 74(4):501–505.

Teas, J., S. Pino, A. Critchley, et al. 2004. Variability of iodine content in common commercially available edible seaweeds. *Thyroid*, 14(10):836–847.

Tipoe, G. L., T. M. Leung, M. W. Hung, et al. 2007. Green tea polyphenols as an anti-oxidant and anti-inflammatory agent for cardiovascular protection. *Cardiovascular & Hematological Disorders—Drug Targets*, 7(2):135–144.

Triantafyllou, A., A. Bikineyeva, A. Dikalova, et al. 2010. Anti-inflammatory activity of Chios mastic gum is associated with inhibition of TNF-alpha induced oxidative stress. *Nutrition Journal*, 10:64.

Triantafyllou, A., A. Bikineyeva, A. Dikalova, et al. 2011. Anti-inflammatory activity of Chios mastic gum is associated with inhibition of TNF-alpha induced oxidative stress. *Nutrition Journal*, 10:64.

Vanschoonbeek, K., B. J. Thomassen, J. M. Senden, et al. 2006. Cinnamon supplementation does not improve glycemic control in postmenopausal type 2 diabetes patients. *Journal of Nutrition*, 136(4):977–980.

Vasto, S., E. Mocchegiani, G. Candore et al. 2006. Inflammation, genes and zinc in ageing and age-related diseases. *Biogerontology*, 7(5–6):315–327.

von Zglinicki, T. 2002. Oxidative stress shortens telomeres. *Trends in Biochemical Sciences*, 27(7):339–344.

Waters, C. M., and B. L. Bassler. 2005. Quorum sensing: Cell-to-cell communication in bacteria. *Annual Review of Cell and Developmental Biology*, 21:319–346.

Willerson, J. T., and P. M. Ridker. 2004. Inflammation as a cardiovascular risk factor. *Circulation*, 109(21 Suppl 1):II2–II10.

Wong, J. Y. Y, I. De Vivo, X. Lin, et al. 2014. The Relationship between inflammatory biomarkers and telomere length in an occupational prospective cohort Study. *PLoS One*, 9(1):e87348.

Wong, C. P. and E. Ho. 2012. Zinc and its role in age-related inflammation and immune dysfunction. *Molecular Nutrition & Food Research*, 56(1):77–87.

Wu, B. J., L. Yan, F. Charlton, et al. 2010. Evidence that niacin inhibits acute vascular inflammation and improves endothelial dysfunction independent of changes in plasma lipids. *Arteriosclerosclerosis, Thrombosis & Vascular Biology*, 30(5):968–975.

Yeh, T. S., N. H. Hung, and T. C. Lin. 2014. Analysis of iodine content in seaweed by GC-ECD and estimation of iodine intake. *Journal of Food & Drug Analysis*, 22(2):189–196.

Young, H. Y., Y. L. Luo, H. Y. Cheng, et al. 2005. Analgesic and anti-inflammatory activities of [6]-gingerol. *Journal of Ethnopharmacology*, 96(1–2):207–210.

Zheltova, A. A., M. V. Kharitonova, N. I. Iezhitsa, et al. 2016. Magnesium deficiency and oxidative stress: An update. *Biomedicine (Taipei)*, 6(4):20.

Index